Food
$f$or
Recovery

May '94

Dear Sue

Vibrant Health

&

Happiness

always

Also by Joseph D. Beasley, M.D.

The Betrayal of Health

Diagnosing and Managing Chemical Dependency

How to Defeat Alcoholism

Wrong Diagnosis/Wrong Treatment:
The Plight of the Alcoholic in America

The Impact of Nutrition, the Environment, and Lifestyle on the
Health of Americans: A Report to the Kellogg Foundation

The Impact of Nutrition on the Health of Americans: A Report to
the Ford Foundation

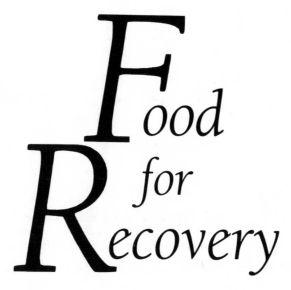

Food for Recovery

The Complete Nutritional Companion for Recovering from Alcoholism, Drug Addiction, and Eating Disorders

Joseph D. Beasley, M.D.
Susan Knightly

Crown Trade Paperbacks
New York

To my wife, Kimley.

Joseph D. Beasley, M.D.

To my mother, Barbara Knightly; in memory of my father, John Knightly; and to S.J. Hawes for his lonely struggle.

Susan Knightly

Published by Crown Publishers, Inc., 201 East 50th Street, New York, New York 10022. Member of the Crown Publishing Group.

Random House, Inc. New York, Toronto, London, Sydney, Auckland

CROWN TRADE PAPERBACKS and colophon are trademarks of Crown Publishers, Inc.

Manufactured in the United States of America

Design by Mercedes Everett

Library of Congress Cataloging-in-Publication Data

Beasley, Joseph D.
    Food for recovery: the complete nutritional companion for recovering from alcoholism, drug addiction, and eating disorders / Joseph D. Beasley, M.D., Susan Knightly.
        Includes bibliographical references and index.
        1. Substance abuse—Diet therapy.   2. Alcoholism—Diet therapy.   3. Eating disorders—Diet therapy.   4. Recovering addicts—Nutrition.   5. Recovering alcoholics—Nutrition.   I. Knightly, Susan.   II. Title.
RC564.29.B43   1993
616.86′0654—dc20   93-25244
                                                                              CIP

ISBN 0-517-88181-0

10 9 8 7 6 5 4 3 2 1

First Edition

ACKNOWLEDGMENTS

Every book reflects the efforts of scores of people besides the authors, and *Food for Recovery* is no exception. Collectively and as individuals, we have many people to thank for the time, energy, and support they have given us in the months it took to bring *Food for Recovery* to its final form.

Dr. Beasley would like to thank:

All the patients and their loved ones who have joined me in a team effort to understand and treat their conditions. It has been a privilege and an honor to work with you all, and my patients continue to be my main teachers.

All those in the basic sciences and health professions who have helped me in the past and continue to provide me with so much help and support.

The staff of Comprehensive Medical Care, who daily give all they have to our patients and their families.

My wife, who has encouraged and supported me in the long hours necessary to complete this book.

Jane Kaplan, R.D., for the years of work she contributed to developing nutritional plans that work for people in recovery.

Mary L. Williams, for her input and suggestions for making the sections on allergy and immunity both accessible and accurate.

Susan Knightly would like to thank:

Jane Littell, who tested all the recipes in my very hot, very tiny kitchen, and who brought with her a sunny disposition that made the work a pleasure.

My research assistants—Patricia Morris, Cynthia Lowry, Catherine Walthers, Ellen Zucker, Nancy Messer, Dianne Lange, and so many others—who were a very effective cheering squad during their many hours of tedious work.

Peggy Levison, Ph.D., for being a great listener and for her help in solving all the "other" problems so the work could progress.

My loving husband, Leonard Yakir, and my stepson, Benjamin, for their encouragement and for putting up with all the papers and people that filled our home for two years.

And we both extend our warmest gratitude to:

Loretta Barrett, a patient, supportive, and inspiring agent.

Erica Marcus, editor extraordinaire, who patiently worked with us to bring it all together.

Catherine Heusel, who gave our very different voices a singular tone and who edited above and beyond the call of duty.

CONTENTS

PART THREE

APPENDIXES

Introduction: *Why We Wrote This Book*

Some years ago, a man named Jim attended his first Alcoholics Anonymous meeting. After more than a decade of heavy drinking and cocaine abuse, he had hit bottom. Like his mother and grandfather before him, Jim was an alcoholic. Unlike them, he took steps to save his life.

From the start, Jim seemed to be doing everything right. He went into an inpatient detoxification program. He continued with outpatient rehabilitation and counseling. He went to meetings and kept in close contact with his sponsor. He "worked the program" with dedication and commitment. But something was still terribly wrong.

Despite the fact that he was dry, Jim was tired, depressed, and plagued by cravings for alcohol and cocaine. He always seemed to have a head cold. Indigestion was a constant companion. He was countering his fatigue and cravings by drinking quarts of coffee and eating several candy bars a day, but it wasn't helping much. By the time we met him, Jim was beginning to despair of ever feeling truly *healthy* again.

As we shall see in chapter 1, Jim's story has a happy ending. He learned that the process of recovery is far more than giving up the drug or behavior you abused. Whether you are a compulsive overeater, an anorexic, a cocaine addict, or an alcoholic, recovery is always a process of renewal and repair of a damaged body, mind, and spirit.

Jim discovered that his recovery was not meeting the repair needs of his *physical* self, and that he was suffering the consequences. While Jim was working on his mind and spirit, his body was crying out for the restoration and care it desperately needed but was not getting.

Jim was actually very lucky to make it as far as he did. The vast majority of people with addictions and eating disorders either drop out of treatment or relapse within the first year of trying to get into recovery. The consequences of such relapse are vast, both for the individual and for society. These disorders cost billions of dollars each year in lost productivity, lost wages, health-care bills, and legal bills. If you or someone you love is battling an addiction or eating disorder, it is imperative to get into recovery as soon as possible. *But* . . . recovery must go beyond simple abstinence or regular attendance of support groups.

Consider . . . if your house were on fire, what would you do? Call someone to talk about your feelings? Sit down and pray? Stay inside and try to conduct business as usual? Of course not! Your first response would be to put the fire out—either by dousing it yourself or by calling the fire department. You might pray while doing these things, or call a friend for support once the immediate crisis were past, but your first response would be to deal with the immediate danger. Anything else would be foolish and dangerous.

Active alcoholics, drug addicts, compulsive eaters, and anorexics/bulimics are living in the biological equivalent of a burning building. Every cell of their bodies is gradually being consumed and destroyed by the effects of their addiction or compulsion. Dousing this fire and rebuilding the ruined "building" from the foundation up must be one of the foremost priorities of any recovery program.

Addictions and eating disorders cause severe and extensive biological and nutritional damage that has permanent long-term consequences. Those of us in recovery are different—our nutritional needs, biological susceptibilities, and risks of certain illnesses (including cross-addictions) are much greater than those of the "average" person. We don't have the luxury of eating pounds of sugar, additives, and other chemicals each year—our already damaged bodies simply cannot take that kind of abuse (in fact, *no one* can take this abuse over time).

As a physician and a professional chef who teaches, both of whom are in recovery, we have always been impressed by the concept of recovery as a process of the body, mind, and spirit. But as we have attended 12-Step and other recovery meetings across the country, we have seen a critical flaw in the movement that has given us so much.

At meeting after meeting we listened to people talk of their spiritual growth as they chain-smoked cigarettes, drank cup after cup of coffee, and ate doughnuts and cookies. We saw people "in recovery" with the pallor of cancer patients, complaining of mood swings and ill health. We observed hundreds of people in "white-knuckle recovery" . . . desperately clinging to abstinence in the face of cravings and anxiety.

We both have had ample opportunity to work with these people, and we have found that many (if not most) of them do not understand the importance of the body in the recovery process. Instead, like Jim, they unwittingly continue much of the abuse and damage of their pre-recovering days. As a result, *they are too physiologically impaired to truly "work" a recovery program.* They are like carpenters with a blueprint but no tools.

Without a recovered *body,* neither the mind nor the spirit can reach its full potential. Recovery programs that do not recognize this fact and thus do not include physiological restoration in their approach are about as effective as firemen who stand in front of a burning building and wish that it wouldn't burn down.

Only when recovery is a complete physical *and* spiritual regeneration can the seeds of recovery blossom into the vibrant beauty of a restored body, mind, and spirit. We know this from personal experience, from the experience of people like Jim, and from hard scientific evidence of the biological impacts of addictions and eating disorders.

If you are battling an addiction or eating disorder and want not only to survive but thrive in recovery, you must counter the toxic and malnourishing effects of your condition. You need to rebuild your body from the inside out, cell by cell. The first and best way to start this process is through *nutrition*. Food truly can work for recovery, when you understand your body's needs and how to meet them. You can give your cells the fuel and tools they require to heal, and build a strong foundation of physical health that will make your recovery a joyous, vital, lifelong process. Only from such a foundation can any of us hope to reach our full spiritual and mental growth.

Although this book is geared specifically to those who are in recovery, its basic principles are applicable to all who care about their health and well-being. In our rushed, stressful, and increasingly polluted world almost everyone's health is being compromised by poor nutrition and toxic effects. The nutritional and lifestyle guidelines in this book are designed to reduce these biological stresses and strengthen the body's natural vitality. They are not temporary measures or a "fad diet" —they are a lifelong plan for restoring and maintaining health.

It has long been said that addictions and eating disorders are a "family affair," passed from generation to generation through genetic predispositions, cultural habits, and environmental conditioning. Recovery, then, should also be a family affair—a process in which every member of the family is healed and strengthened. The recovery program detailed in this book will benefit not only the recovering person, but everyone in his or her household. If you are going to embark on the journey of recovery, bring your loved ones with you. If they don't want to try this approach to food and recovery, implement the measures yourself. Remember, you are in a burning building, you don't have time to negotiate or argue. Get to work on your own recovery, and let your increasing good health and vitality speak for you.

With this in mind, we present this book to everyone—recovering and otherwise—who wants to take up the reins and begin the fulfilling journey to a recovered body, mind, and spirit. May you enjoy the adventure as much as we have.

Part One

1 Body-Mind-Spirit

Recovery from any illness involves the body, the mind, and the spirit. Together, these three elements make up who we are, and true healing includes all these aspects of the self. Like a three-legged stool, recovery cannot stay upright and balanced unless all three "legs" are equally strong.

In many recovering individuals, the body leg of recovery is weak, damaged, or missing altogether. Instead of enjoying the natural high of a healthy sobriety, these individuals teeter on the brink of relapse, battling mood swings, fatigue, cravings, and general ill health even as they "work the program."

Let's return to the case of Jim. As the child of an alcoholic mother, Jim started out with several biological strikes against him, since he was biologically and genetically susceptible to the development of alcoholism (see chapter 9). But since Jim also grew up in a classic alcoholic household, he was ignorant of his unique susceptibility to the disease that had destroyed two generations of his family. Instead of avoiding alcohol, he set out to prove he was different (stronger) than his mother and grandfather, and he ended up a full-fledged alcoholic and heavy cocaine user by the time he was thirty.

After Jim's detoxification and treatment, he resolved to live his life to the fullest without alcohol or drugs. He went to AA meetings regularly, got a sponsor, never had another drink . . . and felt simply awful for two years.

He experienced dizziness, disorientation, and some fainting spells. He was always tired. Whenever he ate he felt bloated and uncomfortable. And he kept craving alcohol and cocaine.

When we met Jim, two years after he had been detoxified, he was drinking twenty cups of coffee a day and living almost entirely on candy, cakes, and cookies. His nose was constantly clogged and his throat was always sore. His fatigue and depression were so constant that he had been placed on disability. He had seen a half dozen doctors and psychotherapists, who had done their best but had been unable to help him. His first words to us were: "I got sober for *this?*"

It was soon revealed that Jim's problems were not "all in his head," as he had supposed. Like many active and recovering alcoholics, Jim was suffering from an abnormality of carbohydrate metabolism called alcoholic hypoglycemia. This condition can cause severe symptoms and even death in some individuals when they are actively drinking. Individuals who continue to eat infrequently, consume high levels of sugar and caffeine, and remain poorly nourished continue to have a form of hypoglycemia even after they stop drinking. The symptoms of this hypoglycemia can be very disabling in recovery.

Glucose (or blood sugar) is the brain's fuel. When the level of glucose in the bloodstream drops below a certain point, the brain is essentially "running on empty." The fatigue, anxiety, depression, and cravings Jim experienced were his brain's way of crying out for more fuel. When Jim was drinking, alcohol served as a substitute. When the alcohol was gone, he started "treating" his severe drops in blood sugar with candy, cakes, and caffeine. These made his blood sugar level rise and fall dramatically, perpetuating the cycle of anxiety, fatigue, cravings, and more sugar binges.

In addition to his disordered glucose metabolism, Jim's years of addiction and his poor diet in recovery had left him very nutrient depleted. A malnourished brain is a malfunctioning brain; the symptoms of this dysfunction include depression, anxiety, concentration problems, and craving.

Jim was also amazingly sensitive to a variety of environmental factors and foods, particularly house dust, house dust mites, regional molds, and other airborne allergens and coffee, corn, rye, wheat, dairy products, and oats (see chapters 8 and 10 for more information on these conditions). Since Jim's diet consisted almost entirely of coffee, sugar, and highly refined forms of wheat, corn, and milk, it was really small wonder that he felt terrible.

Although he had been dry for two years, Jim had never really recovered from his alcoholism. He had tried to care for his mind and spirit only, and had ignored his body, so his physical problems not only remained, but worsened. He was a classic example of the "dry drunk"—the person in recovery who has kicked his addiction (be it alcohol, drugs, or food), but only by gritting his teeth and suffering through constant ill health and discomfort.

For Jim, the first step to physical recovery was understanding how badly his body had been damaged by his alcohol and drug abuse, and what he could do to restore himself to a state of vigorous good health. It was important that Jim realize that *he* had the power to bring about this recovery, and that one of his most important tools (and allies) was food. He needed to learn which foods could help, which foods could hurt, and how and when he should be eating.

Jim was surprised to learn that, for people in recovery, the pattern of "three square meals" a day is not sufficient. Instead, he began to have several smaller meals and frequent healthy snacks—including fresh fruits, nuts, and vegetables. Then Jim began learning how to eat better when he was out, and to choose and prepare foods for himself in his home. Despite his initial trepidation, Jim soon learned to enjoy choosing and preparing his meals, using vegetables, grains, and spices that he had never known existed. He hosted small dinner parties before and after meetings to show off his culinary prowess and share some of the lessons he had learned.

At the same time, Jim began a program of exercise, allergy treatment, and nutritional supplementation to revitalize his body and restore his immunological and nutritional state. Within a few weeks, he lost his feelings of overwhelming fatigue and was sleeping well. The cravings for alcohol and sugar disappeared. For the first time in nearly four years he was able to breathe through his nose. Jim felt he was understanding many aspects of his recovery for the first time. He felt, by his own admission, as if a cloud had lifted from his life.

The cloud that Jim felt hanging over him during the first two years of his recovery was not unusual. It afflicts most recovering individuals, not because they are lazy, or bad, or uncommitted to their recovery, but because they (and often the people treating them) have made the fundamental mistake of underestimating the body part of their recovery.

In recovery, the triad of body-mind-spirit is interdependent. Neglect one aspect, and the other two will also suffer. In pursuing the goals of mind and spirit, all too many of us neglect or actively abuse the body—consuming caffeine by the quart, smoking cigarettes by the carton, and eating junk foods on a regular basis. All this abuse has a definite impact on the mind and the spirit. In Jim's case, his eating habits were not a *symptom* of his depression and fatigue, they were the *cause*.

No one is really in recovery until his or her body is in recovery. The body is more than a receptacle for the mind and spirit, it is *part* of the mind and spirit, and disorders of the body are reflected in our moods, feelings, and thought processes. (If you have ever tried to work when sick with the flu you can understand this concept.)

The conditions that brought so many of us into the recovery movement have devastating effects on the body, from the tiniest cell in the lining of our intestines to the longest nerve connecting our brains and toes. Nothing escapes unharmed. The devastation is so complete because these disorders affect every cell of the body. The billions of cells that carry out the most basic of our bodies' processes have been not only poisoned (by the chemicals we were ingesting) but starved. Damaged and deprived of the raw materials they need, these poisoned and malnourished cells cannot function. Even the most overweight of compulsive eaters is malnourished because the foods he or she compulsively consumes rarely have any real nutritional value.

Even before many of us became addicted, we were probably operating with several strikes against us—biological and psychological factors that contributed to the eventual rise of our addictive or compulsive disorders. We will examine some of these in detail in later chapters, but for the moment let's just consider a few of these primary factors:

1. **Genetics**—Inherited differences in metabolism, nutritional needs, neurochemistry (chapter 7), and the like that can render us more susceptible to the toxic and addictive effects of many substances (including foods).
2. **Allergy**—Unique susceptibilities to various pollens, foods, and other substances that can contribute to overall ill health and many cravings (chapter 8).
3. **Toxicity**—From heavy metals and hundreds of toxic chemicals (such as lead, cadmium, PCBs, DDT) that can contaminate our water, air, and food supplies (chapters 3 and 11).
4. **Malnutrition**—The result of eating a "typical American diet" that is as full of fat, sugar, and chemical additives as it is deficient in the most important nutrients.
5. **Cultural pressures**—From a society that promotes alcohol and many other legal drugs (such as caffeine and cigarettes) as the way to success, popularity, and happiness; that often glamorizes illegal drugs as chic "alternative lifestyles"; and that worships at the altar of leanness even as more than 40 percent of the population is overweight.
6. **Psychological distress/mental illness**—This can exacerbate (and be exacerbated by) the above factors, and sometimes serves as the immediate trigger for using potentially addictive substances, or starting compulsive patterns of behavior.

Once these underlying factors are complicated by addiction, alcoholism, or eating disorders, an already bad situation becomes incomparably worse. Now we are also battling:

1. Cravings
2. Compulsive consumption (despite damaging consequences)
3. Pan-cellular toxicity and malnutrition (chapter 6)
4. Hypoglycemia (chapters 6 and 7)
5. Hyperinsulinism
6. Distorted fat metabolism (chapters 3, 6, and 9)
7. Neurotransmitter imbalances (chapter 7)
8. Increased allergic responses (chapter 8)
9. Decreased ability to fight infection (chapter 8)
10. Gastrointestinal damage (chapter 6)
11. Cross-addiction (often to physician-prescribed medication; chapter 10)
12. Sexual dysfunction

When we view recovery from this perspective, it is easy to see why so many people are not making the most out of existing recovery programs. All too often, these underlying biological factors are never dealt with. Indeed, for most of history addicts, alcoholics, and individuals with eating disorders were considered either weak-willed or moral degenerates who were punished for their failings. With the dawn of psychiatric thought, these individuals went from being bad people to mentally ill people, who were using drugs, alcohol, or food to treat their underlying psychiatric problems. Treatment was geared to identifying and dealing with these underlying problems, using everything from individual counseling to drugs. Taking care of the myriad physical problems of this population was (and is) rarely even considered.

This means that many of the people who enter recovery programs are unprepared, physically and therefore mentally, to really make use of the growth and support these programs have to offer. Some, like Jim, will stick with it and get some measure of comfort and sobriety even as they continue to feel unwell. But many thousands simply give up and fall back into the disorders they were striving to overcome, or become cross-addicted to some other substance.

The hard fact is that most recovery programs don't work particularly well. Statistics on the most studied addiction, alcoholism, all point to something very wrong in the way we are handling addictive disorders. Up to 70 percent of individuals who start treatment drop out before the end of the first year. Indeed, one study of a hospital-based program found that 45 percent of the patients had dropped out of contact within the first month! And data on those who do complete treatment are no more encouraging.

Almost twenty years ago a review of 384 studies of alcoholism treatment programs found that alcoholics who received absolutely no treatment were just as likely to stop drinking for six months (or more) as those who received treatment. Ten years later, in 1985, a study in *The New England Journal of Medicine* detailed the status of 400 alcoholic individuals who had received treatment three years before. The findings were both startling and depressing. Only 15 percent of the patients had maintained their sobriety! And even that outcome is more encouraging than a 1985 story in *Consumers Research,* in which it was reported that sixty out of every one hundred alcoholics will never receive treatment for their disease, and that only five of the forty who do get treated will achieve "measurable sobriety."

Although there are fewer specific studies on the other addictions and eating disorders, what is known is not good. For example, a recent report by a Congressional panel investigating *physician-supervised* weight loss programs found that a whopping 95 percent of the people who lose weight on such programs eventually gain all or more of the weight back! (And that statistic doesn't take into account the hundreds of unsupervised diet plans that are out there.) On the other end of the eating disorder spectrum, anorexia, which afflicts some two million Americans, kills up to 20 percent of those who suffer from the disorder.

It doesn't need to be this way. Thousands of recovering men and women have turned their recoveries into the vital, serene, and abundant joy of a recovering body, mind, and spirit. In addition to our personal experiences, there is hard scientific evidence (accumulated over nearly fifty years of research) that relatively simple nutritional and lifestyle changes can have an enormous impact on the success of a recovery program.

It began in the 1940s and 1950s, when researchers at the University of Texas were investigating the impact of diet on alcohol consumption in animals. Their findings were remarkably consistent. When given a free choice between alcohol and water, nutritionally deficient lab rats chose alcohol far more often than their well-fed counterparts. Roger Williams, the great nutrition pioneer, summarized the findings in his 1956 book, *Biochemical Individuality:*

> When the animals were given well-fortified diets supplemented particularly with vitamins, they all developed wisdom of the body and turned away from alcohol consumption.

Humans also have an innate "wisdom of the body." But our modern lifestyle, from the way we eat to the way we work, play, and sleep, has cut us off from this inborn wisdom. Like those lab rats forty years ago, we are obeying the wrong signals and suffering as a result.

Unlike lab animals, we have the option of improving and supplementing our own diets. We can reconnect with the innate wisdom (and healing powers) of the body and make abstinence a comfortable and enjoyable state.

One of the first studies to demonstrate the power of this type of nutritional treatment in humans was conducted in the early 1980s by another researcher at the University of Texas. Ruth M. Guenther knew from her extensive review of the scientific literature that most alcoholics were malnourished, and that the majority of them return to drinking even after they have been treated. What would happen, she wondered, if nutritional therapy were added to a standard alcoholism treatment program? Could humans regain their "wisdom of the body" in the same way experimental animals had nearly three decades before?

To investigate this possibility, she undertook a study at an alcoholism treatment unit in a local Veteran's Administration medical center. The control group of patients went through the basic program of inpatient alcohol education, AA meetings, AA-oriented group counseling, and work incentive, followed by outpatient follow-up care. The study group went through the same program with the addition of a program of nutrition education, dietary supplements, and therapy. Both groups were in treatment for the same time (28 days), with the same physicians, social workers, nurses, educational program, and counseling. The only difference between the two groups was the nutrition program.

The nutrition program consisted of dietary change, vitamin and mineral supplements, and nutrition education. The normal hospital diet was adjusted to include: wheat germ and bran with each meal, whole-grain bread, decaffeinated beverages, sugar substitutes, and unsweetened canned, frozen, or fresh fruits for dessert instead of pies, cakes, puddings, or sweetened fruits. Nuts, cheese, and whole-grain bread and peanut butter were available for snacks between meals and in the evening.

Education included weekly classes on the basics of nutrition, menu planning, shopping and food preparation, and how to read labels to recognize hidden sugars, alcohol, and preservatives. Patients were taught about the effects of alcoholism on their health and nutritional state, and the importance of maintaining a healthy diet and lifestyle after their discharge. Most importantly, they were given specific, useful information on how they could actively improve their health and well-being in recovery and were encouraged to maintain this regimen after leaving the hospital. From day one through their discharge, patients were told that the nutritional principles were meant to be a lifelong plan.

Six months after their discharge from the hospital, 81 percent of the study group were not drinking. Only 38 percent of the control group had maintained their recovery. Since all the patients had been randomly selected and assigned to either study or control, the only difference between the two groups was the element of nutritional therapy. While some members of the study group admitted to slacking off on their diet and supplements, the difference in recovery rates cannot have been mere chance (in fact, statistical analysis showed the odds of these results occurring by chance were less than 2 in 1,000). As one patient said, "Something has helped, and it may be the diet and vitamins." Another explained it as "You get your health—you get more resistance."

Several years later, researchers at Brunswick Hospital Center and at Comprehensive Medical Care in New York (led by Dr. Beasley), in conjunction with statistical experts at the State University of New York at Stony Brook, applied a similar program to 111 patients with severe and chronic alcoholism. All had long and difficult histories of alcohol and drug abuse, with many failed treatment attempts (one man had been through twenty detoxifications!). All had deficient diets, 80 percent were clinically malnourished, almost two thirds had liver disease, and almost half were also addicted to other drugs. On the whole, they were a difficult group with little apparent chance of achieving long-term sobriety. Would a combined program of nutritional restoration and psychological measures succeed where other primarily psychological measures had not?

The patients spent twenty-eight days in the hospital in a treatment program similar to that designed by Ruth Guenther and her colleagues. In addition to the nutrition education, supplements, and a monitored diet, each patient underwent blood testing to identify potential food allergens. During their inpatient treatment, each patient's diet was individualized to limit exposure to these foods.

At the end of the twenty-eight days, the patients began a twelve-month program of medical follow-up. In addition to aftercare and AA meetings, patients came in for medical evaluations and workups at least once a month, nutrition counseling and supplements, and random urine screens and blood work.

At the end of one year, 91 of the original 111 patients were still in the program. Of these, 74 percent were sober and stable (confirmed by lab work and at least one significant other). The research and treatment teams were pleased. After years of reading about failure rates that hovered around 85 percent, they were finally seeing successful outcomes. And if these results could be achieved by patients with such severe addictions and discouraging histories, the prospects for individuals in the early stage of addiction are truly bright, if they receive the right kind of care. Indeed, it should be possible to turn those 85 percent failure rates to 85 percent success.

We have seen such positive results in thousands of patients— alcoholics, chronic overeaters, bulimics, anorexics, and addicts of all kinds. Although the transition was sometimes difficult, every one of these men and women found that once they had enjoyed the tremendous health benefits and "natural high" of a good nutrition program it was almost impossible to go back to their old eating habits. In the words of one patient: "I had a Twinkie the other day, just for old time's sake, and couldn't even finish the first bite. I can't believe I ate that stuff. What was I thinking of?"

The founders of the 12-Step movement always understood the importance of the body in recovery. *The Big Book,* the primary text of Alcoholics Anonymous, clearly states that the body of the alcoholic is as abnormal as his or her mind, and that any understanding of alcoholism that does not acknowledge its physical aspect is incomplete.

Bill W. knew the pitfalls of ignoring the body from firsthand experience. For many years after giving up alcohol, Bill lived on sugary foods, coffee, and cigarettes—suffering all the while from mood swings, alcohol cravings, depression, chronic insomnia, and a host of other symptoms. It was not until he met Dr. Abram Hoffer of Vancouver, Canada that Bill learned of the dangers of his poor dietary habits and substitute addictions, and completed the process of his physical recovery. (Unfortunately, Bill did not stop smoking for many years, and eventually he died of emphysema.)

Bill worked hard to inform others of the importance of healing the body when recovering from alcoholism; and though many heeded his efforts, the message did not take a firm hold.

One of the reasons that Bill's message did not take hold was a widespread ignorance of the nature of good nutrition. The situation is much the same today. Although we all eat, few of us really think about what we are eating and what it can mean to our bodies. We rely on very incomplete, simplistic, and often incorrect bits of nutritional "knowledge" in making our food choices, and we expect our bodies to cope with whatever we give them. In recovery, this kind of behavior simply doesn't cut it.

Many still believe that "the four food groups" are enough. This is completely untrue. Those simple, industry-promoted guides are only a small part of what good nutrition is about. Others feel that if they eat vegetables they are meeting their nutrient needs. As we shall see, growing, harvesting, transport, and processing practices now make even fresh vegetables less than perfect sources of vitamins and minerals. Still others think that if they "take their vitamins" they can eat whatever they want. Once again, a fallacy at work.

Nutrient needs, like fingerprints, are unique to the individual. The recommended dietary allowances are designed as guidelines for whole populations, not individuals. Most importantly, they do not even begin to address the special needs of people recovering from the long-term damage of alcoholism, drug addiction, or an eating disorder. In order for you to begin "eating for recovery," it is important to understand what addiction has done to your body and what proper nutrition can do to help you recoup your losses. And in order to do that, you must have at least a basic groundwork in the principles of nutrition. The information in this book can affect both the quality and length of your life.

2 *What Is Nutrition?*

Let's go back to the case of Jim for a moment. One of the most important findings of Jim's medical evaluation was his extreme sensitivity to several foods, particularly dairy products. Jim was dismayed when he heard he was going to have to drastically reduce his intake of milk and milk products, but he tried to make the best of it. With a resigned shrug he said, "I guess I'll just have to learn to like yogurt."

If you see nothing particularly wrong with that statement, count yourself among the millions of Americans who have a lot to learn about food and nutrition. Yogurt *is* a dairy product: Yogurt cultures are grown in milk. When told this, Jim looked a bit startled, and then laughed: "Well what do you know? I guess I never really thought about where yogurt comes from."

In these days of ready-to-eat meals, few of us think about where our food comes from, or what it contains, or what it can do. It's easier to just put something into our stomachs to stop those pesky hunger pangs (or nagging cravings) than to think about what our bodies are going to *do* with the food once it's in there.

There is a big difference between being well *fed*—having enough food to fill your stomach—and being well *nourished*—having the right food to fill your needs. If you ate a box of cornstarch you might feel full (and a little nauseated), but you certainly wouldn't be nourished.

Good nutrition encompasses not only the foods we eat, but every aspect of the way we live our lives. It is affected by anything that affects our bodies, including our emotions, our relationships, and the stresses we encounter in day-to-day life. It depends not only on foods, but on our bodies' ability to digest, distribute, use, and store the nutrients contained in those foods. Anything that interferes with the body's ability to carry out these tasks is going to interfere with nutrition.

Addictions, eating disorders, emotional stress, and the many other disorders addressed by the recovery movement interfere with almost every aspect of the body's ability to carry out its nutritional tasks (see chapter 6). Add to this fact the harsh reality of *what* most of us are eating, and it's small wonder so many people in recovery are nutritional disasters. If it can be done wrong, nutritionally, most of us have been doing it.

Food and Nutrients

According to the Random House College Dictionary, food is "any nourishing substance that is taken into the body to sustain life, provide energy, promote growth, etc." Nutrients, on the other hand, are chemicals within foods that our bodies use to conduct the myriad biochemical reactions of life. Given a relatively small number of nutritional building blocks (around 50 at last count), the body can construct an astonishing array of biochemical compounds and conduct thousands of complex biochemical processes. From the killer cells of the immune system to the most delicate reproductive cell, every fiber of our being depends on the presence (and balance) of nutrients within the body.

The degree to which a given food is "nourishing" depends on the number and proportion of nutrients it contains. Food, like gasoline, can be either high- or low-octane. The more nutrients a food contains, the better its ability to sustain life, provide energy, and promote growth.

Ironically (given their overriding importance in the quality of our lives), the significance of nutrients in food has only recently been recognized. For centuries, humans have mistaken quantity for quality when dealing with food . . . and have suffered the consequences.

   *Millions of sailors died horrible deaths from scurvy (a chronic vitamin C deficiency) before the importance of providing fresh fruits (particularly limes) on long voyages was recognized and acted upon.

   *Untold millions in Asia succumbed to beriberi, a thiamine deficiency caused by consuming a diet that consisted primarily of refined white rice.

   *In the American South at the turn of the twentieth century, thousands of individuals were confined to mental hospitals when they were in fact suffering from pellagra, a chronic niacin deficiency characterized by dementia (madness), diarrhea, dermatitis, and eventually death. These men and women had been living on the prevailing diet of fatback pork, molasses, and corn bread, which might have been filling but was also markedly deficient in niacin. When their in-hospital diet was changed to include more nutritionally rich foods (including liver extract and fresh vegetables), these supposedly mad patients were miraculously healed.

Such dramatic cases are the ones that most people think of when they hear the word "malnutrition." But malnutrition has many guises.

2.1 THE KNOWN ESSENTIAL NUTRIENTS

*Water
*Carbohydrates (energy)
*Fiber
*Protein
The Essential Amino Acids

   arginine (for children)
   histidine (for children)
   leucine
   isoleucine
   lysine
   methionine
   phenylalanine
   thereonine
   tryptophan
   valine

*Lipids/Fats
The Essential Fatty Acids

   linoleic acid
   linolenic acid

*Minerals
Major Minerals

   sodium (Na)
   magnesium (Mg)
   phosphorus (P)
   chlorine (Cl)
   potassium (K)
   calcium (Ca)
   sulfur (S)

Trace Minerals

   iron (Fe)   copper (Cu)
   iodine (I)   manganese (Mn)
   chromium (Cr)   zinc (Zn)
   fluorine (F)   selenium (Se)
   molybdenum (Mo)   tin (Sn)
   silicon (Si)   vanadium (V)
   cobalt (Co)   nickel (Ni)
   arsenic (As)

*Vitamins
Fat Soluble

   A (retinol)
   D (calciferol)
   E (tocopherol)
   K (phylloquinone)

Water Soluble

   B_1 (thiamine)   choline
   B_3 (niacin) B_2 (riboflavin)
   B_6 (pyridoxine) B_5 (pantothenic
   folic acid   acid)
      (folacin) B_{12} (cyano-
   biotin   cobalamin)
   C (ascorbic acid)

The woman who binges and purges constantly, the cocaine addict, the alcoholic, the valium addict—all are malnourished to some degree. Even grossly overweight individuals, who seem to have too much nutrition, are almost always critically malnourished. Like the pellagra victims of the past, they are consuming the wrong balance of nutrients, in the wrong amounts.

In the body, nutrients function like an orchestra. In order for a symphony to reach its full expression, all the instruments must perform together. Similarly, in the symphony of human biochemistry, nutrients always act in concert.

If you were attending a symphony and the entire string section went on strike, you would certainly notice the difference. If, however, only one violinist chose to walk out, you might not consciously notice the difference in sound, but something would be missing.

Major nutritional diseases such as pellagra are the equivalent of the entire string section going out on strike. But even in the case of pellagra, niacin is not the sole culprit. Just as the string section consists of many different instruments, so the disease of pellagra involves several nutrients. Lack of niacin is the primary deficiency, but niacin requires other nutrients in order to perform its functions. When niacin alone is used to treat pellagra, many symptoms remain. A full nutritional program that *includes* intensive niacin supplementation is needed to fully restore pellagra victims.

The same is true for all of the single-nutrient diseases. Although one particular nutrient may be missing most conspicuously ("Oh, the violins are missing!"), it is never the only one that has gone ("And I don't hear any cellos, either.").

To take it a few steps further, any nutrient deficiency, no matter how small, is going to have a very wide impact. Like a snowball rolling downhill, a seemingly insignificant nutrient deficiency can grow to enormous significance as its effects spread through the nutritional system.

Although we have learned a tremendous amount about nutritional science in the last century or so, it is still a very young field that is growing by leaps and bounds. Unfortunately, new knowledge still takes a long time to get into mainstream practice. From a recovery perspective, the thing to remember is that the nutrients in food work as a team, and that it is crucial to your body's health to have all the team members present at all times. This means looking beyond the mere appearance or amount of food and considering its contents. For although food is remarkably hardy (grain can be stored for years, wines and cheeses have to be aged, and dehydrated foods can be stored for decades), nutrients are fragile and easily lost or destroyed. This is why eating whole, unprocessed foods is so vitally important in recovery, since any level of processing (be it cooking a raw vegetable or hydrogenating an oil) removes nutrients. As we shall see, many of the wonders of our modern food production system are stripping our foods of most of their nutritional value.

An Introduction to the Nutrients

Before we discuss the various individual nutrients, it's important to get a handle on one of the most misunderstood concepts in nutrition: calories.

Strictly speaking, a calorie is not a specific *thing* at all. It is measurement of how much energy a given food provides. When we talk about the number of calories in a food, we are really discussing how much energy the body gets from that food. Calories are not nutrients, and it is possible for a food to provide plenty of calories without providing many nutrients.

Ideally, we want to have an even balance between the number of calories we consume and the amount of energy we expend. But caloric need can vary a great deal among individuals. If you are a professional figure skater who practices six hours a day and competes ten months out of the year, you burn a lot of energy, and you need a fair number of calories to power all that activity and maintain normal bodily processes. If, on the other hand, you are an accountant who does a lot of detail work behind a desk and exercises only intermittently, your energy needs are a lot less spectacular. If you eat foods that provide more calories (energy) than your body needs at the time, your body will store it away for later use—in fat cells.

Calories, then, are only the most basic and simplistic of nutritional measures. A food such as sugar or bourbon may provide energy in the form of calories, but it won't provide any of the nutrients that the body needs to help run the "furnace" that burns all that energy. The balance of calories to nutrients in a given food is usually referred to as "nutrient density." Nutrient-dense foods provide lots of nutrients in relatively few calories, while low-nutrient-density foods have far more calories than nutrients.

Addicts of all kinds and persons with eating disorders tend to consume low-nutrient-density foods—fast foods, junk foods, and so-called convenience foods that contain huge amounts of refined carbohydrates, artificial additives, and unnatural fats. When this poor diet is compounded by alcohol intake, drug use, or the devastating effects of binging and purging, it provokes an even greater nutritional crisis wherein the already overburdened body must draw on stored nutrients in order to function. If you really intend to nourish your body in recovery, you must give your body not only the nutrients it needs to function right now, but also the nutrients it requires to replenish those lost nutritional stores. And in order to do that, you need to understand what the various nutrients are and how they are processed within the body.

3 The Macro-Nutrients

Not all nutrients are created equal. Some, such as water, must be consumed in large amounts every day. Others, such as arsenic, should only be taken in infinitesimal amounts. But whether we need them by the pound (macro-nutrients) or the fraction of a milligram (micro-nutrients), all of the nutrients are important. The body (and mind) will eventually become just as ill when deprived of a micro-nutrient such as niacin as it does when deprived of a macro-nutrient such as water; just ask all those pellagra victims in the turn-of-the-century South.

The five macro-nutrients are protein, carbohydrate, fat (containing all the essential fatty acids), water, and fiber. Most of the foods we eat come from these five groups. The micro-nutrients (vitamins, minerals, and trace elements) are found within the macro-nutrients.

Protein

Protein is a crucial part of all animal bodies, accounting for 10 percent to 20 percent depending on age and body weight. (Most of the rest is water, fat, and the calcium of bones and teeth.) The human body builds and uses more than 50,000 different proteins in its day-to-day functioning.

In order to carry out this amazing feat, the body requires only twenty-two protein "building blocks"—the amino acids. About half of these are essential nutrients; without them, the body cannot function. With them, the body can build all the other "nonessential" amino acids and function at peak efficiency.

We get amino acids by eating protein foods, which our bodies then break down into their constituent amino acids. The primary protein foods—poultry, fish, soybeans, meat, and dairy products—contain all the essential amino acids and are called *complete* proteins. But the secondary sources—from the vegetable kingdom—usually contain only *incomplete* proteins. Cereals, for example, are low in the amino acid lysine but high in methionine and tryptophan. Beans, on the other hand, have mirror-image amino acid profiles. When foods from the two groups are eaten together, the body gets the full set of necessary amino acids.

3.1 THE ESSENTIAL AMINO ACIDS

arginine (for children)	methionine
histidine (for children)	phenylalanine
leucine	thereonine
isoleucine	tryptophan
lysine	valine

Many cultures have developed meals centered around complementary proteins. In the Middle East, bread and cheese are traditionally eaten together; in Mexico, rice and beans. The recipes later in this book rely heavily on such protein complementarity, as well as on fish and chicken and other low-fat protein sources. The recipes are designed to help you decrease your intake of saturated animal fats (see below), not to turn you into a vegetarian. If you choose to eschew meat entirely it is critical that you eat complementary foods to ensure that you get enough dietary protein. We have seen many vegetarians who believed they were eating healthy when they were in fact quite malnourished and protein deficient.

Protein foods are among the first to fall by the wayside in addictions and eating disorders. Primary protein sources (such as meat and fish) are either too expensive or too time-consuming to prepare for an individual in the throes of an addiction, while anorexic and bulimic individuals often avoid them because of the calories they contain. And most protein foods do not provide the unique emotional and biological satisfaction that compulsive eaters derive from the next nutrient group: carbohydrates.

Carbohydrates

Carbohydrates are the primary source of calories (fuel) for the body's cells. They burn fast and easily to produce energy and heat. Carbohydrates are found almost exclusively in the vegetable kingdom—in fruits, vegetables, and grains.

Carbohydrate foods range from the complex—called *starches*—to the simple—called *sugars*. Starches are potatoes, rice, corn and other vegetables, bread, cereal, and pasta. Sugars include table sugar, fruit, syrups, and honey. Actually starches and sugars are part of a continuum in which the molecularly complex starches degrade into the more simple molecules of sugar. We see this process every time a fruit ripens, as the starches of the young fruit gradually break down into the sweet sugars of ripeness.

The individual cells of the body cannot use carbohydrates until they have been reduced to their simplest form: glucose. During digestion, starches are broken down into complex sugars, complex sugars are broken down into simple sugars, and simple sugars are absorbed into the blood, chiefly as glucose. The bloodstream carries the glucose (along with oxygen from the lungs) to all the body's cells, where it fuels all life processes. Energy provided by carbohydrates that is not needed at the time of digestion is processed and stored as fat.

The body needs a constant supply of energy—in the form of blood glucose—to carry out its myriad functions. As we saw in the case of Jim, when this need is not properly met a host of physical, emotional, and psychological problems can result.

The specific form of a carbohydrate has a tremendous influence on its effect on our bodies. The more refined the carbohydrate, be it rice, sugar cane, or wheat (see chapter 11 for details on refining), the fewer nutrients it contains and the more abruptly it enters the system as blood sugar. The body's metabolism is designed to convert complex and "natural" sugars into glucose in a slow, steady process that keeps blood glucose levels stable so that cells are constantly and steadily nourished. When refined sugars are dumped into this system, blood sugar levels rise to abnormal levels, and the body reacts by trying to *decrease* blood sugar levels. It does this by releasing extra adrenaline and insulin, and over time this biochemical overcompensation affects the production of critical brain chemicals, causing fatigue, depression, and mood swings.

Fats

Although they may be the most dreaded of the macro-nutrients, fats (or, to use the technical term, lipids) are basically good for the body. Dietary fats are essential to the absorption, transport, and use of the fat-soluble vitamins A, D, E, and K; and the body's fat cells serve as insulation (to help maintain proper body temperature), as storage (for fat-soluble vitamins), and as a source of energy in times of caloric need.

Like proteins, fats occur in all animal foods, from sirloin steak to yogurt. But like carbohydrates, they are also found in the vegetable kingdom, particularly in seeds and nuts and related foods such as grains, and in beans (hence corn oil, peanut oil, olive oil, and so forth).

Carbohydrates, proteins, and fats all contain carbon, hydrogen, and oxygen. Fats, however, have a much higher concentration of carbon and hydrogen, which take much longer to burn than oxygen. As a result, high-fat foods provide more long-term energy (calories) than carbohydrates or protein foods. Both proteins and carbohydrates provide about four calories per gram. Fat provides nine. So an ounce of butter or olive oil will give you about 255 calories to burn, where an ounce of carbohydrates or pure protein will provide 113 calories.

The basic structural components of dietary fats are the fatty acids. Nutritional science is still discovering the many roles these substances play in human health. At least two fatty acids—linoleic acid and linolenic acid—are known to be absolutely necessary to the functioning of the body's cells, and they are known collectively as the *essential fatty acids* (EFAs). The body can also derive EFAs from some of the more complex fatty acids. *Essential fatty acid deficiencies have been linked to several biological and emotional disorders, including alcoholism and depression* (see chapter 9).

Fatty acids are differentiated on the basis of saturation—that is, the balance of carbon and hydrogen in the molecule. In saturated fatty acids, every carbon bond is occupied by a hydrogen atom. The molecule is thus "saturated" with hydrogen. Unsaturated fatty acids are missing one (in monounsaturated fatty acids) or more (in polyunsaturated fatty acids) hydrogen atoms, so the carbon atoms form double bonds to make up for these "missing links." (See table 3.2 for visual comparisons.)

These seemingly simple molecular variations made a tremendous difference in both the form of the fat and the way it behaves in the body. Saturated fatty acids molecules are very straight, rigid, and molecularly stable. They stick together and resist chemical and temperature changes, both inside and outside of the body. Dietary fats that contain a lot of saturated fatty acids remain solid at room temperature and gel together quickly even after being heated. Lard and other animal fats contain primarily saturated fatty acids, as do cocoa butter, palm kernels (and oils), and coconut products.

In unsaturated fatty acids, the molecule bends at the site of the carbon double bond, making it flexible and sensitive to heat and chemical influences. Since the double bond also gives the molecule a slightly negative electrical charge, unsaturated fatty acids not only don't stick together, they actually repel each other. Most vegetable oils (with the exception of palm and coconut) are composed of unsaturated fatty acids, and they remain liquid at room temperature.

And what about cholesterol? Despite cholesterol's bad reputation, it too plays an important part in the body's normal functioning. Cholesterol is a hard, waxy substance that is a critical component of all cell

3.2 DEGREES OF SATURATION IN FATS

Saturated—Stearic Acid (found in beef and lamb fats)

Chemical Formula:

Molecular Model:

Monounsaturated—Oleic Acid (found in olive oil)

Chemical Formula:

Molecular Model:

Polyunsaturated—Linoleic Acid (found in safflower oil)

Chemical Formula:

Molecular Model:

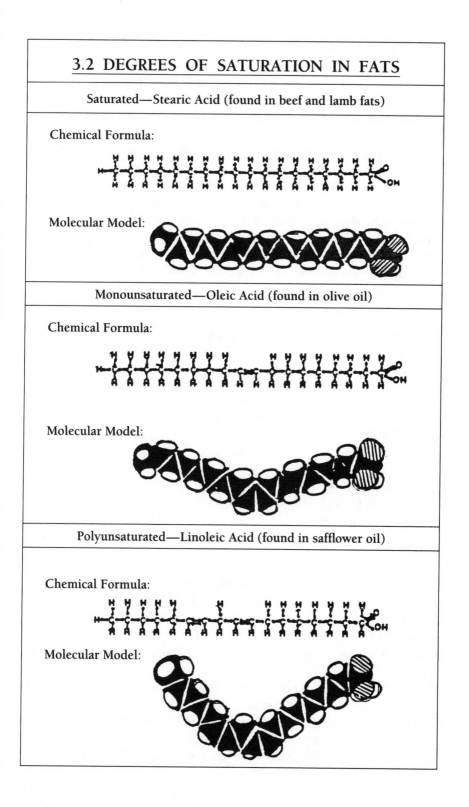

walls. It is part of the bile acids that digest fats, a major component of brain and nerve tissue, and a forerunner of many hormones, particularly the sex hormones. As nutrition researcher Dr. Henry Schroeder has noted, without cholesterol "the skin would dry up, the brain would not function, and there would be no vital hormones of sex and adrenal."

Because cholesterol is crucial to so many of the body's functions, the body makes cholesterol all the time. The building blocks of cholesterol are carbon fragments that the body derives primarily from dietary fats (once the essential fatty acids have been metabolized), carbohydrates (when they have been broken down into simple sugars), and occasionally proteins. In foods, "ready-made" cholesterol is found only in the saturated fats of animal foods (meats, whole milk products, lard, and so forth). All vegetable oils are cholesterol-free.

3.3 EXAMPLES OF DIETARY FATS (by saturation)

Saturated	Monounsaturated	Polyunsaturated
Chicken fat	Olive oil	Safflower oil
Lard	Canola oil	Corn oil
Beef tallow	Peanut oil	Soybean oil
Palm oil	Sunflower oil	Cottonseed oil
Butter		Sesame oil
Cocoa butter		Sunflower oil
Palm kernels/oil		Fish oils
Coconut meat/oil		

The cholesterol controversy stems from the fact that cholesterol is a major component of the plaques that clog arteries and kill millions of people each year. This fact led many eminent researchers and health authorities to conclude that we are eating far too much dietary cholesterol, and that this overload is the cause of arterial plaque and heart disease.

This explanation seems logical, but the situation is a bit more complex than most people realize. The relationship between cholesterol in the *diet* and cholesterol in the *blood* is debatable, at best. There are some human groups—most notably Eskimos still living above the Arctic Circle in traditional fishing and whaling communities—who consume a diet composed almost entirely of saturated fats and protein. Yet these people have virtually no incidence of atherosclerosis (or many other chronic diseases). However, members of this same group who live below the Arctic Circle, and who consume a diet similar to ours, do suffer from these conditions. As we shall see, similar patterns hold true in several other regions. Heart disease, cancer, and other degenerative diseases rise precipitously whenever a natural, wholefoods diet—even one that is high in saturated fat—is replaced with a modern diet high in refined carbohydrates and processed foods.

Such evidence indicates that more than dietary cholesterol is at work in the development of heart disease. Refined carbohydrates are prime suspects, since dietary excesses of these simple sugars prompt the body to build more cholesterol. And research has indeed shown that sugar and other refined carbohydrates cause significant increases in blood cholesterol. Lifestyle factors—including cigarette smoking, lack of exercise, alcoholism, and addiction—are also implicated. Some researchers theorize that the arterial walls themselves have been damaged, and that arterial plaques are the body's attempt to "patch" these damaged regions.

The perpetrators of this arterial damage are thought to be *free radicals*—that is, hyperactive molecules that are destructive by-products of many chemical reactions. Once released in the body, free radicals damage cell walls, break apart other molecules, and generally create havoc. In addition to heart disease, free radicals are thought to be involved in many other degenerative diseases, including cancer.

Free radicals are always present in the body but are kept in control by the action of a variety of micro-nutrients, including vitamins E, C, and A and antioxidant enzymes. Deficiencies in these nutrients are now suspected as potential factors in the development of heart disease, and promising research is being done on using nutritional supplementation in the prevention of heart disease.

The problem of fat, then, is far from simple. To borrow an old cliché, we can't live with it, and we can't live without it. Since dietary fat comes in many forms, we must concentrate on quality as well as quantity when making choices about this particular macro-nutrient. There is no doubt that the vast majority of us consume far too much saturated fat, in the form of red meat and dairy products. Cutting back on these forms of dietary fat is a sensible part of any recovery program. But we must also be careful when choosing unsaturated oils.

Although food oil companies (and some scientists) would have us believe that all vegetable oils are perfect, heart-healthy alternatives to saturated fats, there are some very serious drawbacks to many processed mono- and polyunsaturated oils. The carbon bonds in unsaturated fat are actually weak links that can be attacked by oxygen, turning the oil rancid and actually producing free radicals. Most polyunsaturated oils on the market today are so highly processed that they bear little resemblance, nutritionally or molecularly, to the original product (see chapter 12). So while polyunsaturated oils may indeed be better for us than saturated oils, the ones we find on our supermarket shelves are often pale and toxic shadows of their original, nutritionally sound selves.

For people in recovery (and others who care about their health) the best sources of dietary fat are natural whole grains and seeds, various fish, and unsaturated oils that are as fresh and unprocessed as possible. Dairy and meat products should be used sparingly. For those of you who are worrying about calcium, keep in mind that calcium is found in many foods other than milk (see chapter 15).

Our recipes and specific dietary guidelines rely heavily on such alternative sources of dietary fat, and fit the various guidelines for low-fat diets, with two important caveats. Unlike some health experts, we advise against using both processed polyunsaturated oils and any form of hydrogenated fat (such as margarine). We've already noted the drawbacks of polyunsaturated oils, and in chapter 12 we will examine the significant health risks of the hydrogenated fats, which are now found in everything from cupcakes to potato chips.

Fiber

In the strictest sense, fiber isn't really a nutrient at all. Instead, it is the part of some foods that our bodies *cannot* digest—the hard outer shells of seeds and grains and the peels of certain vegetables and fruits. Bran, one of the most familiar fiber foods, is the outer shell of the wheat grain (or germ). High-fiber foods include oatmeal, whole grains of any kind, and any raw fruit or vegetable.

Fiber is generally found in the plant kingdom, where it serves as a form of defense, protecting the more delicate inner tissues of plants and their fruits, seeds, and grains. In the body, these protective shells retain their toughness, so that even after they have been broken up by our teeth and the physical action of the stomach, they still resist being dissolved by the enzymes and acids of our digestive system.

As a result, these hardy bits of food pass through the digestive tract virtually unchanged. Although they may have been ground down a bit, they retain their basic structure, giving form to solid wastes and giving the muscles of the intestinal tract something to work on. This mechanical effect of fiber is the basis of many of its positive health effects. For example, fiber is known to:

> *Alleviate diarrhea and constipation by keeping bowel contents moving smoothly

> *Reduce pressure within the intestinal tract that can contribute to the development of diverticular diseases (splits and pouches in the tract), appendicitis, hiatus hernias, hemorrhoids, and varicose veins

> *Prevent cancers of the bowel and intestinal tract by shortening the time potential carcinogens are actually in contact with the cells of the bowel, colon, and intestines.

In addition to its helpful physiological effects, some forms of fiber may also be beneficial biochemically. Research on several forms of fiber has shown that increased fiber intake can lower blood levels of LDL (low-density lipoprotein, sometimes called "bad" cholesterol) cholesterol, often as effectively as the cholesterol-lowering drugs currently in use. In addition, fiber is thought to bind other toxic substances and speed them out of the body, like a biochemical detergent.

Whatever the mechanisms, it's clear that the fibrous parts of our food supply—be they apple peels, cucumber seeds, wheat bran, or the hulls of brown rice—are an integral part of the nutritional spectrum and should not be discarded. The body needs fiber, both for its physiological action and its still-to-be-understood chemical properties. For this reason, you will find that most of the recipes in this book call for using whole fruits and vegetables, peels and all, rather than selected parts. To get the most out of our foods nutritionally, it is important not to waste any of their life-giving nutrients.

Water

Water is the one nutrient that no living creature can do without. There are bacteria and viruses that can live without air, but no life form (on this planet, at least) can survive without water.

Not only is water a nutrient in and of itself, it also often contains other nutrients, particularly minerals. Groundwater absorbs minerals from the rock and soil surrounding it and passes these absorbed minerals on to us.

Water purification plants and improved health standards have largely eliminated most bacterial threats to our water supply. But now a range of chemical substances imperil our water, including lead from old pipes, pesticides and chemicals from agricultural runoff, and toxic substances from landfills and illegal dumping. These threats to our most "essential" essential nutrient are becoming an increasingly present problem. In general, it is best to assume that most drinking water in the United States is polluted (until proven otherwise) and rely on bottled, distilled, or filtered water (see chapter 11).

The five macro-nutrients are the most familiar nutrients—the basis for the much-vaunted "four food groups." But one of their primary functions, nutritionally, is to serve as "hosts" for the micro-nutrients—that is, vitamins and minerals. When raw fruits, vegetables, fats, grains, or meats are made into prepared jellies, oils, flours, or sandwich meats, their original stores of micro-nutrients are depleted and destroyed (see chapter 12). For those in recovery, who are already in the red when it comes to their nutritional balance, it is important to look beyond the macro-nutrients when choosing foods, and consider their micro-nutrient content as well.

4 *The Micro-Nutrients*

Vitamins and minerals are a source of confusion to many people, recovering and otherwise. Health food stores and pharmacies are full of various "nutrient formulations" designed to strengthen the immune system, help you sleep, help you stay awake, make you more virile, make you less anxious, cure menstrual cramps, ease headaches, and so forth, ad infinitum. We've gone from an era when vitamins and minerals were completely unrecognized to one in which they are viewed as either miracle cures or snake oils. While some scientists (and food faddists) tout various individual vitamins and minerals as the "cure" for everything from acne to cancer, many physicians are telling their patients they don't really need supplements. What's a person to do?

Far too many people are looking at the micro-nutrients the same way they look at drugs. ("Got a cold? Take two Cs and call me in the morning.") Nutrients—all nutrients—are *not* drugs, and vitamins and minerals are not instant cure-alls for any disease or disorder, be it alcoholism, anorexia, or cancer. The micro-nutrients, like the macro-nutrients in which they are found, are players in a much larger nutritional "game." In tandem with the other elements of good nutrition, they help the body maintain its internal healing processes. Vitamins and minerals won't "make you better," but they will, in the right balance and amounts, help your body make itself better.

Minerals

The first group of micro-nutrients, the minerals, is generally divided into two categories: major and trace. The major minerals are those we need in grams down to tenths of a gram per day. The trace minerals are required in only minute amounts, often measured in millionths of a gram.

As a group, the minerals play several fundamental roles in maintaining the overall structure and balance of the body. Among other functions, minerals:

*form the basis for our entire skeleton, giving bones rigidity and strength *activate many enzyme systems

*control the balance of fluids within and around individual cells

*affect the electrical impulses by which cells communicate

*regulate the pH balance.

4.1 THE ESSENTIAL MINERALS

Major Minerals		Trace Minerals
sodium (Na)	iron (Fe)	molybdenum (Mo)
magnesium (Mg)	copper (Cu)	tin (Sn)
phosphorus (P)	iodine (I)	silicon (Si)
chlorine (Cl)	manganese (Mn)	vanadium (V)
potassium (K)	chromium (Cr)	cobalt (Co)
calcium (Ca)	zinc (Zn)	nickel (Ni)
sulfur (S)	fluorine (F)	arsenic (As)
	selenium (Se)	

The pH balance (literally, "power of hydrogen") is the balance of hydrogen in the fluid surrounding the body's cells. Just as the body as a whole needs the correct concentration of oxygen in the air in order to survive, so individual cells need the right concentration of hydrogen in order to function. When hydrogen levels drop too far—a condition known as acidosis—the body's systems become depressed; mental activity slows, consciousness is lost, and the person can progress into a fatal coma. When levels go too far up (alkalosis), the body becomes hyperreactive and severe muscular contractions and potentially fatal convulsions can result. Even relatively minor fluctuations in pH balance can critically influence cellular function.

Alcohol abuse, drug addictions, anorexia, and bulimia all have profound effects on these critical minerals, and therefore on the body's all-important extracellular environment. As we shall see in chapter 6, all of these disorders cause severe fluid imbalances, with a corresponding loss of minerals.

Vitamins

Up until the turn of this century, it was generally assumed that a diet that contained carbohydrates, protein, fat, minerals, and water was enough to sustain life. Despite the hard lessons of scurvy, beriberi, and pellagra, medicine, governments, and society at large had not caught on to the difference between the quality of a food supply and its quantity. This critical difference did not become generally recognized until scientists began nutritional experiments with lab animals. When researchers tried to raise animals on diets made up of relatively "pure" nutrients—consisting solely of protein, or fat, or carbohydrates—they had amazingly consistent results. Not only did the animals not thrive on these purified diets, but if they were kept on the diets for too long they invariably died—and often of diseases that looked remarkably like the diseases seen in man, such as scurvy. Obviously, calories alone were not enough to sustain life. What was missing?

During the first half of the twentieth century, scores of researchers around the world embarked on a search for the mysterious "missing factors" of nutrition. Within a forty-year period, all fourteen known essential vitamins were discovered and then chemically synthesized in laboratories.

4.2 THE KNOWN ESSENTIAL VITAMINS

Fat-Soluble	Water-Soluble
A (retinol)	B_1 (thiamine)
D (calciferol)	B_2 (riboflavin)
E (tocopherol)	B_3 (niacin)
K (phylloquinone)	B_5 (pantothenic acid)
	B_6 (pyridoxine)
	B_{12} (cyanocobalamin)
	folic acid (folacin)
	biotin
	C (ascorbic acid)
	choline

Vitamins hold a unique position in the nutritional universe. They do not serve as building blocks, sources of energy, or basic elements. Instead, vitamins are *co-enzymes* in the body's metabolic processes, fitting like keys into the thousands of chemical "locks" to free the body's enzymes to carry out their tasks. Enzymes control every biochemical reaction in the body by bringing together all the necessary ingredients for each individual reaction. They are the all-important catalysts for the body's most basic and integral functions.

Like a key for which there is no master, no vitamin can substitute for another in a given metabolic system. At the same time, no vitamin carries out a basic function all by itself. As with the orchestra referred to earlier, every component of the vitamin–enzyme system must be in place for the symphony of life to proceed in harmony.

Since the body cannot produce vitamins on its own, we have to turn to foods to obtain these vital "missing factors." Although animal tissues—particularly organ meats such as liver—are rich sources of the B group and other vitamins, our primary source of vitamins is the plant kingdom.

Like most of the nutrients we have discussed thus far, the vitamins are divided into two distinct groups, based on their ability to dissolve in water. The water-soluble vitamins (vitamin C and the B vitamins) are absorbed more easily by the body and are not kept in long-term storage in any appreciable amounts. Water-soluble vitamins that are not needed by the body are "flushed out" in the urine. Because of this, it is virtually impossible to overdose on these vitamins and we need to have a fairly steady and constant supply of them in the diet.

The fat-soluble vitamins (A, D, E, and K), on the other hand, can only be absorbed from the intestinal tract in the presence of fat (hence the importance of having *some* fat in the diet). Because of their affinity for fat tissue, these vitamins can be stored in the fatty deposits of the body. As a result, it is possible (albeit unlikely) to consume toxic levels of the fat-soluble vitamins.

The vitamins and minerals that comprise the micro-nutrients are the most vulnerable members of the nutritional team. We have never met a recovering alcoholic, bulimic, anorexic, chronic overeater, or any other addict who was not deficient in vitamins and minerals—both as a result of their abysmal diets and because of addiction-induced damage to the organs that process nutrients. Because of this, most recovering individuals at first need fairly intensive supplementation just to recoup their losses.

Although there are many good reasons to take vitamin supplements (see chapter 11), they are not the way to ensure good nutrition. For one thing, we have yet to identify all the "missing factors" required for human life. Supplements based on incomplete knowledge simply cannot provide us with everything we need. For another, supplements are, by definition, designed to *augment* a good diet, not replace it. Even in the best of all possible worlds, vitamins are lost during the harvesting, transportation, and preparation of foods; and we are living in anything but the best of all possible worlds (see chapter 12). High-quality, *comprehensive* nutritional supplementation (as opposed to single vitamins) can offset these losses and help ensure that the body has the necessary balance of vitamins and minerals to function well. Appendix I outlines some of the basics of such a supplementation program.

Table 4.3 lists the major micro-nutrients and their biological functions, as well as good dietary sources and some of the effects of deficiency and toxicity. Although several of the nutrients (such as vitamin E) have no specific toxic effects listed, this does not mean that you should take them in massive doses. A complete balance of nutrients is essential to proper physical functioning. Overdosing on any nutrient can upset that balance and stress the liver and kidneys. In many cases an overdose will cause acute nausea and vomiting. So treat all vitamin and mineral supplements with the respect they deserve.

4.3 MAJOR MICRO-NUTRIENTS AND THEIR FUNCTIONS

Nutrient	Sources	Functions	Signs of Deficiency	Signs of Toxicity
VITAMINS				
Vitamin A	fish, fish oils, eggs, green and yellow vegetables, dairy products	maintains health of skin and photoreceptors in the retina	night blindness, rough skin, dry eyes, corneal softening and clouding	headaches, peeling skin, enlarged spleen
Vitamin B$_1$ (thiamine)	whole grains, meats, nuts, legumes, potatoes	carbohydrate metabolism, nerve function, heart function	nerve damage, heart failure, brain damage (Wernicke-Korsakoff syndrome)	
Vitamin B$_2$ (riboflavin)	milk and milk products, eggs, liver, meat	energy and protein metabolism, maintains integrity of mucus membranes	dryness, scaling, and splitting of lips and mouth, corneal changes, dry and inflamed skin	
Vitamin B$_6$ (pyridoxine)	fish, liver and other organ meats, whole grains, legumes	crucial to metabolism of linoleic acid, helps convert tryptophan to niacin, important in formation of blood cells and blood clotting	anemias, skin lesions, neuropathy, convulsions (in infants). Contributes to development of dependency syndromes	
Vitamin B$_{12}$ (cobalamin)	liver, meats, eggs, milk and milk products	maturation of red blood cells, nerve function, DNA synthesis, folate and methionine metabolism	anemias, psychological disorders, loss of visual acuity. Contributes to development of dependency syndromes	

Nutrient	Sources	Functions	Signs of Deficiency	Signs of Toxicity
Biotin	liver, kidney, yeast, egg yolk, cauliflower, nuts, legumes	amino acid and fatty acid metabolism	inflammation of the skin and tongue. Contributes to development of dependency syndromes	
Niacin	dried yeast, liver, meat, fish, legumes, enriched whole-grain products	carbohydrate metabolism, oxidation-reduction reactions	inflamed, peeling skin and tongue, gastrointestinal disorders (including severe diarrhea), central nervous system dysfunction (dementia)	
Folic acid	fresh green leafy vegetables, fruit, organ meats, liver, dried yeast	maturation of red blood cells, synthesis of components of DNA	anemias, red blood cell abnormalities, neural tube defects (in infants of folic-acid-deficient mothers)	
Vitamin C	green peppers, citrus fruits, tomatoes, potatoes, cabbage	bone formation, collagen formation, vascular function, tissue respiration and repair	inflammation of the gums and mouth, tooth loss, hemorrhaging	
Vitamin D	sunlight, fish liver oils, egg yolk, liver, fortified dairy products	absorption and utilization of calcium and phosphorous, bone formation	rickets	anorexia, kidney failure, calcification of soft tissues
Vitamin E	vegetable oils, wheat germ, green leafy vegetables, egg yolk, legumes	stability of cellular membranes, anti-oxidant	loss of hemoglobin from red blood cells, muscle damage	

Nutrient	Sources	Functions	Signs of Deficiency	Signs of Toxicity
MINERALS				
Sodium	in most processed foods, naturally in seafood, sea vegetables and cheeses	fluid balance, nerve transmission, muscle contractility	dehydration	mental confusion, coma
Potassium	bananas, prunes, raisins, milk	nerve transmission, muscle activity, fluid retention	cardiac disturbances, paralysis	same as deficiency
Calcium	milk and milk products, meat, fish, eggs, whole grains, beans, fruit, vegetables	bone and tooth formation, blood clotting, cardiac function, muscle function	neuromuscular hyperexcitability	diarrhea, renal failure, psychosis
Phosphorus	milk and milk products, meat, poultry, fish, whole grains, nuts, legumes	bone and tooth formation, part of DNA, energy production	irritability, weakness, blood cell disorders, gastrointestinal and renal problems	kidney failure
Magnesium	green leaves, nuts, whole grains, seafoods	bone and tooth formation, nerve conduction, enzyme activation, muscle contraction	neuromuscular irritability	low blood pressure, respiratory failure, cardiac disturbances
Iron	widely distributed in most foods other than dairy products, but less than 20% is absorbed by the body	blood formation, enzyme function	anemia	liver damage, skin pigment changes, diabetes. May contribute to the development of heart disease
Iodine	seafoods, sea vegetables, dairy products	thyroid function, energy control mechanisms	goiter, brain damage (in infants)	skin changes, swollen lips and nose
Fluorine	widely distributed	bone and tooth formation	tooth decay, osteoporosis	pitted teeth, spinal spurs
Zinc	widely distributed in vegetables, but not well absorbed	wound healing, growth, enzyme and insulin formation	growth retardation, gastrointestinal problems, skin disorders, liver damage	
Copper	organ meats, oysters, nuts, legumes, whole grains	component of enzymes	anemia, Menkes' kinky hair syndrome	liver damage

Nutrient	Sources	Functions	Signs of Deficiency	Signs of Toxicity
Cobalt	green leafy vegetables	part of B_{12} molecule	anemia	cardiomyopathy
Chromium	brewer's yeast, widely distributed in most foods	glucose metabolism	impaired glucose tolerance in malnourished children and diabetics	

Source: *The Merck Manual of Diagnosis and Therapy,* 15th ed. (Rahway, NJ: Merck Sharp & Dohme Research Laboratories).

5 Making It Work: Digestion, Absorption, and Utilization

As we noted earlier, nutrition depends not only on the food you eat, but on how your body handles that food. The most nutrient-rich foods in the world won't do you much good if the nutrients don't get out of the foods and into the cells of your body. In order for this to happen, your body must:

1. extract the nutrients from food (digestion),
2. get the nutrients into the bloodstream so they can reach the body's cells (absorption), and
3. actually put the nutrients to work in biochemical processes (utilization).

Disrupt any part of this process, and malnutrition (to varying degrees) is the result. Nutrition is a remarkably complex process, and addictions (particularly alcoholism) and eating disorders of all kinds cause disruptions throughout this system. (We'll discuss these effects in detail in chapter 6.)

Digestion and Absorption

The work of extracting nutrients from food, breaking them down into usable form, and absorbing them into the body is carried out in the gastrointestinal (or GI) tract—a convoluted tube that begins at the mouth and continues down through the rectum. As food passes through this tube it is physically and chemically broken down into its component parts, which are then processed by various organs (particularly the liver and pancreas) for use or storage within the body's cells.

Digestion begins in the mouth, where food is ground up by the teeth and mixed with enzymes in saliva that begin breaking down the molecular structure of the food particles. From the mouth, food moves through the tube of the esophagus into the muscular bag of the stomach, where powerful digestive enzymes (including hydrochloric acid) continue to break down the food particles. The delicate lining of the stomach is protected from these corrosive juices by a layer of mucus. Without this protective layer, the stomach would digest itself.

From the stomach, partially digested food empties through the pyloric sphincter into the duodenum and small intestine, the primary site of digestion and absorption of nutrients. The inner walls of the small intestine are convoluted and covered with millions of fingerlike projections called villi. As the intestinal muscles contract and mix the partially digested food with digestive enzymes from the pancreas and gallbladder, the villi absorb nutrients and pass them into the bloodstream.

Whatever remains after all this breakdown and absorption continues on into the large intestine, where water is removed and solid matter moves slowly through the intestines and finally out of the body. (Liquid wastes are processed through the kidneys, which filter waste products out of the blood and pass them to the bladder for excretion.)

Utilization

Digestion and absorption only make nutrients *available* for use by the body. The actual process of *using and storing* these nutrients (metabolism) is performed by the liver, the pancreas, and other organs, which break nutrients down into components that can be absorbed by individual cells.

Nestled alongside the stomach and above the intestines on the right side of the body, the liver is one of the body's most remarkable organs. Nutrient-rich blood from the digestive tract flows through the liver's microscopic canals and pockets, where nutrients are metabolized and given their "marching orders" for distribution to the body's cells.

The liver is also a storage site (for vitamins and carbohydrates) and a detoxification plant. The cells of the liver break down poisonous (or potentially poisonous) compounds such as alcohol and drugs into less toxic products that can be eliminated from the body. As a result, the liver bears the brunt of many toxic assaults on the body, and it is particularly susceptible to the damaging effects of alcohol and drug abuse.

The pancreas is one of the body's most crucial glands, and it is also one of the most susceptible to the ravages of alcoholism and drug abuse (see chapter 6). Through its secretions into the duodenum and the bloodstream, the pancreas controls blood glucose levels, helps break down fats and cholesterol, helps break down starch, and maintains pH balance by releasing minerals.

The pancreas releases its digestive enzymes, minerals, and hormones (insulin and glucagon) in response to a variety of biological signals, including the level of glucose in the blood, the pH balance, gastric acids, the presence of dietary factors such as fatty and amino acids, and nerve impulses from the brain.

The most well-known disorder of the pancreas, diabetes, is characterized by the failure of the pancreas to produce insulin and by the inability of the body's cells to absorb/use insulin and glucose. Without insulin, the body's cells cannot absorb glucose from the bloodstream and are left without fuel even as blood glucose levels rise. Unless controlled with proper treatment, diabetes causes extensive biological damage that includes a greatly increased rate of circulatory disorders, atherosclerotic disease, nerve damage, and a potentially fatal form of acidosis (ketoacidosis) commonly referred to as a diabetic coma.

Addictions (particularly alcoholism) and eating disorders damage the pancreas both by their direct toxic effects and by disrupting many of the biological "cues" on which the pancreas depends. Pancreatitis (inflammation of the pancreas) is one of the most severe manifestations of advanced alcoholism.

Appetite vs. Hunger: The Importance of the Brain

Nutrition, even poor nutrition, cannot occur unless we eat something. But the process of deciding to eat, and of choosing particular foods, is really quite complicated.

Why do we eat? The simplest answer is "Because we're hungry." But the process of eating (or of wanting to eat) is not just a matter of full stomach versus empty stomach. If it were we would never have "just enough room" for dessert after a huge meal, or "not feel like having" a particular food even though we had not eaten in a while.

Although the actual handling of nutrients is done by the organs of the gastrointestinal and digestive tracts, the impulses to start and stop eating come from much higher up: the brain. And when it comes to eating, the hypothalamus is command central—a command central that is all too easily confused and circumvented.

Within the body, the hypothalamus is the nutritional equivalent of an air traffic controller, monitoring information coming in from various pathways and giving out orders accordingly. From its vantage point within the brain, the hypothalamus receives information both from the organs that digest and absorb nutrients and from the contents of the bloodstream itself. For example, it is the hypothalamus that signals the pancreas to secrete insulin when blood glucose levels get too high.

Whenever we eat a meal, an intricate communications network is activated within the body. All along the gastrointestinal tract, receptors monitor the contents of the food being digested. If the brain had to wait for nutrients to be entirely digested and circulating in the bloodstream before issuing the "stop eating" signal, our meals would be unending. But because of its ability to monitor the content of our food as we are consuming it, the brain (through the hypothalamus) can make an "educated guess" about when we have eaten enough, and tell us to stop. This signal that we have had enough is referred to as "satiety."

Different foods can have very different influences on satiety. For example, numerous researchers have found that there is a longer period of satiety after a protein-rich meal than after a carbohydrate-rich meal. Low-nutrient-density foods, on the other hand, may leave us feeling full but still wanting more, since the brain "knows" that we have not taken in enough nutrients. It is this satiety effect of different foods that may be responsible for the phenomenon of "being hungry an hour later" after certain meals.

Of course, it is always possible to ignore the cues being sent from the hypothalamus. We can continue to eat when we are no longer really hungry, or ignore the desire to eat when we are. We can eat nutrient-poor foods (such as cookies, candy, or booze) when the brain is really signaling for something nutrient-rich (fruit, chicken, or some vegetables). Every day we are surrounded by social and environmental cues, from television commercials to aggressive hosts, that can override the inherent wisdom of the body. And if we override it long enough, we can actually change the delicate chemical balance of the brain.

When we look at the whole spectrum of nutrition, it is clear that good nutrition—the kind needed by all people in recovery—is a lot more than just getting enough of the four food groups. It's getting the right balance of nutrients, in the right number of calories, eaten at the right times. It's having a healthy, functional gastrointestinal tract—from the muscles of the tongue to the caniculi of the liver. And it's being in touch with the "wisdom of the body" so that we eat what we *need* rather than what we *want*. (Of course, when we are in proper nutritional balance, what we want usually *is* what we need!)

When we become enmeshed in an addiction, eating disorder, and even some compulsive and emotional disorders, all of these components fall to pieces. Indeed, as we shall see in the next chapter, nutrition is one of the first things to go in these disorders, which is why it needs to be one of the first things restored in recovery.

6 The Impact of Addictions

Nutrition is one of life's most intricate and amazing processes. It is also at once incredibly vulnerable and remarkably resilient. Although any nutritional deficiency—no matter how small—can disrupt the balance of nutrition and the functioning of our cells, the body will hang in there for quite a while even in the face of severe want. It will draw on its nutritional stores (such as the calcium in bones), shift gears so that it expends less energy (the lethargy seen in malnourished Third World children), and generally make every adjustment it can in order to survive.

This resilience may be one of the reasons that so many people (doctors included) underestimate or ignore the nutritional impact of addictions and eating disorders. They assume that the absence of obvious symptoms of malnutrition (such as the bleeding gums of scurvy or the madness of pellagra) equals good nutrition. Nothing could be farther from the truth.

Drug addiction, alcoholism, anorexia, bulimia, and even compulsive overeating all have devastating effects on nutritional status. As we have seen, when these nutritional impacts are addressed and restored, recovery is a relatively smooth and comfortable experience. When they are not, recovery often becomes a long battle against the ongoing symptoms of pancellular (affecting all cells) malnutrition, symptoms of which can include:

heartburn	dental decay	fatigue
nausea	cravings	frequent minor illnesses
diarrhea	anxiety	insomnia
loss of appetite	depression	impotence

Think of these symptoms as biological distress signals—an ongoing SOS from the body's starved and poisoned cells. It is not enough to treat the symptoms (by taking an antacid, or a tranquilizer, or an antidiarrheal); you've got to repair these systems from the inside out. And in order to do that, you have to understand what went wrong in the first place.

41

Some Common Denominators

One of the problems with discussing the nutritional impact of drug addictions, alcoholism, and eating disorders is the very uneven state of research in these fields. The nutritional impact of eating disorders has been very well studied, and that of alcoholism has received some attention, but the impact of drug addiction has been largely ignored. The reasons for this are complex. Part of the problem is that many patients are addicted to substances that are illegal, so systematic study of their physical condition is difficult. Another (and perhaps larger) obstacle is the widespread perception of all drug addicts as criminals and deviants. Who cares if they're malnourished? They deserve whatever they get.

Although the research on specific drugs may be scant, we do know a lot about the general nutritional impact of addictions of any kind. And while the drugs of abuse have very different effects, there are several unifying nutritional themes that are common to most drugs (from cocaine through valium), alcohol, and even eating disorders. These nutritional effects are seen regardless of the specific drug or behavior being abused.

First and foremost, these disorders completely disrupt the brain mechanisms that control eating behavior. Alcohol suppresses the hypothalamic regions that prompt eating behavior. Stimulant drugs (such as cocaine and speed) suppress the brain's appetite control center, which is why some stimulants were once widely abused as diet pills. Marijuana and other forms of cannabis also disrupt the appetite control center, prompting food cravings (most notably for carbohydrates) that are popularly known as "the munchies." Heroin and other opiates slow down the action of the gastrointestinal tract and interfere with nutrient absorption. This effect is reversed during opiate withdrawal, when heroin addicts experience severe cramps, diarrhea, and vomiting that drain the body of nutrients. In essence, drug and alcohol addictions (and anorexia) tell us *not to eat.* Food loses its normal, healthy position in day-to-day life and is replaced by the drug. For example, it has been estimated that alcoholics consume up to one half of their total caloric intake in the form of alcohol. These individuals literally have "liquid lunches." And breakfasts. And dinners. And everything in between. Eating comes in a poor second (or third) in the life of an addict or alcoholic.

Food takes on an inappropriate role in eating disorders, as well— except that instead of being ignored, eating becomes the center of the universe. For anorexics and bulimics, food is the enemy, a trap waiting to be sprung. Eating is a failure of will that must be atoned for through purging (vomiting, taking diarrhetics or diuretics) or excessive exercise to burn the hated calories. For compulsive overeaters, on the other hand, food is a panacea, a comforter and friend in time of need. Eating is a fix.

In eating disorders and addictions, the quality of the food consumed is invariably abysmal. Compulsive overeaters tend to choose foods high in refined carbohydrates such as sugar, which are known to have dramatic emotional and psychological effects (see chapter 7). During binges, bulimics make similar food choices, sometimes consuming gallons of ice cream or boxes of cookies in one sitting. We have already noted that alcoholics consume 50 percent of their calories as alcohol, and when they do eat more solid foods alcoholics (anu most drug addicts) tend to pick "fast foods" that are high in sugar, fat, caffeine, and additives.

In sum, then, eating disorders, addictions, and alcoholism all share the following characteristics:

*Food takes on an inappropriate role in life.

*Food is consumed at the wrong times.

*Food is consumed in the wrong amounts.

*The foods that are consumed are nutritionally deficient.

These factors alone would be enough to render the addict or individual with an eating disorder malnourished. When you add in the toxic effects of the drug or behavior itself, however, the nutritional stakes increase geometrically. (The specific impact of alcoholism and eating disorders will be addressed in detail a little later in this chapter.)

Whenever you consume a drug, be it alcohol or heroin, it is broken down (metabolized) by the liver. As we saw in chapter 5, the liver is critical to the processes of nutrition. When the liver (and its coworkers in the body's metabolic factory) is overloaded and toxified by addictive drugs, its nutritional functions are also damaged. The body loses its ability to digest, absorb, and utilize the few nutrients it is getting, leading to a fairly consistent pattern of addiction-induced nutritional damage:

*Ingested nutrients aren't well absorbed.

*Absorbed nutrients aren't well utilized.

*Normal metabolism becomes deranged, from the cellular level on up.

Without proper fuel to carry out the most basic life processes, the toxic and malnourished cells of our bodies become damaged and dysfunctional. From the brain to the skin, every cell in the body is fighting to stay alive (with an ever-shrinking supply of ammunition) in the face of an ongoing chemical assault. In this state the entire body is more susceptible to illnesses of all kinds, from the mildest cold virus to the most aggressive cancer cell.

While all addictions and eating disorders are associated with major malnutrition and its resultant dysfunctions, alcoholism has some of the most spectacularly damaging effects on the bodily systems involved in nutrition.

Alcoholism

Have you ever thought about the *ways* in which most drugs of abuse are taken? Some are snorted. Some are injected. Some are smoked. Some are swallowed. Of those that are swallowed only one also has the distinction of being (technically) a food: alcohol. This means that the body processes alcohol through the same mechanisms it uses for other foods, much to its own detriment.

Alcohol is, first and foremost, a poison. As it passes through the digestive tract, it leaves a trail of destruction that is unparalleled among the addictions. The direct negative effects of contact with alcohol include (organ by organ):

*Esophagus—tissue irritation and damage to the sphincter muscle connecting the esophagus and stomach. Can lead to nausea, vomiting, and a reflux (backup) of stomach acid into the esophagus that causes chronic heartburn.

*Stomach—irritation of the stomach lining and a thinning of the protective mucus layer, which leads to further irritation from stomach acids and eventually to ulcers and internal bleeding.

*Intestines—cellular damage in the intestinal wall and villi makes them more porous, allowing large, incompletely digested food particles to pass directly into the bloodstream. Quite literally, alcoholic patients develop "leaky guts." (See chapter 8 for other ramifications of this condition.)

The digestion of alcohol causes a series of unique and disruptive biochemical messages to be sent throughout the nutritional system. These messages prompt a wide range of potentially destructive reactions, including substantial decreases in the enzymes needed to digest carbohydrates, absorb and activate vitamins and minerals, metabolize amino acids, and oxidize (burn) fatty acids.

Physiologically, the muscles of the intestinal tract respond to alcohol by moving more rapidly, causing diarrhea. Urinary output is also increased.

In the liver, the detoxification system is working overtime, trying to break the alcohol down and get it out of the body as fast as possible. One of the products of this breakdown, acetaldehyde, is a toxin in its own right. The liver continues to break acetaldehyde down into its component parts, but if the flow of alcohol is too swift and too great the liver simply can't keep up. As a result, some of that acetaldehyde gets into the bloodstream, where it can poison every cell with which it comes in contact.

If the flood of alcohol is long-term and constant, the liver may finally try to adapt to the situation by kicking into overdrive. It will set up an additional system to process all that alcohol: the microsomal ethanol oxidizing system, or MEOS. Unfortunately, it *won't* set up a similar system to break down acetaldehyde, and as a result even more of the toxic chemical will find its way into the body's cells. Even worse, the MEOS, once it has kicked in, will actually *need* alcohol in order to maintain its existence. Hence addiction.

Of course, the liver has better things to do than just process alcohol, and all this alcohol processing and acetaldehyde poisoning isn't helping any of those functions. Protein metabolism is altered, and the liver begins burning its own protein stores even as it fails to eliminate fatty acids. As a result, fat begins to build up in the liver itself. This replacement of healthy liver cells with fat damages the liver's ability to detoxify poisons (including alcohol) and process nutrients, and can eventually lead to fatal conditions such as cirrhosis.

The pancreas, on the other hand, is suffering the effects of all those misguided biochemical messages. As serum blood glucose levels rise (because alcohol is the ultimate refined carbohydrate), the pancreas responds by dumping insulin into the bloodstream in an attempt to bring things into balance. Its ability to absorb and process the essential fatty acids and fat-soluble vitamins is impaired. And if the alcohol intake continues, pancreatic enzymes can actually begin to digest the cells of the pancreas itself—a potentially fatal complication of advanced alcoholism.

The hypothalamus, in its position of biochemical air traffic controller, is also running into problems. The signals coming in from the GI tract and the bloodstream are anything but normal, and acetaldehyde is starting to have a damaging effect on the cells of the brain. The end result is a *suppression* of normal hunger and an increase in messages to consume more alcohol. Every drink the alcoholic takes is telling his or her brain that it doesn't want any other food.

The end product of all this is, of course, a nutritional disaster. The liver and the pancreas are so "out of it" that normal digestion, absorption, and utilization of nutrients has come to a virtual standstill. Fat metabolism becomes very distorted, increasing the risk of heart disease and damaging other systems dependent on the essential fatty acids and the fat-soluble vitamins. Important nutrients such as zinc, magnesium, potassium, and calcium are actually being flushed out of the body in the urine. The body's ability to absorb thiamine, B_{12}, folic acid, and even glucose (the brain's only source of fuel) drops dramatically. In a desperate attempt to make up the deficit and fuel the efforts to process the alcohol, the body starts drawing on its stored nutrients, including the calcium stored in bones and teeth. (This is why alcoholics are exceptionally prone to tooth decay and broken bones.) Overall, the alcoholic becomes seriously deficient in all of the major nutrients.

Eating Disorders

Eating disorders—whether undereating or overeating—may well be the most difficult of addictive disorders to treat, not just because the substance being abused is food, but because of the biological impact of these conditions.

If you have ever been chronically under- or overweight, you know how difficult it can be to change. We've lost count of the times we have heard the sad refrain: "No matter what I do I just can't seem to lose [gain] any weight!"

Eating disorders do more than just disrupt the normal processes of nutrition; they reprogram the body's internal thermostat. For example, if you gain weight and remain at that weight for an extended period of time, the appetite control mechanisms in the brain "believe" that weight is the norm. When you go on a diet to lose weight, that internal thermostat is going to disagree with you. Although you think you are dieting, your body thinks it's being starved. When you restrict calories, it will slow the rate at which you burn them (resting metabolic rate). When you try and avoid fatty foods, sweets, and so forth, it will prompt cravings—since as far as the brain is concerned you are *supposed* to have all those fat cells filled to capacity. This is the central reason that diets that rely on caloric restriction alone often fail.

In the case of anorexia, the body *is* being starved—and the metabolic response is the same. As anorexia progresses, the hypothalamus, through its connections to the pituitary gland and gonads, sends out emergency orders of a different kind. Since the body isn't receiving enough nutrients to cover even its own needs, it takes steps to prevent any additional drains on its resources—specifically pregnancy. In anorexic women, menstrual cycles eventually stop altogether.

The starvation of anorexia is a state of extreme physiological stress, and as we shall see in chapter 7, this stress prompts the release of several potent and addictive brain chemicals. Anorexic individuals become as addicted to these brain chemicals as heroin or cocaine addicts are to their drugs of abuse—and often have even more difficulty "withdrawing" from them.

We have already discussed the poor nutritional quality of the food consumed by most individuals with eating disorders. In the case of people who binge and then purge, this is exacerbated by the devastating effects of purging.

The gastrointestinal tract is essentially a one-way street. Food comes in, goes down, and eventually goes out. Purging either reverses (vomiting) or radically speeds up (enemas, diuretics) this process. Both methods are anything but good for the gastrointestinal tract.

Vomiting brings corrosive stomach acids up into the delicate tissues of the esophagus, throat, and mouth, damaging the lining of these organs and eating through tooth enamel. (Long-term bulimics invariably have extensive dental damage.) The strain of forcing the stomach contents back up through the tract also causes veins within the throat and esophagus to become distended, and ruptures and internal bleeding can occur. Diarrheals damage the lining of the intestines (much as alcohol does), so that bulimics often develop "leaky guts" similar to those found in alcoholics, even as much-needed nutrients are rushed out of the body. Diuretics, meanwhile, put excessive strain on the kidneys and cause critical nutrients to be flushed out in urine.

When individuals with eating disorders get into recovery, they are faced with the formidable task of both repairing this gastrointestinal damage and "reprogramming" brains that have become seriously disordered. For persons battling obesity, there is the stubborn internal thermostat, while for anorexics and bulimics there is the seductive and addictive call of stress-induced brain chemicals.

Fortunately, there are ways to combat these problems and help the brain and the organs of the digestive system to achieve a normal balance once again. As we shall see in the next chapter, food can be a potent ally in bringing the brain back "on line."

7 Diet and the Mind: The Relationship Between What We Eat and How We Feel

We know that drugs and alcohol change the way we think and feel. (That's why we did them in the first place!) Yet foods—from the humble baked potato to the most expensive filet mignon—also affect the brain, and hence our thoughts and feelings. But since the impact is often both delayed and subtle, we do not notice it.

Almost everyone remembers the balm of hot chicken soup during a miserable head cold. Or the soothing effect of a cup of warm milk on a cold winter's night. For generations, mothers have told their children to "eat, you'll feel better," and for generations children have benefited from their wholesome (if unscientific) advice.

The calming effects of certain foods is not an illusion; it is a biochemical effect that we can harness and use in the recovery process. Strange though it may seem, food can be an extraordinarily effective "tranquilizer" in times of stress. A friend of ours likes to tell a story that dramatically illustrates this fact.

She was sponsoring a woman we shall call Karen in her local AA group. One evening, Karen called her in a state of distress. She had just had a fight with her boyfriend, was very upset, and was worried that she might relapse. Could our friend please come over?

After talking with Karen for a while, our friend told her that she would be able to go over, but not right away. But while Karen waited, she wanted her to do something to keep her hands and mind occupied. Instead of watching television or worrying about her boyfriend, our friend told Karen to have a glass of juice and then make some fresh mashed potatoes—using real potatoes. She gave Karen detailed instructions on how to make them, and asked her to eat them, out of a bowl, while sitting in her favorite comfortable chair. Karen was puzzled, but she promised to give it a try while she waited.

A little while later, as our friend was starting out, the phone rang. It was Karen. "This is so strange!" she said. "I did as you said and I actually feel a lot better! I mean, I'm still angry at my boyfriend, but I feel a lot calmer."

In recommending that Karen drink some juice and then cook mashed potatoes, our friend had made use of several of the potentially healing powers of food. The juice had given Karen a quick blood sugar boost and the process of preparing the mashed potatoes had given her something concrete to do while waiting for her sponsor to arrive. Eating the potatoes out of a bowl, in a comfortable chair, had allowed her to relax and enjoy the texture, temperature, and flavor of the food. And, most importantly, the potatoes themselves had provided nutrients that actually changed the chemical balance in her brain.

Our friend, and all those generations of concerned mothers and grandmothers, were far from the first to believe in and use the healing powers of food. In fact, they are only part of a long line of physicians, healers, and scientists who have used food for recovery.

Historical Precedents

Long before the discovery of psychiatric drugs, doctors of all cultures used food as part of their treatments. Although its popularity has waxed and waned (replaced over time by more dramatic interventions such as leeches, purges, surgery, and drugs), food has always been one of the safest and most effective ways of preventing and healing disease.

The importance of diet in conditions such as heart disease, gout, and even cancer has been well recognized for many years. But there are equally compelling scientific and historical arguments for diet's impact on psychological conditions. In the 1790s, when most asylums were chaining their inmates to walls and dousing them with ice water, a devout and humane man named William Tuke, along with his family, revolutionized the care of the mentally ill. Horrified at the cruelty and squalor of England's asylums, the Tuke family established the York Retreat in the English countryside. As part of their humane approach to mental illness, the Tukes used food to calm manic patients. Noting that a full stomach induced tranquillity and even sleep, the Tukes fed their more excitable patients meat, cheese, bread, and port at bedtime. Instead of shackling patients to their beds or the walls, the Tukes fed them to sleep. Though the Tuke family did not know it, they were manipulating the very chemistry of their patients' brains.

Some Basic Brain Biology

It is easy to think of the brain as something completely apart from the body, but everything we see, hear, smell, taste, think, and feel is processed through this remarkable organ. We take these abilities for granted—until something catastrophic, such as a stroke or other severe brain injury, deprives us of them. Or until the brain is devastated by the effects of drugs, alcohol, or eating disorders.

The highs and lows we feel from drugs, alcohol, and even certain behaviors such as binging and purging are all the result of their impact on the brain. These substances and behaviors exert their addictive effects by replacing, interfering with, or speeding up the brain's normal chemical processes.

Brain cells communicate via highly specialized chemicals known as neurotransmitters. Through the release of neurotransmitters, the brain responds to signals from every cell, organ, and system of the body and sends out controlling signals of its own.

The production and release of neurotransmitters is a special electrochemical process that has evolved as a result of the brain's unique structure. Although the brain may look like a unified mass, its individual cells are not directly connected. Instead, each nerve cell in the brain is separated from the others by infinitesimal gaps known as synapses. Cells communicate by ejecting neurotransmitters into these gaps, where it floats across and "docks" into waiting receptor sites on neighboring cells. This prompts an electrical charge within the receptor cell, triggering the production and release of more neurotransmitters—sort of an electrochemical domino effect. Once all the neighboring receptor sites have been filled, whatever chemical is left in the gap is reabsorbed into the cell and is recycled for later use (a process known as re-uptake). It is an extremely efficient and highly specialized system. Each neurotransmitter is associated with a specific region of the brain, where it governs highly specific activities.

The fuel that powers all these nerve impulses and neurotransmitter releases is serum glucose, or blood sugar. Like a delicate and finely tuned engine, the brain needs a steady supply of this fuel in order to function efficiently. As Jim found out, when the supply of blood glucose becomes irregular, brain function suffers accordingly—the neurological equivalent of engine knocks.

The brain gets glucose from the foods we eat, so the quality and frequency of the food supply is a critical determinant of the quality of brain function. With too much blood glucose (as in the case of diabetes), extensive nerve damage occurs. With too little (as in the case of insulin shock and alcoholic hypoglycemia), headaches, confusion, anxiety, weaknesses, and sometimes convulsions and comas ensue. The body maintains a stable supply of blood glucose through a complex regulatory system that monitors glucose levels and releases biochemicals (including insulin) to either increase or decrease the rate at which glucose is absorbed and used. It is an elegant system, but, like everything about the brain's chemistry, it is easily disturbed.

The Impact of Addictions and Eating Disorders

Most of what we now know about the brain and its chemicals has come to us courtesy of research on the very drugs that disrupt its balance. Some of the first research on the drugs of dependency dealt with the effect of opiates such as heroin and morphine. These drugs, like so many others, were originally thought of as miraculous gifts that could relieve man of pain. It didn't take long to realize that the "gift" had a price tag: a ferocious physical addiction. The question was, why?

In their efforts to find an answer, researchers discovered something rather amazing. Morphine and its chemical relatives actually *look like* some of the brain's chemical transmitters! These neurotransmitters— the endorphins and enkephalins—are released in times of physical or emotional stress and, among other things, suppress pain in crisis situations. Soon it was discovered that the brain produces not only natural painkillers, but natural stimulants (epinephrine and norepinephrine), natural tranquilizers (serotonin), and undoubtedly many more, all with unique duties in the functioning of the human body and mind.

At first it was thought that the effect of drugs is limited to mimicry —neurotransmitter "look-alikes" fit into receptor cells and stimulate brain cells. This certainly seems to be the case with heroin, for example. But it is only part of the story.

Some drugs, such as cocaine, interfere with the re-uptake of excess neurotransmitters, so that it stays in the synapse and continues to stimulate receptor cells. Others, including alcohol, combine with other natural chemicals to form substances that can either block re-uptake or stimulate receptors (and sometimes both). In essence, a drug's potency and addictive potential depends on its ability to interact with or mimic a chemical already produced by the brain. The drugs of abuse are simply accelerating or prolonging the brain's natural processes.

On the surface, this may not seem like much of a problem. After all, if it's a basically natural process, what does it matter if it goes on a little faster or longer? But even natural processes have their limits.

When properly nourished and left to its own devices, the brain will naturally maintain a proper balance of neurotransmitters, producing a surplus when necessary (such as during an accident or a terrible fright), and then going back to the norm. When it fails to maintain this balance, problems develop. Parkinson's disease, for example, is in part the result of a chronic deficiency of the neurotransmitter dopamine; and some forms of depression have been linked to a deficiency of serotonin.

When we add an outside chemical to this subtle balancing act, all hell breaks loose. Although we may initially experience an intense and pleasurable response (a cocaine "rush," heroin euphoria, added pep from a cup of coffee), when the drug wears off we often feel far worse than we did before. This is because the brain interprets the presence of that outside chemical as a message to stop producing the natural one. It "reads" the chemical as a neurotransmitter surplus, and slows things down accordingly. In cases where re-uptake is blocked, the brain may literally run out of the raw materials it needs to produce neurotransmitters, so that when the outside drugs are used up the brain simply can't resume production fast enough to make up the difference.

This problem isn't limited to drugs and alcohol. Research on eating disorders—particularly the binge–purge and starvation syndromes of bulimia and anorexia—has shown that these abnormal patterns are accompanied by an increase in several neurotransmitters, including the endorphins. In addition to the nutritional and organ damage caused by eating disorders, people with these problems may actually be addicted to their own abnormally high levels of natural opiates!

Over time, drug abuse, alcoholism, and eating disorders cause chronic disturbances in neurotransmitter activity and deplete the brain's reserves so badly that it becomes dependent on the outside drugs (or, in the case of eating disorders, excessive stimulation) in order to maintain even a semblance of balance. Take away the drugs, and the brain is left "empty-handed"—its reserves exhausted, its ability to produce neurotransmitters severely impaired. At this point, the addicted person starts feeling the symptoms of withdrawal, and often rushes back to the drug or behavior that will make him or her feel normal.

Sugar, Caffeine, and the Brain

For those in recovery and battling eating disorders, two of the most common sources of (temporary) relief are sugar and caffeine. At meetings across the country you can see recovering alcoholics, cocaine addicts, and drug addicts of all kinds drinking coffee and eating doughnuts as they work on life without their drug of choice. Little do they know that they have simply exchanged it for another addiction.

Sugar and caffeine, for all their charms, are traps for the unwary recovering person. The poor nutritional habits of all addicts, and the particularly severe nutritional abnormalities of alcoholics and eating disorder patients, disrupt the normal regulation of blood glucose. In the absence of a consistent, high-quality food supply, the normal processes of blood glucose maintenance become completely "out of whack," and the addition of sugar (or very highly refined carbohydrates such as white flour) only makes matters worse.

Research has shown that alcoholism, eating disorders, and many drug addictions are associated with abnormal glucose metabolisms. Simply put, the body is not able to maintain a stable concentration of glucose in the blood, so that the brain is alternately flooded with and starved of fuel. When blood glucose levels drop (hypoglycemia), the addicted person can experience drastic mood changes—particularly depression. Every time blood glucose levels drop below a certain point, these individuals feel depressed, anxious, and moody and experience cravings for their drug or behavior of choice.

The effects of this blood glucose roller coaster can continue even after the drinking (or drug use, or binging and purging) stops. The recovering person continues to feel fatigued, depressed, anxious, headachy, and beset with cravings, and soon learns that a candy bar, soda, or cake can make him or her feel better, at least for a little while. Of course, it doesn't take long for the symptoms to return. Hypoglycemia is an "up one/down two" proposition. For every degree you go up by consuming some sugary food, you go down two when the sugar wears off.

Bill W. understood the problem of alcoholic hypoglycemia better than most. In a 1968 communication to AA's physicians, he noted that "we alcoholics try to cure these conditions [of hypoglycemia], first by sweets, and then by coffee . . . In exactly the wrong way, we are trying to treat ourselves for hypoglycemia."

Caffeine, meanwhile, not only boosts blood sugar levels, it also counteracts feelings of depression through its stimulant effect. Since caffeine is present in many sugared foods, particularly soft drinks and chocolate, people who treat their blood sugar drops with soda, chocolate bars, or a doughnut and coffee are getting a nutritional "double whammy."

The problem with such quick fixes is that they perpetuate the cycle of "feast or famine" that has been disturbing the brain all along. Highly refined sugars raise blood glucose levels dramatically, prompting the pancreas to release extra insulin in an effort to normalize blood sugar. The extra insulin then causes blood sugar levels to *drop* dramatically, and the cycle starts all over again. Obviously, this particular form of "diet therapy" is exactly the wrong one for a healthy recovery.

Modern Evidence: The Tukes Were Right!

So if sugar and caffeine are wrong, what foods are right? Well, as we noted at the beginning of this chapter, mashed potatoes are always an option. Indeed, Judith Wurtman, Ph.D., a nutrition researcher at the Massachusetts Institute of Technology and author of *The Carbohydrate Craver's Diet,* has noted that a plate of freshly baked apple pie or hot mashed potatoes can be just as calming as a shot of whiskey. But we never see the hero of an action film being told "You need a stiff shot of mashed potatoes." In Dr. Wurtman's words, "Even though eating is incomparably safer (for you and society) than drinking [or drug use] during stress, it is not a socially favored behavior."

Actually, scientific validation of the old folk remedy of "eat, you'll feel better" has been relatively late in coming. It was only in the last two decades or so that scientists began to make serious progress in understanding food's influence on the chemistry of the brain. Researchers such as Judith Wurtman and her colleague and husband Richard are now unraveling the complex relationship between what we eat and how we feel.

The building of a neurotransmitter takes a lot more than an electrical impulse and some blood sugar. In fact, it requires a range of raw materials that the body gets from the foods we eat. These building blocks (or *dietary precursors*) of neurotransmitters have dramatic, measurable effects on neurotransmitter production and balance. Like those patients in the York Retreat two centuries ago, we experience these effects as changes in mood.

Two of the most studied dietary precursors are the amino acids tryptophan and tyrosine. Although the specific mechanisms are complex, research has shown that foods high in tryptophan (including such old favorites as warm milk, mashed potatoes, and bread) are likely to slow you down, while foods high in tyrosine (fish and other high-protein foods) are likely to perk you up. The greater the concentration of a specific dietary precursor in a given food, the more noticeable and dramatic its effects.

The influence of diet on brain function does not end with these dietary precursors, however. In order to use these building blocks, the brain requires all of the essential nutrients—particularly the B vitamins (including thiamine, niacin, and riboflavin) and the essential fatty acids. Without the proper amounts of these nutrients, in just the right balance, the brain cannot maintain its internal equilibrium. For example, deficiencies in the B vitamins (particularly thiamine and niacin) can cause many seemingly psychological symptoms, including paranoia, hyperactivity (mania), confusion, confabulation (elaborate lies to cover mental deficiencies), and depression.

Research on the relationship of food and mood has shown just how important our diet is to the health and well-being of our brains, and how much we have yet to learn about this marvelous and sensitive organ. With each passing year and each additional research development we are discovering that we can actively nourish and care for "the home of the mind," just as the Tukes nourished and cared for their patients so many years ago.

Learning from the Past: Eating for Recovery

The Tukes, the Wurtmans, and the long line of mothers and grandmothers in between have an important lesson for people in recovery: *You can change the way you feel by changing what you eat.* By tailoring your diet to include the dietary precursors of your damaged neurotransmitters, you can give your brain the raw materials it needs to resume normal production. By eating a high-quality diet at regular intervals you can ensure that your brain is properly fueled to carry out these processes. And by engaging in a balanced and comprehensive nutritional supplement program you can be sure that your brain has the materials it needs to catalyze (or jump start) neurotransmitter production.

Conversely, eating infrequently, or eating lots of sugary, caffeine-laden foods, will perpetuate the cycle of deficiency, depression, fatigue, mood swings, and anxiety that characterizes withdrawal and incomplete recovery or relapse.

This book is intended to provide you with specific information —in the form of shopping and cooking techniques, recipes, lifestyle guidelines, supplement recommendations, and hard scientific facts— to make the changes that can help your brain (and the rest of your body) reach a full and fulfilling recovery. The choice, and the power, are yours.

8 Adverse Food Reactions and Food Addictions

While it is easy to understand allergies to cats or to roses, the concept of having a negative immunological reaction to food can seem incomprehensible. Food is such an integral part of life, how could one have a bad reaction to it?

Strange though it may seem, food allergies (or *adverse food reactions,* as they are known to most medical practitioners) have been recognized for centuries. Hippocrates treated the first recorded case of an adverse reaction to food: a man who broke out in hives after drinking milk. Since then, the literature has been filled with references to individuals who suffered unpleasant symptoms in response to various foods. Today, some 17 to 20 percent of Americans are known to suffer from adverse food reactions, and allergic diseases in general are responsible for up to 10 percent of visits to doctors' offices each year. It has been estimated that up to 7.5 percent of children have adverse reactions to cow's milk alone.

Adverse food reactions are complex phenomena that defy easy characterization. Some manifest themselves immediately after the food is ingested, while others can be delayed for hours or even days. The symptoms can range from such classic allergic symptoms as sneezing and hives to emotional reactions (such as depression) to severe and potentially fatal respiratory collapse (anaphylaxis). To complicate matters even further, persons with food sensitivities are often responding to the very foods that they love and eat the most. "Oh, come on!" they say. "I feel fine when I eat this stuff." Little do they know that when the body is constantly exposed to some substances it can actually become *addicted* to their presence.

While some adverse food reactions may be present from birth, many develop over time, the result of chronic exposure or biological damage. In the latter category, alcoholism, eating disorders, and addictions of all kinds are prime culprits, due to their damaging effects on the gastrointestinal tract.

A Brief Introduction to the Immune System

The immune system is a truly awe-inspiring surveillance/defense network with links to every organ and system of the body—particularly those of the gastrointestinal tract, the neurochemical network, the respiratory system, and the systems that govern hormone release. The immune system monitors and responds to stimuli coming in from all these systems—stimuli ranging from a grain of pollen, to a molecule of milk protein, to a severe emotional shock, to sexual arousal. If it has an impact on the body, it has an impact on the immune system.

The immune system responds to these stimuli in a variety of ways, many of which are still unknown. In the classic allergic response, for example, the body mistakes some relatively benign substance (such as pollen) for something far more harmful (such as a bacterium). These perceived threats are generically known as "antigens." When an antigen is detected, the immune system unleashes various types of immuno-globulins (more popularly known as antibodies).

The immunoglobulins are the body's "shock troops," rushing to capture and isolate the invading substance before it can do any harm. Along with these shock troops, a variety of inflammatory substances are released (most notably histamine), which allow fluid to accumulate at the invasion site and further "wall off" the invaders. (It is this in-flammatory portion of the immune response that gives us the runny nose, watery eyes, and congestion of allergies and colds.) Once the invaders have been captured, other immune cells can either destroy, break down, or bind them for removal from the body.

One of the most amazing things about the immune system is the fact that once immunoglobulins (or antibodies) are formed, they re-main in circulation forever, ready to attack an invader at any time. This is why, in general, once you've had mumps or chicken pox, you will not get them again. The antibodies to the virus have been lying in wait for another invasion; they can attack and disable subsequent "invading forces" before they can get a foothold.

Given the number of very real biological threats that surround us, the comprehensive coverage provided by the immune system isn't overkill. Without its constant surveillance and protection we would be prey to every passing toxin, bacterium, virus, microbe, or microscopic beastie that came our way. But there are drawbacks. The ubiquitous nature of the immune system's coverage—and the equally ubiquitous threats that naturally surround us—means that it is under constant assault. Under optimal conditions, in a well-nourished, properly bal-anced body, the system copes remarkably well. Even in less than opti-mal conditions, the immune system can hang in there for quite a while before serious breakdowns start. But physical, chemical, nutritional, allergic, and psychological stresses will eventually undermine the body's standing army. In these instances, the immune system's vigilance can go disastrously wrong.

*It can start producing antibodies to the body's own tissues, mistaking them for hostile invaders (as in rheumatoid arthritis).

*It can lose its ability to recognize and respond to actual threats (seen most dramatically in the case of AIDS, and also in the uncontrolled growth of cancer cells).

*Or it may become hyper-reactive, overreacting to alien substances, so that the response causes more damage than the substance itself would have (as in the case of most allergies).

When the body is constantly assaulted by drugs, alcohol, or the ravages of binges and purges, the delicate balance of the immune system is disrupted. The malnutrition that accompanies all these disorders weakens the immune system, depressing its ability to respond to threats. As a result, these individuals are more susceptible to a variety of ills, from head colds to wound infections, and their bodies are less able to heal themselves after injuries. Even more ominously, a malnourished immune system is less able to recognize and destroy cancerous cells. This decreased ability to fight cancer makes alcohol and many drugs of dependency "co-carcinogens"; that is, when combined with known carcinogens (including those found in tobacco), they contribute to the development of potentially fatal cancers. Cancer is one of the primary causes of death among alcoholics—particularly cancers of the liver, lungs, pancreas, breast, cervix, throat, and all the organs of the digestive tract.

Food and the Immune System

Like millions of Americans, we once thought that food was food, and allergies were allergies, and never the twain would meet. We were wrong. Foods can have dramatic and occasionally fatal immunological effects—and immunological reactions to foods are far more prevalent than many people (including physicians) realize.

There are two types of adverse reaction to a food. One of them is immediate: A person goes into a restaurant, unwittingly eats something with shrimp in it, and promptly starts to swell up with generalized hives. In these cases there is no doubt whatsoever that a food allergy exists, and the food-sensitive individual has no choice but to avoid the food.

The other, more common type of allergic response to a food is a delayed reaction. It can appear hours or even days after the food has been eaten, making it easy to miss the connection between the food and the symptoms experienced. The woman who always seems to have a stuffy nose a few hours after dinner, or the man who always seems to be "gassy" after lunch may be suffering from delayed reactions to some part of their meals. In general, there are several "clues" that may indicate a delayed reaction to foods. They include:

*a history of childhood allergies or colic that you later "outgrew"

*chronic or episodic diarrhea

*discomfort or "gassiness" after eating

*constipation

*chronic postnasal drip

*unexplained rashes

*sleepiness after eating

*mood swings (highs or lows) after meals.

One of the most paradoxical things about adverse food reactions is that reactive people can actually become *addicted* to the foods to which they are sensitive. In these cases, the body responds to the continual presence of the food by "shifting gears" in order to accommodate it. It is almost as if the body says, "Okay, if you're going to keep eating this stuff, I'll just have to adjust."

Over time, this "new order" becomes so entrenched that the body needs the substance, and when it is removed the body actually craves its presence. We have seen this allergy/addiction cycle countless times —in adults who practically live on peanut butter sandwiches when they are allergic to peanuts, in children who refuse to eat anything but macaroni and cheese when they are allergic to cheese and wheat, and in countless other patients who have told me they "couldn't live without" the very foods to which they are most allergic. The most common reactive foods include peanuts, milk, eggs, grains (wheat, rice, corn), tomatoes, citrus fruits, yeast, soy, and chocolate.

Ironically, in some (perhaps many) of these cases the reaction may have developed over time, as a result of a limited or repetitive diet. Our bodies are not designed for a monotonous diet, and when bombarded with the same food (or any other substance) day in and day out an adverse response can evolve.

There are many drawbacks to this adjustment, however. This cycle involves the immune system's learning to ignore a substance that it perceives to be a threat. This "down-regulation" of the immune system's normal vigilance can cause other immune effects, including increased susceptibility to other illnesses and autoimmune disorders (because the immune system's ability to differentiate threats accurately is impaired).

This allergy/addiction cycle has some pretty serious ramifications. We know of one young woman (a recovering bulimic) whose adverse food reactions almost derailed her marriage.

One year after her wedding, she and her husband were in counseling because he was convinced she was having an affair. Several nights a week, she would wake up, get dressed, and leave the house, returning up to an hour later. At first she would not tell him where she went, until finally she admitted that she was going out to drink a quart of milk. She just had to have it, she said, and she only went out when they didn't have any in the refrigerator.

This seemed improbable, at best, to her husband, and he began to badger her about these nocturnal trips. She, meanwhile, was becoming increasingly upset and frustrated—and she decided that her frequent colds and headaches were related to the stress of her marriage. They went to a counselor, who listened to their story and suggested that, in addition to counseling, she have a complete immunological workup.

It was soon discovered that she was indeed reactive to milk—and some half dozen other foods that she frequently craved. While on a specialized diet prior to being tested (see appendix J), she thought she would go crazy from the cravings, anxiety, and all-around illness she experienced. Like any other addict, she was experiencing withdrawal. And like any other addict, she had to learn to live without some of the substances to which she was addicted.

Did allergy testing and treatment save the woman's marriage? Not exactly, but it did take a tremendous strain off of her and her husband and make her a healthier, more functional partner.

Alcoholism

In addition to generally weakening the immune system via addiction-induced malnutrition, many drugs of dependency have direct toxic effects on specific organs and cells of the immune system. Alcohol is a primary culprit in this regard.

Since alcohol must be absorbed through the normal processes of digestion, it affects every organ of the body. Each of these organs has links to the immune system, but several—particularly the liver and the cells of the bone marrow—are crucial to the production and regulation of immune cells.

Alcohol-induced damage also interferes with the production of immune cells that are normally manufactured in the bone marrow, causing a potentially critical shortage of immunological "troops" for the body's ongoing fight against illness and infection.

Since so many alcohol- and drug-dependent individuals engage in a wide range of unhealthy behaviors, from unsafe sexual practices to cigarette smoking, they can least afford this kind of immune dysfunction. Chemically dependent individuals are therefore facing an immunological double threat: a poorly armed immune system continually threatened and undermined by a range of toxins and stresses.

William B. Silkworth, M.D., who was one of Bill W. and Dr. Bob's medical advisors in the early days of AA, wrote in the preface to *The Big Book* that chronic alcoholics are allergic to alcohol, and that the ferocious cravings of alcoholism are limited to persons with this allergy. Dr. Silkworth was a man ahead of his time. Some of the most intriguing research of recent years has been done in the area of allergy and alcoholism, and all of it indicates that something unusual is going on in the immune systems of many alcoholic individuals.

Several studies have shown that alcoholic patients have an unusually high degree of allergic responses, both to "classic" allergens such as pollen and to various foods. Among foods, grains (the primary ingredient of many alcoholic beverages) are particularly common culprits.

The cause of these adverse food reactions, and their importance in the development of alcoholism, is subject to a lot of debate, most of it of the "which came first, the chicken or the egg?" variety. It is possible that adverse food reactions in alcoholism are acquired as a result of alcohol's damaging effect on the digestive tract.

When alcohol passes through the stomach and intestinal tract it causes subtle cellular damage in the linings of these crucial digestive organs. Over time, alcohol damages these delicate tissues so much that they become more porous and allow large, incompletely digested food particles to pass directly into the bloodstream.

When improperly digested food particles enter the bloodstream, immune cells identify them as foreign and attack with specially designed antibodies. Once these antibodies have come into existence, they are always there, waiting for the next invasion. Unfortunately, food particles "invade" all the time—every time the alcoholic eats. This kind of continuous assault is an ideal environment for the allergy/addiction cycle. The immune system is always on "red alert," fending off invaders that are actually part of the food supply as well as alcoholic beverages.

We have yet to discover whether alcoholic individuals are highly allergic from day one—before they ever tried an alcoholic beverage—or whether their immune responses develop as a result of alcohol-induced digestive and liver damage. It is possible (indeed, likely) that a combination of factors is at work, and that the situation gets progressively worse as drinking continues.

Eating Disorders

People with eating disorders, like recovering alcoholics, are remarkably prone to adverse food reactions/addictions. They have uncontrollable urges to eat specific foods (most often sweets, although, as we saw earlier, other foods are also culprits), which they go to extraordinary means to control. A close look at their medical histories almost invariably reveals colicky infancies, childhoods punctuated by frequent colds, coughs, and runny noses, and other signs of immunological dysfunction. And we have yet to meet an eating disorder patient—whether obese or anorectically thin—who did not say there was at least one food they consistently craved or "could not live without."

The roots of these adverse food reactions/addictions are unclear. Given the immunological clues found in so many of these patients' medical histories, it is likely that many eating disorder patients were born with adverse food reactions to specific foods (or developed them at a very early age) that were never detected. Over the years, the allergy/addiction cycle became entrenched, prompting ever more intense cravings.

Individuals who binge and purge may actually intensify (or cause) adverse food reactions through the gastrointestinal damage caused by purging (see chapter 6). In these cases, a "leaky gut" syndrome similar to that seen in alcoholism can develop. The damaged lining of the intestinal tract allows food proteins to pass into the bloodstream and prompt an immunological reaction.

The immunological overdrive that occurs when offending foods are eaten on a regular basis (as in the case of compulsive overeaters) can also injure the lining of the gut. In these cases, the damage may allow not only undigested proteins to be absorbed, but additional calories as well.

The fact that a "leaky" intestinal lining can encourage weight gain is nothing new. When it was found that antibiotics kill not only bacteria but the normal intestinal microorganisms of the gastrointestinal tract (thereby increasing the permeability of the intestinal lining), some farmers used the fact to their advantage. They began giving their cows, pigs, chickens, and other livestock high doses of antibiotics (far more than was needed to prevent illness), thereby weakening the intestinal lining and making it possible for the animals to gain more weight on less feed. Obese individuals with adverse food reactions may unwittingly be doing the same thing, by assaulting their digestive tracts with immunologically reactive foods.

Whether you deal with a food allergy/addiction by avoiding the food altogether, eating as much of it as possible and then throwing up, or simply overeating, it is critical that adverse food reactions and sensitivities be identified. Until they have been, the cycle of craving and disordered eating is likely to continue, making recovery an uphill battle.

Adverse food reactions and addictions are one of the least recognized common denominators in addictive and eating disorders. This is unfortunate, since these conditions can be major stumbling blocks on the road to recovery. The immunological impacts of food allergy/addiction are widespread, and they make themselves known in the form of repeated low-level illnesses, gastrointestinal problems, and ferocious cravings. Indeed, food cravings—particularly for sweets and the various grains that are components of alcoholic beverages—have derailed many a budding recovery.

This is why it is so very critical that you investigate possible adverse food reactions when starting out in the recovery process. In chapter 9, we will discuss some of the techniques for identifying and coping with adverse food reactions, and in appendix J you will find more specific guidelines and references. As always, remember that your situation is unique. In recovery, your *biological individuality* determines every aspect of what you need to heal and thrive.

9 Biological Individuality

The physical and nutritional damage that we have discussed thus far happens fairly consistently in everyone who develops addictions or eating disorders. This is because the toxic nature of these chemicals and behaviors is nearly universal: Alcohol is poisonous to every cell in every body, drugs interfere with neurotransmitters found in every brain, and compulsive binging and/or vomiting will always disrupt normal hunger/satiety patterns.

But there is a lot of variation among individuals with these disorders. A group of friends can grow up in the same neighborhood, go to the same schools, attend the same parties, seem to share the same drinking patterns, and only one may develop alcoholism. Two friends might both try cocaine at the same time, and only one might go on to become a compulsive user.

The prevalence and course of these disorders can differ greatly between specific persons and groups. One person may become a full-fledged addict after only one or two encounters with a drug, while another may go for years before becoming completely enmeshed. This is particularly true when it comes to alcoholism. Women, for example, tend to develop alcoholism later in life than men, and the progression of the disease is faster and more severe. Some ethnic groups (such as the Chinese) have such severe negative reactions to alcohol that alcoholism is almost completely unknown among them, while other groups are particularly vulnerable to alcoholism. Even apparently "emotional" disorders, such as depression and schizophrenia, seem to be more prevalent in certain areas and cultures than others.

This variability led to many misconceptions about those who suffer from these disorders. Alcoholism has been viewed as everything from a crime to moral degeneracy to a form of madness. Addicts are still generally looked upon as evil, drug-peddling criminals who should be punished. Obese individuals are fair game for every comic in the Western Hemisphere. Anorexics and bulimics are often viewed as spoiled children seeking attention. Almost across the board, medicine, psychology, government, and society at large have assumed that people with these disorders made some conscious choice to "get this way," and that the only reason they don't change is because they don't want to.

Perhaps somewhere, in some dark corner of the world, there is an addict, anorexic, bulimic, or obese person who made a conscious, considered decision to become addicted and stay that way. But we doubt it. The mechanisms involved in developing these disorders are just not that simple. "Coming down with" any of these conditions involves a combination of social conditioning, environmental cues, and —most importantly—the particular biochemical "programming" of the individual.

Each of us was born with a unique genetic inheritance. This genetic programming determined the color of our eyes and hair, the shape of our faces, and myriad other surface characteristics. It also contained the instructions for producing enzymes, controlling metabolism, and building new cells. It is these subtle cellular aspects of our genetic inheritance that influence both our unique nutritional requirements and our susceptibility to addictions, obesity, anorexia, and many other diseases. The importance of this biological individuality has yet to be fully appreciated by many in the medical profession, but it is a critical concept for those of us in recovery.

The History of Biological Individuality

The fact that taste in music, in art, and in food varies greatly between individuals has been recognized for ages. Long before the birth of Christ, Lucretius noted that "What is one man's meat is another man's rank poison." Although the phrase has been repeated for centuries, science has only recently begun to unravel the truth behind the cliché.

One of the first clues to the true extent and significance of individual differences came at the turn of the twentieth century, when an Austrian scientist named Karl Landsteiner was investigating the problem of blood transfusions. Although physicians had been performing transfusions for many years, each transfusion was a risk. Some patients would inexplicably die from the technique that saved so many others. The cause of these fatal reactions confounded physicians. After all, blood is blood, isn't it?

As Landsteiner found out, this wasn't the case. Instead, he showed that human blood is not at all uniform. He discovered three distinct blood types (A, B, and O), thereby allowing physicians to make appropriate matches before giving transfusions and saving the lives of countless patients.

Landsteiner's discovery was just the beginning. Shortly afterward, an Englishman named Archibald Garrod demonstrated that biochemical differences go far beyond blood types. In a 1902 letter to the British medical journal *Lancet,* Garrod wrote that "just as no two individuals in a species are absolutely identical in their bodily structure neither are their chemical processes carried out along exactly the same lines."

Garrod had uncovered a fundamental biological truth: Metabolism —the complex biochemical processes that fuel and run the body— differs as much as fingerprints between individuals. Sometimes the differences are obvious: People with lactose intolerance, for example, are missing the enzyme needed to digest the natural sugar in milk. But it is the other, more subtle manifestations of biological individuality that are of importance in recovery (and human health in general).

Whenever you go for a physical or blood tests, your results are judged against a variety of hypothetical "norms." Normal body temperature is assumed to be 98.6 degrees Fahrenheit. Normal blood pressure: 110 over 80. When dealing with blood tests, normal *ranges* are used, in recognition of the natural variability that can exist among people.

Nutritional guidelines such as the Recommended Dietary Allowances operate under similar principles. They take the amount of a nutrient (such as vitamin C) that will prevent symptoms of deficiency (such as scurvy) in most people, and add a little for good measure.

All of these norms are based on the assumption that most people are pretty much alike. Sure, they may have minor differences, but serious metabolic deviations such as lactose intolerance are rare, right?

Wrong. As Archibald Garrod pointed out in 1902, it is variation, not consistency, that is the norm among living creatures. For example, have you ever wondered what your stomach looks like? If you go by most medical textbooks, you would assume it looks pretty much like figure 9.1.

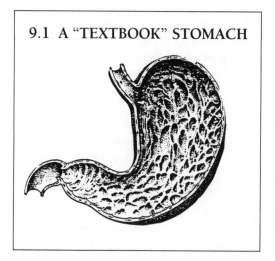

9.1 A "TEXTBOOK" STOMACH

Dr. Barry Anson of Northwestern University and his research team thought much the same thing when they began compiling the *Atlas of Human Anatomy* in the late 1940s. What they found was remarkably different. The "average" stomach proved pretty difficult to come by. Instead, stomachs seemed to vary as much as eye color (see figure 9.2).

9.2 ACTUAL STOMACH VARIATIONS

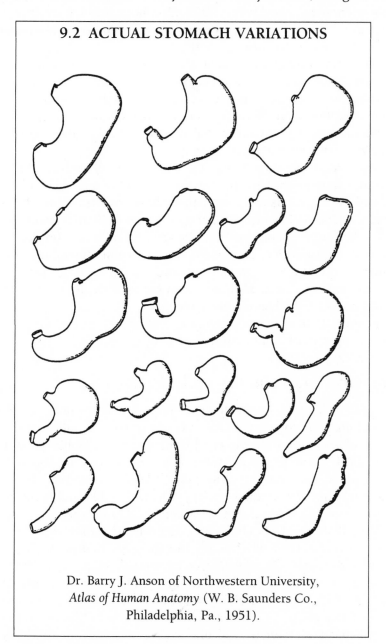

Dr. Barry J. Anson of Northwestern University,
Atlas of Human Anatomy (W. B. Saunders Co.,
Philadelphia, Pa., 1951).

So your stomach may look nothing (or exactly) like the illustration in your doctor's medical textbook. Similarly, your stomach and the rest of your gastrointestinal tract may *act* nothing like those described in medical texts. The same holds true for your brain, your heart, and every other organ of your body. While there are certain *probabilities,* such as "normal" body temperature, that hold true for most people, when dealing with an individual human it's important to remember that he or she may be very different.

Nowhere is this more true than in the area of nutritional needs. The fuel requirements of a diesel eighteen-wheeler truck are very different from those of a subcompact car. The same is true for humans. Our genetic heritage, our mothers' health while we were in the womb, childhood illnesses, environmental toxins, and, of course, addictions all pattern what we need nutritionally.

We have already discussed the importance of getting the right nutrients, in the right balance, if we are to achieve robust good health. But what if our needs are greater than those set forth by the Recommended Dietary Allowances? What if our genetic inheritance is missing the "code" for producing a particular enzyme that in turn breaks down a particular nutrient? What if our disease has compromised our bodies to such an extent that we will always need more than the average levels of some nutrients? Standardized measures such as the RDAs simply cannot take all these factors into account.

Biological individuality, therefore, can be a critical factor in both the development of illness and its course or recovery.

Biological Individuality and Alcoholism

Although biological individuality is an important factor in the development of many, if not all, diseases, it is of particular significance in the disease of alcoholism. As the late biochemist Roger Williams pointed out in 1981, alcoholism is a disease of *individuals.* It is not contagious. It does not attack families, towns, cities, states, or countries. It attacks individual members of these groups. Alcohol, unlike influenza, does things to some people it doesn't do to others. The big question is why.

More than 100 studies have been published that show that alcoholism can actually "run" in families, and that the children of alcoholic parents are far more likely than their peers to develop alcoholism. For a time it was assumed that these children simply learned to drink by observing their parents or had some intrinsic mental defect that made them become alcoholic. Then a series of research studies on adoptees showed that the children of alcoholic parents were four times more likely to become alcoholic than those of nonalcoholic parents, regardless of where they were raised. Soon after, another series of studies on twin children of alcoholic parents showed that identical twins (who carry the exact same genetic code) are far more likely to both develop alcoholism than fraternal twins, even if raised apart. In addition, when another study had psychologists evaluate the children of alcoholics and children of nonalcoholics (without letting the psychologists know which group was which), they found no significant psychological and behavioral differences between the two groups. In other words, research has shown that the closer you are, genetically, to an alcoholic, the greater your risk of developing alcoholism, and this risk has nothing to do with some inherited psychological defect.

The question that remains, of course, is why. While identical twin children of alcoholic parents are more than twice as likely to both become alcoholic, alcoholism is not inevitable, and the concordance is not perfect; not every twin sibling of an alcoholic develops alcoholism. Recent research has shed some light on what it is that makes the children of alcoholics unique, and how it may contribute to their later succumbing to alcoholism. In a series of studies throughout the 1980s researchers at the University of California found that, when compared to control subjects, the sons of alcoholics have:

*less intense responses to alcohol, with less feelings of drunkenness and fewer hormonal changes, and actual *improvements* in hand-to-eye coordination and muscle control

*significant differences in brain wave activity, both before drinking and in response to alcohol.

Other researchers have found that sons of alcoholics have higher serum levels of acetaldehyde (alcohol's toxic by-product) after drinking than do the sons of nonalcoholic controls.

These findings, and scores of others like them, indicate that in some individuals alcohol produces an abnormally positive response (specifically improved performance, better hand–eye coordination, less feeling of drunkenness), even as it produces a toxic and addictive biochemical response (increased acetaldehyde levels). The individual enjoys drinking more, increases his or her consumption, and speeds up the biochemical processes of addiction.

Once again, these subjective differences don't shed much light on *why* at-risk individuals seem to be responding so differently. Whatever the genetic coding that predisposes an individual to alcoholism, it is likely that the code is at least partially reflected by exceptional nutritional needs. Just as different engines require different octane fuels, so the unique nature of the body is reflected in *its* fuel requirements.

Long before the genetic link in alcoholism had been established, Roger Williams and his coworkers at the University of Texas did extensive work on the problem of individual differences in alcohol metabolism, primarily in animal studies. As we noted in chapter 1, these researchers found that they could actually change an animal's drinking behavior by manipulating its diet! In scores of studies, Williams and colleagues found that deficiencies of vitamin A, thiamine, riboflavin, pantothenic acid, and vitamin B_6 caused increased alcohol consumption. Returning the vitamins to the diet, on the other hand, caused alcohol consumption to fall.

Based on this work and the growing body of evidence on the nutritional, metabolic, and structural individuality of humans, Williams theorized that individuals who are particularly vulnerable to the addictive effect of alcohol have unusual nutritional needs, which are not met by diets that are perfectly sufficient for other people. When vulnerable people drink alcohol, they aggravate their already marginal nutritional situation. And if they drink heavily, they suffer extensive metabolic breakdowns.

The full implications of Roger Williams's animal research to the world of human alcoholism was not fully appreciated until recently. More modern research on ethnic and individual differences in the development of alcoholism and its biological effects now lends support to his early theories.

For example, science has known for many years that the Korsakoff syndrome is the result of severe thiamine deficiency. This condition, which consists of personality disintegration, memory dysfunctions, and a withdrawal from reality, afflicts only a small percentage of chronic alcoholics. Why is it so selective?

In 1977, researchers found that patients with this disorder have a unique enzyme that requires high levels of thiamine in order to perform its functions in the brain and nervous system. As a result, individuals with this enzyme have an unusually high requirement for thiamine. The metabolism of alcohol (and, interestingly enough, sugar) drastically depletes the body's thiamine reserves—reserves that the Korsakoff-susceptible person simply cannot do without. Over time, these individuals suffer the severe and often irreversible brain impairments of Korsakoff's syndrome.

Another nutritional angle that has generated considerable research interest is the possible influence of essential fatty acid metabolism in susceptibility to alcoholism. This theory rose out of the odd fact that alcoholism (and depression) seems to be far more prevalent in certain northern countries—particularly in areas of northern Europe—than it is in more southern climes. What is it about these areas, researchers wondered, that makes people so much more susceptible to alcoholism? In their search for answers, several researchers (most notably Dr. David F. Horrobin of Oxford University) began to look closely at the natural dietary patterns of these areas, and they found a possible answer to the riddle.

In many regions of the world, including high up in the Arctic Circle, fatty fishes such as mackerel and salmon have been dietary staples for generations. These foods are rich in essential fatty acids, which the body uses to construct a variety of crucial substances including prostaglandins, hormone-like substances which are important to the functioning of the cardiovascular, immune, and nervous systems. Deficiencies in prostaglandins have been linked to symptoms such as depression, gastrointestinal distress, headaches, and, perhaps, a craving for alcohol.

Alcohol has a unique effect on the prostaglandins. On the one hand it speeds up the body's impulses to produce prostaglandins. On the other, it slows down the action of the enzyme responsible for processing the essential fatty acids of which prostaglandins are made. In essence, alcohol increases the demand for prostaglandins even as it cuts off the supply. If a person were suffering from a prostaglandin deficiency, alcohol would seem to be a miracle cure for many of his symptoms, such as depression, since for a short time prostaglandin production would increase. But the cure would be short-lived. In a short while the supply of raw material for prostaglandins would be exhausted, and he would be left craving more alcohol.

Researchers theorize that centuries of consuming a diet high in naturally occurring essential fatty acids (EFAs) caused the people of certain seafaring areas (including Scandinavia, Norway, British Columbia, and parts of Ireland) to lose the enzymes necessary to build EFAs (and therefore prostaglandins) from other fat sources. The sea provided them with all the essential fatty acids they needed. For a time.

As the Industrial Age dawned and our modern diet of highly refined and processed foods infiltrated these regions, the natural dietary pattern was disrupted. When these people abandoned their natural dietary patterns, their bodies simply could not keep up. The denatured, processed, and highly saturated fats of the modern food production system did not provide the essential fatty acids of their old diet, and their bodies had lost the ability to extract EFAs from other fat sources. The process of essential fatty acid metabolism was blocked, and prostaglandin production was seriously damaged.

Not surprisingly, this dietary shift was followed by a disease shift. Within a decade or so of "modernization" a host of diseases began to rear their ugly heads in areas that had once rarely known such troubles: cancer, heart disease, diabetes . . . and alcoholism.

This problem was not limited to the first generation to experience the dietary shift. Evolutionary development takes millions of years, technological development mere decades. The problem of essential fatty acid/prostaglandin deficiency appears to have persisted in many individuals whose ancestors were from these areas.

Does this mean that everyone whose parents or grandparents are from Norway (or a similar northern clime) is EFA-deficient and is going to develop alcoholism? Of course not. Alcoholism is a complex disease, and the genetics of alcoholism are undoubtedly far more complex than today's researchers even dream. But if you are of Celtic Irish, Welsh, Scottish, or Scandinavian descent and in recovery from alcoholism or some other addiction, there is a good chance that you have unique EFA needs that are not being met by your current diet. Addressing these needs could have a significant effect on the comfort and success of your long-term recovery.

Eating Disorders

Fat runs in families. This bit of folk wisdom was usually chalked up to the fact that people in the same family tend to eat alike and hence gain weight alike. But research on the genetics of obesity (and on other eating disorders) has shown that eating behaviors and weight patterns may also be genetically determined. If so, individuals with a family history of obesity or other eating disorders, like children of alcoholics, need to be exceptionally careful and intelligent in their dietary choices.

Perhaps the strongest recent research on this topic was a 1990 study of 673 fraternal and identical twins, some of whom had been raised apart and some of whom had been raised together. This study found that genetic inheritance, and *not* environmental influences, was the predominant influence on weight and body mass later in life. Twins ended up with much the same body mass regardless of where they were raised, and the similarity between identical twins was stronger than that between fraternal twins.

Such genetic influences are not limited to obesity. Researchers investigating anorexia among twins and triplets discovered similar patterns and theorized that anorexia, like obesity, has a genetic component. The question that remains to be answered is what, specifically, is this genetic component? Could it be an inherited personality type? A hypothalamic disorder? Some sort of neurochemical disorder that leads to a distorted body image? Or all of the above?

Most of the theories on these disorders focus on the body's internal thermostat system, which determines what "ideal" weight is and enforces that ideal weight come hell or high water (see chapters 5 and 6). In anorexia, it has been suggested that there is a weakness in the natural mechanisms that prompt the body to gain weight after a period of weight loss. In obesity, it is thought that the body "believes" that it is meant to be fat. In both cases, however, once the pattern is established it takes heroic efforts to change.

This does not, of course, mean that it is impossible to change (read "recover from") eating disorders. But the fact that genetics—the most basic programming of the body—is such a major component of these conditions also means that the body itself will initially resist our efforts. This resistance, in the form of cravings, lowered metabolic rates, urges to exercise excessively (or not exercise), and so forth, is *not* "all in your head," and being discouraged by the resistance is not a loss of will. Like the alcoholic or the drug addict, the patient recovering from an eating disorder is battling strong biochemical cues and fighting to restore a radically disordered body. Every pound gained or lost should be considered a major victory, and each day of healthy eating and a balanced lifestyle brings the eating disorder patient closer to a lifelong pattern of health and well-being.

Determining Your Needs

Individual human beings are unique in *every* way. What is right for your neighbor may not be right for you, and some of the best clues to what you need can be found in your family medical history. If you are the child of an alcoholic, you should not assume that beer-chugging contests are harmless diversions. For you, alcohol may be a time bomb. If you come from a long line of overweight people, you need to be careful about keeping your activity level up and your empty calorie level down, to combat genes that may "want" you to have more fat than you'd like. And if your family has a history of anorexia (or unusually thin people who "eat like birds"), you may want to avoid dieting at all, and concentrate on eating a balanced and natural diet that will meet your nutritional needs.

Determining nutritional needs is the great dilemma presented by biological individuality. Norms based on "average" people (such as the RDAs) are, at best, loose guides by which to determine the actual needs or sensitivities of individuals. Although the RDAs and most other norms attempt to take individual variability into account, it is clear they are not going far enough.

The slow pace of human evolution puts us at real biological risk in our rapidly changing world. But since we can't speed up evolution (or slow the advance of technology), we must do the best we can to accommodate our ancient biological needs in our very modern world. To do so, we must understand how our biology works and what we really need—nutritionally, environmentally, and in the way we live our day-to-day lives—in order to maintain good health.

Over the last twenty years, Dr. William Shive of the Clayton Foundation for Biochemical Research at the University of Texas at Austin has developed a technology that will permit individualized nutritional analysis. By analyzing the growth and efficiency of lymphocytes (immune cells that circulate within the bloodstream), Dr. Shive and his colleagues have been able to determine individual differences in nutrient needs and gauge long-term nutritional status (since lymphocytes are dormant until roused into action by a threat, and therefore reflect the nutritional state of the body at the time they were formed). This technology will make it possible to determine the unique nutritional needs of individuals in recovery and will allow them to select the foods and nutritional supplements that will best meet these needs.

Until this technology becomes widely available, however, there are several things you can do on your own to get a better idea of your unique needs. To begin:

> *Find out your family medical history, particularly of illnesses such as alcoholism, allergies, cancer, heart disease, or stroke.

> *Undergo allergy testing to determine the inhalants (pollens, etc.), foods, or chemicals to which you may be sensitive.

> *Carefully evaluate your diet (and your reactions to foods) to identify possibly reactive foods.

If you suspect you have food sensitivities or allergies (and if you are in recovery from alcoholism or an eating disorder it is very likely), there are several ways in which you can find out for sure:

> *Skin testing measures the "wheal" (a welt or hive) response to various food proteins that are injected under or scratched into the skin. This testing should only be carried out by medical

professionals who have been properly trained, since severe allergic reactions can be life-threatening.

*Various *blood screens* can detect the presence of antibodies to foods within your bloodstream. Blood screens often serve as a first step before skin testing.

*Or you can carry out an *oral food challenge* to determine if a specific food or foods causes a reaction after you eat it. (Oral food challenges are often used as a final confirmation of results found via the other two testing methods.)

We have found that skin testing followed by supervised oral food challenges is the best way to work out adverse food reactions and identify various levels of reactivity to foods. However, it is possible to carry out the oral food challenge on your own, if you suspect a particular food or foods of causing a reaction. The first step is to "clear the decks" by going on a specialized diet that will give your body a respite from the foods and chemical additives that are most likely to prompt an immunological reaction. At the end of the detoxification period, you will then "challenge" your body by eating the suspect food in its purest form and monitoring your body's reactions. Both the detoxification diet and the oral food challenge procedure can be time consuming, but they are excellent gauges of food sensitivities and allergies. Appendix J provides specific instructions for both procedures.

Assuming you have a reaction to a test food, what are you supposed to do about it? To begin, avoid the food completely for one month. At the end of one month it is time to begin rotating the food back into your regular diet, checking your reactions just as you did during the oral food challenge. Learning to diversify and rotate your food choices is the foundation of learning to live with food allergies and sensitivities, and it opens a whole new world of foods and cooking techniques.

Basically, a rotation diet is one in which no food is eaten more than once every four to seven days. That may sound simple, but when the food in question is milk, or wheat, or sugar—all of which are ubiquitous in almost every prepared food on the market—setting up a rotation diet becomes a little more challenging. In these cases, in particular, switching to whole foods is critical. The recipes in this book use a variety of grains, few dairy products, and little to no sugar to accommodate those who have such food allergies or sensitivities. An example of a four-day-cycle rotation diet can be found in appendix J.

An integral part of learning to rotate foods is learning to recognize *food families*. In chapter 2 we noted that Jim was unaware of the fact that yogurt is a dairy food. This misconception could have caused plenty of problems for Jim, since his immune system would have reacted to yogurt just as it did to milk. When dealing with food allergies and sensitivities, it is crucial that we understand which foods are chemically similar, so that we can avoid immunological cases of mistaken identity. If, for example, you know that you have problems with brewer's yeast, you may want to avoid eating too many mushrooms—since mushrooms, like yeast, are members of the "fungi" family. We know a woman who complained of having terrible breathing problems at night, even when it was not allergy season. She couldn't understand what the problem was, since she normally only had such symptoms during goldenrod season. It turned out that she had been drinking an herbal tea that contained chamomile flowers—which are in the same botanical family as goldenrod. When she stopped the tea, her breathing problems were relieved. Cases such as these show that understanding food families can help us avoid accidental immunological overloads or irritations and more effectively rotate the various aspects of our diets. Appendix K lists the major food families and their most common members.

Although it is possible to evaluate certain aspects of your individual biological needs entirely on your own, using methods like the oral food challenge, a good physician can be invaluable in helping you determine your unique biological risks and/or needs. Once you have identified potential genetic, immunological, and nutritional risks to your health, consult with your physician about the ways in which you can adjust your diet and lifestyle to optimize your health and meet your needs. If your physician downplays the importance of such measures, don't be discouraged. An increasing number of doctors are recognizing the importance of health promotion and disease prevention. Seek out a physician who practices such comprehensive medicine. You'll be amazed at how much of a difference relatively minor (although not necessarily easy!) changes can make in your overall health and well-being.

10 *Putting It Together:*
The Main Components
of a Diet for Recovery

Now that you know what your body needs in recovery, it's time to start fulfilling those needs. As we noted in chapter 1, eating for recovery encompasses not only what we eat but how we live. A true diet for recovery calls for many lifestyle and behavioral changes. Basic rules of thumb include:

1. *Eat a variety of foods.* Broaden your food selections. Try new fruits, vegetables, fish, etc.
2. *Rely on wholefoods.* Get to know and enjoy foods that haven't been processed to within an inch of their lives (see chapters 12 and 13 for more information).
3. *Eat more often.* Instead of doing "three square meals a day," have three small meals and healthy snacks in between.
4. *Clean up your food.* Avoid nutritional pitfalls such as sugar and other refined carbohydrates, chemical food additives (preservatives, colorings, etc.), processed and hydrogenated oils, saturated fats, salt, caffeine, and alcohol.
5. *Make the best use of food.* Learn to purchase and prepare foods in a way that makes optimum use of their nutritional value.
6. *Clean up your water supply.* Protect yourself by drinking bottled water and/or by putting a good water filter between yourself and your water supply.
7. *Clean up your air.* Commercial air filters are relatively inexpensive and can make a tremendous difference in the air quality in your home or office, particularly if you suffer from inhalant allergies. (Also see appendix L.)
8. *Get on the move.* Begin an exercise program and rejuvenate your body through activities you enjoy, while you achieve and maintain a healthy weight.
9. *Learn to relax.* Decrease your stress through counseling, relaxation techniques, biofeedback training, or any of the other legitimate methods of stress reduction.
10. *Start a nutritional supplement program.* Learn to replenish nutritional stores depleted by addiction or eating disorders, and to make up for nutrients lost during food harvest, transport, storage, and processing. (See chapter 12 and appendix I.)

11. *Avoid unnecessary medications.* Although medications are necessary for some conditions (including certain psychological problems), people in recovery should be wary of taking drugs they do not need. Recovering addicts of all kinds are highly susceptible to cross-addiction. Avoid potentially addictive prescription and over-the-counter medications, and when you do need to take medication, always take it as prescribed.

12. *Give up smoking.* And, in general, extend your recovery to all aspects of your life. Become educated about health promotion and develop an overall awareness of the many factors that can damage (and strengthen) your well-being.

You've learned much of the information you need to follow these guidelines already in this book, but for the purpose of getting started let's review some specifics.

Balance and Variety

Most Americans believe that they eat both a balanced and a varied diet, and most Americans are dead wrong. Despite the fact that almost every type of meat, fruit, and vegetable is available at all times of the year, most of us eat the same basic foods day in and day out. Not only that, we tend to rely on canned, frozen, or otherwise processed foods rather than fresh items.

As we shall see in the next chapter, processed foods of all kinds rely heavily on the "malevolent seven" of the food production industry: sugar, refined carbohydrates, hydrogenated oils, salt, caffeine, preservatives, and chemical additives. So no matter how "varied" you think your diet is, if you are depending on processed foods (from frozen entrées to apple pies) for your meals, you are by definition getting a huge helping of these items every time you eat. It has been estimated that up to 50 percent of the average American's caloric intake of food by weight consists of these additives.

A diet that is both *healthy* and varied needs to consist of whole, fresh foods rather than processed, packaged ones. To achieve a proper balance of nutrients, your daily menu should include a selection of foods from the groups delineated in table 10.1.

The Importance of Timing

In addition to choosing the right foods, you need to choose the right times to eat them. As noted in chapters 6 and 7, problems of blood

10.1 BREAKDOWN OF A BALANCED DIET		
Complex Carbohydrates 65% (4 calories per gram)	Proteins 20% (4 cal./g)	Fats 15% or less— only ½ sat. (9 cal./g)

Vegetables and fruits (fresh,
  preferably locally and/or
  organically grown)
Grains and cereals
  (minimally processed and
  refined)
Legumes (particularly in
  combination with grains)
	fish
	poultry
	lean meats*
	grain/beans
	dairy foods*
		nuts
		seeds
		oils (cold-
		pressed)
		lean meats*
		fish (cold
		water)
		dairy
		foods*
		some grains
		and beans

* These foods are high in both protein *and* fat, so don't forget to consider both factors when making food choices.

sugar metabolism are common among those in recovery. It is critical that the body receive a steady supply of fuel. Three meals a day are generally *not* enough to keep blood sugar regulated throughout the day.

Since it isn't always possible to time when precisely you will feel the need for a snack, make a habit of carrying healthy snacks with you. Good forms of "carryall" fare include:

*nuts or seeds

*dried fruits (such as raisins or apricots)

*sliced carrots.

Carrying such snacks will help you avoid the trap of going for a candy bar or bag of potato chips when a craving hits. In general, it is wise to eat something every two to three hours, before cravings or hypoglycemic slumps occur.

Clean Foods: Avoiding the Chemical Snare

When you stop by your local fast food restaurant to have a quick burger and fries, you are also getting a none-too-healthy serving of chemicals and additives. This is because every serving of processed food (such as those offered at your average fast food outlet) has been treated with one or more of the following: acidifiers, antifoaming agents, bleachers, buffers, curers, defoliants, deodorants, disinfectants, emulsifiers, extenders, flavor enhancers or fortifiers, hydrogenators, hydrolyzers, moisturizers, neutralizers, preservatives, thickeners, and artificial colors, flavors, and sweeteners.

Some of the items on this rather unappetizing list are necessary to protect the food supply from spoilage and contamination. But for the most part these additives are the price we pay for having a food supply that can be zapped, boiled, baked, or toasted into instant, attractive, but not particularly nutritious meals. Most of these additives are unnatural, many are potential carcinogens, and—despite the assurances of various companies—few are examples of "better living through chemistry."

As we shall see in the next two chapters, much of our modern diet is nutritionally deficient and occasionally toxic—particularly for those who are nutritionally and physiologically compromised. The very old, the very young, the chronically ill, and those in recovery all fit into this category. And we will never have our nutritional needs met as long as we rely on the kind of prepared and chemically loaded foods that most of us have been eating for years.

If you are to achieve a true nutritional restoration, it is important to switch from this type of processed food diet to a diet that relies on *wholefoods* (see chapter 11), while avoiding the various "chemical snares" that are found throughout our food supply. Despite the claims of the food industry, most of these additives are not necessary and do nothing to improve human health. And for those in recovery—who may be more susceptible to the toxic and immunological effects of these substances—the question of what is safe to eat is anything but academic.

Clean Water

Water, as we noted in chapter 2, is our most essential macro-nutrient, and it is also one of the most endangered. Throughout the nation and the world, fresh water supplies are threatened by a range of contaminants, including:

*pesticides (from agricultural runoff)

*chemicals (from industrial pollution)

*acid rain (courtesy of industrial air pollution)

*heavy metals (from old lead pipes and industrial pollution)

Most municipal water systems were developed at a time when the primary worry was the spread of disease through water contaminated by human or animal waste. As a result, the average water purification plant is designed to filter out or purify bacterial contaminants and other biological threats, not the scores of chemicals that are being dumped into the world's water supply by the billions of gallons each year. In fact, the U. S. government has set "acceptable levels" for many of these potent carcinogens—which should not be in our water supply at all!

People in recovery are already suffering from the toxic effects of their addictions and may have a compromised ability to detoxify these chemicals. This is why we strongly recommend that you *do not* rely on your local water purification plant for a healthy water supply. Instead, we suggest that you:

*Drink bottled spring water.

*Install a water filter, for your entire home or at least one specific tap. Make sure you change the filter regularly. Some sources for water filters are Springtime Water Distiller, Midi Still, Katadyne, Multipure, Brita, and Seagull IV.

For more information on oases and allergy-free products:

Book

Coping with Your Allergies. Natalie Golos and Frances Golos Golbitz (New York, Simon & Schuster, 1979).

Resource Group

The Human Ecology Action League
P.O. Box 49126
Atlanta, Georgia 30359-1126

Mail-Order Companies:

Allergy Control Products	Allergy Resources, Inc.
96 Danbury Road	745 Powderhorn
Ridgefield, CT 06877	Monument, CO 80132
1-800-422-DUST	1-800-USE-FLAX

Clean Air

When people in recovery are allergic to environmental factors such as pollen, dander, and dust—with severe hay fever, asthma, chronic nasal congestion, or difficulty breathing—the presence of these factors can further tax an already overburdened immune system. One way to reduce this load is to set up an oasis within your home—a place where your body can have at least eight hours of respite from the barrage of environmental and allergic insults that surround us each day. Most people find that the oasis works best in the bedroom, where they spend eight hours sleeping each night. Books and resources on environmental control are listed in the box below, and appendix L gives specific guidelines for establishing an oasis in your home.

Getting on the Move: The Importance of Exercise

We live in a very sedentary society, and the effects of this sedentary lifestyle are seen in the high rates of obesity, heart disease, atherosclerosis, and certain respiratory disorders that afflict Americans. The benefits of exercise are well known, if often ignored. They include:

* *Increased metabolic rate*—so that calories are burned more efficiently even when we are at rest.

* *Burning of fat stores and buildup of muscle tissue*—(Muscle cells are metabolically active and burn calories, whereas fat cells are inert.)

* *Increased free fatty acids*—which better enable the body to process and utilize dietary fats.

* *Decreased total serum cholesterol and increased levels of high-density lipoproteins (HDLs)*—the "good fats" associated with lower risk of heart disease.

* *Lowered blood pressure.*

* *Increased levels of mood-elevating neurochemicals*—such as the endorphins, so that we feel better mentally as well as physically.

Exercise, like all things in recovery, should be taken in moderation. If you have been a couch potato for the last ten years, don't start out as if you're in training for the Olympic long-distance team. If you are over forty years old, have any history of heart problems, or have respiratory difficulties, see a qualified physician and have a complete physical. If your physician recommends it, also have a stress test, which will demonstrate your work capacity and the response of your cardiovascular system to physical stress. Plunging into an unsupervised exercise program without knowing your limitations is both foolish and dangerous.

Despite the old axiom of "no pain, no gain," becoming physically fit should not be a painful and unpleasant experience. The goal of your exercise program should be optimal physical health—not looking like Cindy Crawford or Arnold Schwarzenegger. As you become increasingly fit you will indeed start looking (as well as feeling) better—but let that be a welcome side effect, not your primary motivation.

In order for an exercise program to work, it needs to be both *consistent* and *frequent*. Pushing yourself to the limit every day for a week and then not exercising at all for a month is not a fitness program. If you really want to improve your cardiovascular and overall fitness, get into an "exercise rhythm." Make time to exercise at least four times a week, and give yourself at least an hour per session.

There are two basic forms of exercise, aerobic and anaerobic. There is a lot of confusion about the nature of each.

> *Aerobic exercises* are those that cause the body to use large amounts of oxygen (and burn calories) and prompt the heart and pulse rate to rise through steady, constant movement. Aerobic exercises tend to involve the large muscle groups, such as those of the legs and arms. They include:
> —walking
> —jogging
> —cycling
> —swimming
> —rowing
> —"step training"
> —cross-country skiing
> —Stairmaster work
> —other active sports such as tennis or volleyball

> *Anaerobic exercises* develop muscular strength and flexibility and do not necessarily increase the pulse or heart rate. Anaerobic exercises include:
> —yoga
> —weight training
> —calisthenics

Both forms of exercise are important for overall fitness. Many of the exercise benefits discussed earlier are functions of aerobic activity. Anaerobic exercise helps keep the muscles toned and limber, and can also be very relaxing.

Contrary to popular belief, you do not have to run a ten-minute mile in order to enjoy the benefits of aerobic exercise. Indeed, trying to run a ten-minute mile when you are out of shape would be both dangerous and demoralizing. While you should ideally break a sweat and get your pulse rate up when doing aerobic exercise, you should not push yourself too hard at first.

1. *Choose an activity you like.* Did you hate jogging around the track in high school? Then don't try to force yourself to like it now. Remember, you are setting a lifelong pattern: Choose an activity you can actually look forward to each day.

2. *Choose your location.* If you are going to work out in your home, choose a room that has a wood or carpeted floor (not one over poured concrete) and that is well heated and ventilated. Make sure you have room to move around freely.

   If you are going to try a gym, choose one that has properly trained exercise physiologists. Choose a facility with a supportive and qualified staff, where you can feel comfortable no matter what you wear or how much you weigh.

3. *Start slow.* If the thought of forty minutes of jogging makes you cringe, try a brisk walk around the block at first. Then make it two blocks, or three, and so on. Make a game of setting new goals for yourself.

4. *Dress the part.* Comfortable clothes can make a tremendous difference in your exercise experience. In general you should wear clothes that allow plenty of freedom of movement (loose-fitting T-shirts, sweatpants, etc.) and good-quality sneakers or running shoes that provide good arch support and cushioning.

   Your muscles should be kept warm during exercise, so wear layers of clothes (a sweatshirt over a leotard, for example) that can be removed or added as you warm up or cool down.

5. *Listen to your body's cues.* Exercise should *improve* your health, not undermine it. The body gives off some very clear signals when it is being overstressed, and you should heed these signals and either slow down or stop exercising when they occur:
   *sharp pain in any muscle or joint
   *excessive fatigue
   *lightheadedness or faintness

    *pain in the teeth, jaw, arms, ears, chest, stomach, or back
    *heart palpitations
    *nausea and/or vomiting
    *headache
    *shortness of breath/wheezing

6. *Stick with it.* The greatest risk in any exercise program is the "inertia factor." You let one day go by without exercising and suddenly it snowballs into a week, a month, or a year, and you find yourself back at square one. Make exercise a part of your life, not just an occasional chore.

Relaxing

In addition to their biochemically addictive properties, almost all addictions and compulsive behaviors are unhealthy ways of coping with stress. When we give up these dysfunctional stress-relievers, it is important to find other ways to deal with life's ups and downs. Fortunately, there are many healthy ways in which we can learn to relax and cope with the stresses of day-to-day life.

Psychological and emotional stresses—both negative (the death of a loved one) and positive (winning the lottery)—prompt a distinct physiological reaction that is known as the stress response. The stress response is a complex hormonal and neurochemical event that affects everything from heart rate to (in the long run) how effectively our immune systems fight foreign invaders. The malnutrition and toxicity that accompany addictions, eating disorders, and related compulsive disorders magnify the stress response, causing even greater havoc. Biological restoration of the type advocated in this book can help repair much of the damage caused by these combined stressors and help the body resist the effects of future stress. But it is also important to learn to recognize and control stress before it gets a strong foothold.

People have been controlling the stress response for centuries through a variety of relaxation techniques, including yoga and meditation. As medical science came to understand the physiological nature of the stress response, the validity of these and other forms of stress reduction came into focus, and additional techniques were developed.

Today, there are several specific stress-reduction techniques that can induce a "relaxation response"—the stress response's biological opposite. Where the stress response revs us up, the relaxation response slows us down, triggering the release of hormones, neurochemicals, and other substances that slow heart rate, respiration, and pulse and make us feel calmer and more serene. Specific techniques that can invoke this response include meditation (including prayer); yoga, t'ai chi, and similar disciplines; and biofeedback.

Biofeedback is a scientific technique that is rooted in many ancient forms of meditation. When receiving biofeedback training, the client is hooked to a machine that monitors one or more of the biological parameters of the stress response (heart rate, muscle tension, brain wave activity, etc.) and converts it into an audible or visual signal. The person then tries to bring the signal within an ideal range, thereby learning to control a normally unconscious physiological response.

Research has shown that recovering alcoholics can learn to increase the frequency and amplitude of certain brain waves through the use of biofeedback, with significant psychological effects including relief of depression. Several studies carried out at the University of Colorado have shown that this particular form of biofeedback training, known as alpha-theta biofeedback, can greatly improve the prospects of long-term recovery.

It is not enough to know how to nip the stress response in the bud; you should also develop a sense of perspective and balance, to keep from getting "stressed out" in the first place. There are several ways to prevent stress buildup:

1. Get adequate rest.
2. Break up your work day with regular "rest stops" to eat, relax, or just take a walk around the block.
3. Take time off from work; let your weekends be weekends, and learn to leave your job behind at the end of the day.
4. Prioritize; differentiate between what is really critical and what is not.
5. Maintain your social life; make the time to play, as well as work, with the people you care about.

Perhaps the best way to achieve such a balance is to reopen lines of communication with the people around you. For those in recovery, silence and secrecy have often been a way of life, and overcoming this unwritten code of silence is an important part of reducing the stress load. Two of the greatest aids in this quest are meetings (where the fellowship and comfort of other recovering persons provide a safe place for honest communication) and psychological counseling (where sensitive personal issues can be addressed in a safe and nurturing environment).

The Problem of Medications

The natural high of good health comes from a life free of the influence of addictive chemicals of all kinds, including prescription drugs. Once you have been addicted to one substance—be it alcohol or the neurochemical "cascades" produced by binging and purging—you are always going to be more susceptible to other addictions. For this reason, abstinence from *all* addictive substances is a critical part of maintaining your recovery. Cross-addiction (from alcohol to food addiction, for example, or from cocaine to alcohol) is a serious threat to recovery and almost always eventually leads to renewed use of the original addictive drug. Abstinence is more than just avoiding your old drug of choice; it is steering clear of any foods, medications, or activities that can start an addictive response.

The importance of total abstinence from addictive substances and activities is one of the cornerstones of 12-Step programs, with good reason. But some individuals in recovery can become so rigid in their adherence to this doctrine that they inadvertently become a danger to newly recovering individuals. For although addictive drugs of any kind should indeed be avoided like the plague, there *are* times when medication and medical treatment are absolutely necessary. *Well-meaning friends who blindly advise others to give up physician-prescribed medications or to go "cold-turkey" from drugs or alcohol may unwittingly endanger the life of the addicted individual.*

Over the years we have both known people who believe that addicted individuals should be able to tough it out through withdrawal. For these people, overcoming addiction is a matter of willpower, not biology. They are dead wrong; and naive individuals who follow their advice may well end up dead, period.

Medical care is critical when *any* addict is entering recovery. "Cold turkey" withdrawal from any drug of abuse—particularly alcohol—is not only painful, but potentially deadly. The extreme physical and neurochemical dysfunctions caused by addictions are not to be taken lightly. If a person is physically addicted, telling him to "just say no" is roughly equivalent to telling him to drive his car off a cliff. Cold-turkey withdrawal can destroy a person's life as irreversibly as the addiction itself.

The first step in embarking on a healthy recovery should always be a good, medically supervised detoxification program (inpatient or outpatient), followed by long-term, medically monitored rehabilitation. In appendix F we delineate some of the basic components of such a biological/behavioral treatment plan.

The underestimation of medications is not limited to those who are just beginning recovery. Many practitioners are only just becoming aware of the prevalence of addictions and still tend to overlook their importance in many "psychiatric" as well as medical conditions.

There are many medical and psychiatric practitioners who prescribe potent and addictive medications when they should be investigating the underlying physical (and perhaps addictive) causes of supposedly psychological problems. Alcoholism and other addictive disorders can mimic mental illness. If not properly identified, addicted individuals may well continue their addiction even as they are being "treated" for their supposedly psychological problems. We have both seen many such cases. Thankfully, there is now an organized effort to train physicians in the detection and treatment of addiction, and we may soon see far fewer cases of misdiagnosis.

On the other side of the coin, *some addicted and recovering individuals do suffer from serious underlying psychological disorders.* Serious mental illnesses, from manic depression to schizophrenia, afflict some 12 percent of the general population, and a similar incidence can be expected among those in recovery. *In these cases, recovering individuals must balance their abstinence from addictive drugs with responsible maintenance of their medication.* Failure to do so can be disastrous.

The big dilemma from a doctor's perspective is when to make a diagnosis of mental illness in these cases. *All* addicted individuals will seem "mad" when they are in the throes of their addiction. They will exhibit symptoms of paranoia, violence, delusional thinking, hyperactivity, depression, and just about any other psychological symptom you can imagine. These symptoms are likely to persist, to some degree, until the person has been completely detoxified and physiologically restored.

This is why we advise the physicians, families, and friends of individuals in early recovery not to make snap judgments about the psychological "wellness" of the recovering person. No patient in early recovery should be labeled mentally ill until he has been detoxified and biologically restored. If mental illness is suspected, the person should be medicated only when it is necessary to prevent him from harming himself or others. A final diagnosis should not be made until the person has been detoxified and in comprehensive treatment for at least a month, and even then the diagnosis should be reevaluated at least every three months during the first year of recovery.

It is clear that the issue of medication in recovery is a complex one, and this is why individuals in recovery must be vigilant about avoiding addictive medications of all kinds and must inform their physicians, dentists, therapists, and so forth of their addiction history. It is not safe to assume that your doctor will ask all the right questions. You must give him or her the information.

Always ask about the possible side effects and addictive potential of a prescribed medication, and ask if there are any nonaddictive alternatives. Find out how long you should be taking the medication, and make sure there is a time and dosage limit. If your doctor or dentist makes light of your concern, try to educate him or her about the realities of recovery. Give him or her the information contained in the Sources section of this book, or recommend *Diagnosing and Managing Chemical Dependency,* Joseph D. Beasley, M.D. (available from the Medical Tribune Bookstore, 257 Park Avenue South, 19th Floor, New York, New York 10010, 1-800-937-8876; or call Comprehensive Medical Care's information helpline, 1-800-787-0230).

If your doctor continues to disregard your concerns, it's time to find another practitioner. The American Society of Addiction Medicine (see appendix G), your local Council on Alcoholism, and local AA chapters can give you the names of physicians in your area who are knowledgeable in the area of addictions.

Prescription medications are not the only risks for recovering individuals. Many over-the-counter medications contain alcohol and other psychoactive substances that can be a problem for those in recovery. Appendixes A, B, and C list the most common addictive drugs, medications that contain alcohol, and medications that are known to be alcohol-free, respectively. If you are considering taking a medication not listed here, always read the label and avoid products that contain alcohol and pseudoephedrine hydrochloride (a decongestant that is also a potent stimulant and appetite suppressant).

Food for recovery, then, is much more than the substances we consume to fuel our bodies' cells and activities. It is also the behaviors, attitudes, environments, and actions that provide nourishment to our lives as a whole. A commitment to recovery is a commitment to a life of balance, variety, and heightened awareness and respect for our needs and limitations, both physical and emotional. The measures discussed in this chapter are all ways in which we can "feed" our recovery and provide a healthy body to support our expanding minds and spirits.

Part Two

11 *Wholefoods and Their Importance*

The nature of food, like that of beauty, is often in the eye (and appetite) of the beholder. Chocolate-covered ants and grasshoppers are considered by some to be delicacies. Many of our favorite foods were once considered too revolting (or dangerous) to even consider eating. The now popular tomato, for example, was "known" to be poisonous until a bold few, Benjamin Franklin among them, took fate by the hand and ate the dreaded "love apples" in public. Needless to say, they did not die, and tomatoes became a dietary staple here in America.

Regardless of these differences, there are certain dietary commonalities among most preindustrial/indigenous cultures. One of the most notable is that foods of all kinds are generally consumed *whole*. All edible parts, from peels or skin to internal organs, are included in the diet. This "waste not, want not" approach makes optimal use of every food's nutrients.

Not every part of every food is edible, of course, but there is an intrinsic balance in the nutrients within most foods. Eggs, for example, despite their load of the dreaded cholesterol, also contain just the right balance of nutrients to process and use that cholesterol. In fact, there is no strong scientific proof that eggs have any effect on blood cholesterol levels! When wholefoods are broken up—"refining" bran out of wheat, rice, and other grains; discarding peels and rinds; and so forth —the inherent harmony of the nutrients is destroyed, and we lose the benefits of their synergistic effects. There is a vast nutritional difference between a fresh, tree-ripened pear and canned pears in sugar syrup.

Wholefoods, then, are those that have been tampered with as little as possible. They haven't been peeled, cored, "refined," or chemically augmented any more than is absolutely necessary to ensure their safety. Ideally, they have also been grown, harvested, and stored with a minimum of pesticides, antibiotics, fumigants, waxes, dyes, or the other chemical indignities usually inflicted on our food supply. The optimal carrot, for example, would be grown in healthy soil free of pesticides and chemical fertilizer, pulled up precisely when it was ripe, shipped, and rinsed briefly before eating.

In the days of our hunter-gatherer ancestors, that's how most plants *were* harvested and eaten. Even when humans discovered farming, the distance between the soil (or, in the case of meats, the pasture) and the dinner plate was relatively short. Today, however, the food on our tables can come from anywhere in the world. Fruits and vegetables are harvested (before they ripen) anywhere from California to the Caribbean, treated to prevent them from ripening (or rotting) too quickly, and shipped over long distances to our local markets. Others are used in a variety of prepared foods that we can thaw, boil, microwave, blend, or bake to have "a complete meal in minutes." Given the fact that so many of our meals come from cans, boxes, and jars, it's small wonder that there are some city-raised children who do not know that milk comes from a cow.

Some foods need to be at least a bit refined before we can eat them. Raw grains of wheat, for example, really aren't of much use as a food until their hulls have been removed. But there is an enormous qualitative difference between whole foods eaten as close as possible to their peak of freshness and processed, prepared, or artificial foods that have been brutalized and stripped of their nutritional value.

Unfortunately, much of the food industry would have us believe exactly the opposite. Each year, the food production industry spends billions of dollars to tell us that candy and caffeinated drinks will give us energy and satisfaction; that alcoholic drinks will make us more social, sexy, and athletic; and that various food "substitutes" are better for us than the real thing. In reality, the products they promote are often high in fat, almost always highly processed and filled with additives, and rarely of any nutrient value at all.

By the time most Americans reach eighteen years of age, they have seen more than a quarter million commercials promoting this drivel. Faced with such a barrage of misinformation, it's hard to know what to think. But in the realm of nutrition (as in most things) knowledge is power, so let's start with the basics.

The Biological Importance of Wholefoods

We live in bodies that were designed long before the technological advances of the last several centuries, and although human technology has changed at a breakneck pace, human biology has not. While our current environment offers us a highly processed, sometimes completely artificial, and always abundant food supply, our bodies are *built* for an unrefined, all-natural, and often scarce food supply.

The current "design" of the human body came into being when our ancestors were still roaming the veldt as hunter-gatherer nomads. Eggs, meats, and sweets (such as honey) were treats, not regular meals. Alcoholic beverages were nonexistent or rare indeed. For many human groups the bulk of the diet consisted of foraged plants, and for all the diet consisted of natural foods in an unadulterated, unprocessed state.

Beneath our civilized trappings, we have retained the biology of our itinerant hunter-gatherer relatives, who consumed food "on the hoof" and were hungry much of the time. When our prehistoric biology runs head-on into our postmodern food supply, it is almost inevitable that problems will ensue. In chapter 9 we discussed the problem of essential fatty acid deficiencies (and alcoholism) in persons living in areas where fresh, coldwater fish was once a dietary staple. Numerous researchers have looked at the changing disease patterns of other areas in the modern world and noted disturbingly similar trends. When traditional, wholefoods diets are usurped by the type of processed, high-sugar, high-fat diets most of us consume, the rates of chronic diseases such as heart disease, diabetes, atherosclerotic disorders, cancer, and even addictions rise precipitously within a couple of decades.

This pattern has held true across populations ranging from Eskimos above the Arctic Circle to Native Americans on the plains of the American Southwest. Much as eighteenth-century European contacts with Pacific Islanders resulted in devastating epidemics of measles, syphilis, and other infectious diseases, the adoption of twentieth-century Western eating patterns seems to be correlated with a rise in chronic diseases.

For example, shortly after World War II the federal government began providing food subsidies to the Pima Indians living on reservations in Arizona. These processed food products, particularly those containing sugar and white flour, quickly replaced the Pimas' traditional wholefoods diet. Within one generation, obesity, diabetes, and alcoholism became serious health problems for the Pima Indians. Today, nearly 90 percent of the population has diabetes, and alcoholism has nearly destroyed the Pima culture.

Research evidence such as this indicates that despite the tremendous advances and changes of the last several generations, we are still bound by the inherent limits and needs of our biology. For example, the "sweet tooth" that seems such an integral part of most humans was instilled when sweets were hard to come by. Today, with sugar and other sweeteners present in almost every food, we must learn to curb this natural craving for sweets and adjust our diet to one that more closely approximates the natural, varied, and wholefoods diet of our ancestors.

Of course, not *everything* about the modern food supply is evil and deadly. Most of our foodstuffs are as appetizing to bacteria, molds, insects, and parasites as they are to us, and these food-borne beasties have caused untold miseries over the centuries. Agricultural advances and various food processing techniques have all but eliminated such food-borne illnesses in industrially developed countries, although they still wreak havoc in many underdeveloped regions. But these valid and *healthy* food processing methods have been joined by scores of unnecessary and potentially dangerous techniques and chemicals that are supremely unsuited to our biology.

Ironically, the technology that makes almost every possible food available at any time of the year also prompts many of us to eat incredibly monotonous diets. When our prehistoric ancestors went "shopping" they had to settle for what was in season, be it roots, grubs, fruits, vegetables, or nomadic animals. Variety was a biological imperative. In our modern world, where almost nothing is out of season if you are in range of a truck, plane, or train, we have been freed from the tyranny of the seasons, and bound by our often unimaginative taste buds. When you look over the lists of fruits and vegetables in the next chapters, don't be surprised if you've never heard of some of them. You have lots of company. Few of us realize just how varied our food choices can be.

Ultimately, the biggest problem with our modern diet is that although it supplies plenty of *food* it rarely supplies a corresponding number of *nutrients*. Without the proper nutritional tools and raw materials, our prehistoric (and damaged) body chemistry is often at a loss. And, like those rats in Roger Williams's lab nearly half a century ago, we lose our "wisdom of the body" and become dysfunctional and unwell.

So what is a modern human with an ancient biochemistry to do? Well, no one expects you to start chasing down your pot roast with a spear, or to plant a wheat field on the terrace of your condo. But you can learn to recognize and use wholefoods, and to avoid processes and chemicals that do nothing to improve food and are often harmful. This is particularly important for individuals in recovery, since our bodies desperately need food of the highest nutritional value, and our livers are frequently unable to process and detoxify chemicals and additives.

So, let's take a look at some of the ways in which wholefoods can be damaged by modern food processing and production.

Produce: Vegetables and Fruit

Fresh vegetables and fruits are among the most important wholefoods in recovery. Lightly cooked, raw in salads or in soups and stews, their high vitamin and mineral content is low in fat, calories, and cost. In fact 90 percent of our vitamin C comes from fruits and vegetables as do 50 percent of vitamin A, 35 percent of vitamin B_6, 25 percent of magnesium, and 20 percent of niacin, thiamine, and iron; but they provide only 10 percent of our calories and 1 percent of fat.

The problem with produce, from a logistical perspective, is that fruits and vegetables are at their most nutritious when they are fully ripened—on the vine, tree, etc. Back when most people grew their own, harvesting produce when it was at peak ripeness was no problem. But when fruits and vegetables became an industry, ripeness became a drawback, not an asset.

Farming today is big business, and the goal is high yields for low cost. Instead of picking vegetables when they are ready to eat, today's farmers pick them when they are ready to ship. Harder, greener vegetables and fruits travel better and do not spoil as soon during long transportation and storage periods. They also don't have anywhere near the nutrient density of their vine-ripened counterparts. A tomato that is ripened on the vine has more than twice as much vitamin C as one that is machine-picked while still green.

In order to keep these early pickings from rotting or becoming infested with bugs, many fruits and vegetables are treated with hazardous fumigants, fungicides, and sometimes irradiation. Other chemicals are used to slow or speed up the ripening process, preserve fruits and vegetables once they are ripe, or change their color to make them *look* more ripe. These chemical additions are used with little or no regard for taste or nutritional quality, and they remain on much of the produce we find in our supermarkets. In fact, it has been estimated that 94 percent of commercially grown produce contains pesticides. Chronic pesticide exposure puts a tremendous strain on the body, compromising the immune and detoxification systems and increasing the body's requirements for certain vitamins, particularly A and C.

We recommend that you buy locally grown fruits and vegetables when they are in season, rather than relying on out-of-state or international imports. When it is necessary to buy such produce, try to choose items that are organically grown (see below).

In general, beware of imported produce. Many chemicals that are banned in the United States are still shipped and sold to foreign countries that have very little monitoring of these toxic chemicals. These toxins find their way back to our tables via imported produce.

Organic Versus Conventional Farming Methods

Just as the quality of our health is determined by the quality of the food, air, and water that support us, so the quality of our food is determined by the quality of the soil in which it is grown. Nutrient-rich soil with a healthy population of earthworms and other soil microorganisms produces healthy, nutrient-rich crops. Over-farmed, nutrient-depleted soil that has been heavily treated with chemicals produces nutrient-depleted crops that contain residues of these chemicals. Unfortunately for consumers, most produce in the United States is grown in just such soil. The combined effects of malnourished soil, early harvesting, chemical tampering, and interstate/international shipping lead to produce that is inexpensive and large, but also waterlogged, tasteless, and stripped of much of its nutrient potential. In the world of produce you definitely get what you pay for.

As we have seen, those in recovery can be highly susceptible to the ill effects of toxic chemicals, and also need the maximum amount of vital nutrients in food. In general, fresh produce is always a better nutritional bet than processed fruits and vegetables. But to get produce that provides optimal nutrition without chemical contamination, increasing numbers of people are turning to fruits and vegetables that are grown on organic farms.

Organic farming relies on the art of balancing the ecological environment. It does not use any of the synthetic chemicals, herbicides, and pesticides of conventional farming methods, relying instead on biological controls, such as the introduction of predatory insects to help eliminate harmful ones. Soil is enriched with organic materials such as fish meal, cover crops, bone meal, and kelp. Crops are rotated, which allows the soil to "rest" and helps control weeds, diseases, and pests.

The most ecologically sophisticated form of organic farming is biodynamic farming, an independent sustainable farming system that utilizes the forces of nature to maximum advantage. Everything on the farm that is not sold is recycled into the earth to build the soil (and therefore the nutrient value of anything grown in it).

Organic produce is picked when close to full ripeness, often by hand. Great care must be used in packing and shipping these fruits and vegetables. They are generally transported, processed, and packaged without chemicals, artificial additives, preservatives, or irradiation. This labor-intensive process makes the price of organic foods somewhat higher than that of their conventional counterparts. However, as the demand for organic foods grows, prices should drop. Organic foods are not only best for humans in recovery, they are also best for the recovery of the earth.

Meat and Poultry

Meat (beef, pork, lamb, etc.) and poultry (chicken, turkey, pheasant, etc.) are excellent sources of protein and of many of the essential vitamins and minerals that are vital for those in the initial stage of recovery. But both food groups have some serious health drawbacks as well.

The downside of red meat is its load of saturated fat and cholesterol, which has led many health experts to recommend that people eat less of it. Poultry products are far lower in both saturated fats and cholesterol, but they, like red meat, can conceal a different, more insidious health threat.

Raising livestock has become as much of a business as farming produce. Many ranchers and breeders have learned to use hormones, antibiotics, and other drugs to raise as many animals as possible in the least amount of space on the least amount of feed. In addition, animal feed (such as grains) that has been raised on conventional farms is often contaminated with the same pesticides found on the produce consumed by humans.

These drugs, hormones, and contaminants have serious implications for human health. Overuse of antibiotics has led to the development of potentially lethal antibiotic-resistant strains of salmonella that are now a significant health threat. Hormones ingested in meat, milk, or poultry can upset the delicate balance of our bodies and brains. And pesticide residues found in meat, poultry, or milk are just as toxic as those found on our produce.

Public outrage over the contamination of our meat and poultry supply (some European markets have actually banned American beef) has prompted a move toward less intensive methods of raising cattle and poultry. Instead of packing thousands of chickens into hangar-like buildings, some farms are returning to a free-range approach, in which the birds have room to move and there is less risk of epidemic illness (which is the usual justification for the use of antibiotics). Similarly, several cattle ranches have returned to free-range methods and guarantee that their beef is free of hormones and other contaminants. Some major supermarket chains, including Grand Union, now carry these products. (See chapter 14 for more information on sources of free-range beef, poultry, and eggs.)

Seafood

Seafood (fish, shellfish, etc.) is probably among the best foods for individuals in recovery. In addition to providing complete proteins and vitamin B_{12}, fresh fish is a vital source of the essential fatty acids (specifically the Omega-3 group), which have been shown to reduce the likelihood of atherosclerosis, to lower serum cholesterol levels, and to relieve some immunological disorders (most notably arthritis and asthma).

Seafood also provides us with important trace minerals, such as iodine, fluoride, selenium, zinc, and copper, and several of the major minerals. Calcium is supplied by eating small fish with their bones such as anchovies, sardines, and canned salmon. Phosphorus, magnesium, sodium, potassium, and iron are other major minerals we obtain from fish.

For all their benefits, however, there are also potential problems with fish and other seafoods. Our oceans and waterways have become dumping grounds for humanity's chemical and biological wastes. These poisons are taking their toll and are now showing up in various foods we gather from the sea.

Some fish retain or actually collect toxins in their fatty tissues, including such known carcinogens and mutagens as mercury, DDT, BHC, PCBs, DCPA, lindane, chlordane, dieldrin, and dioxin. When we consume fish contaminated with these poisons, the toxins are incorporated into our bodies and stored in our own fat cells. Our bodies make an effort to process many of these toxins by stimulating drug-detoxifying enzymes in the liver, greatly taxing our livers and playing havoc throughout our systems. This weakens the immune system and makes us more susceptible to the harmful effects of toxins of all kinds.

Fish generally provides a high nutritional return for our caloric investment, but in today's world fish must be chosen with caution. Despite the rather dire condition of the oceans and many freshwater fishing grounds, it is possible to find relatively safe fish and enjoy its nutritional benefits. As we shall see in chapter 14, all it takes is some informed consumerism and a lot of label reading.

Fats and Oils

Back when humans were running around on the veldt, dietary fat came from natural sources: nuts, seeds, vegetables, fish, and of course meat that had to be hunted and killed.

Today, the bulk of our dietary fat comes from animal products (including dairy products such as whole milk and cheese) and a range of commercially produced oils that are found in everything from cupcakes to potato chips.

If you consider the amount of saturated fat our ancestors probably consumed, you can see why we are advised to cut back on fat in the diet. Prior to the domestication of animals, human breast milk was primarily for babies and young children. Even after we domesticated cows, we had to make our own butter and cheese. Similarly, it took work to get steak for our supper when the steak was on the hoof and running away from us at top speed.

Unfortunately, most polyunsaturated, cholesterol-free oils are not only worthless but harmful. The intensive processing of these oils not only strips them of most of their nutritional value, it renders them almost unrecognizable to our "old-world" biology.

The clear, golden, pure-looking cooking oils that line our market shelves have been bleached, deodorized, and processed at temperatures exceeding 300 degrees Fahrenheit. Once in the body, they form the dangerous free radicals we discussed in chapter 3. When oils are hydrogenated to form solid products such as vegetable shortening, the situation is even worse. By forcing hydrogen atoms back into the oil, food processors alter the original shape of the oil molecules ("cis" fats) and make them stiffer and unrecognizable to the body. The new molecules ("trans" fats) are not properly broken down and absorbed by the body, and they actually contribute to the development of arterial deposits!

In addition to these molecular changes, oil processing destroys vitamins A, K, B_{12}, and E, as well as chromium, manganese, cobalt, and copper. The essential fatty acids are rendered either inactive or toxic as a result of oxidation.

Since we do need some fat in our diets, the quality and source of that fat is a key part of the recovery program. The best source of such fats are the original sources of many oils: nuts, seeds, fish. When choosing cooking oils, go for those that are as close to their natural state as possible. Cold-pressed oils have been extracted using only pressure, which reduces some of the negative effects of processing. Light and oxygen degrade oils and make them rancid, so buy oils in opaque containers and keep them refrigerated. Margarines and vegetable shortenings made with hydrogenated oil are not whole foods and are not a good part of a recovery diet. Small amounts of unsalted butter are preferable.

Finally, be alert to the many processed fats hiding in prepared foods. If the label says "hydrogenated" or "partially hydrogenated" vegetable oil, beware. Palm and coconut oil (sometimes referred to as tropical oils) are a particular pitfall, since they are highly saturated, even if they don't contain cholesterol.

Processed and Prepared Foods

As the nature of our food supply has changed, so have our food choices and our eating patterns. Between 1909 and 1976, Americans' intake of processed fruits went up by 913 percent. Processed vegetables, up 306 percent. Fats and oils (largely processed), up 139 percent.

During those same years, despite the increasing and year-round availability of fresh fruits and vegetables, our yearly consumption of these foods dropped, respectively, by 61 and 41 pounds per person.

In other words, we have drifted away from fresh produce, whole grains, natural fats and oils, and fiber-rich foods—the foods for which we are designed—and toward treated fats, sugar, and highly processed foods—the foods our bodies barely recognize. American children now drink more soft drinks than fruit juice. Is it any wonder that our health is suffering?

Processed and prepared foods pose a real dilemma for those in recovery. Some of the better brands (see chapter 15) can be very useful in the early days of recovery, when it is often all we can do to maintain our abstinence and get to meetings. But as recovery progresses, we must wean ourselves *off* such food products. When we do buy prepared foods, it is important to read labels and to avoid the additives, colorings, and other artificial substances that pose a unique risk to recovering persons.

Food additives are nothing new, of course. Foods have been preserved with sugar, salt, woodsmoke, and the like for centuries. Strictly speaking, the spices used in pickling and other home cooking techniques are all food additives. But the myriad chemicals that are poured into our modern food supply have very different biological effects than their natural predecessors, and therein lies the problem.

Many additives that were once considered safe (red dye #4 and cyclamates, for example) were later discovered to be harmful and removed from the market. The Federal Drug Administration, in allowing additives, relies on information provided by the manufacturer—information that is not always correct and occasionally is fraudulent. Although the FDA is reviewing its list of additives that are "generally recognized as safe" (GRAS), the process is long and complex, and there are many known or suspected carcinogens in our food supply. Indeed, only a small fraction of the thousands of chemicals that pervade our food have been adequately tested. (See appendix N for a table of particular additives and their risks.)

The major problem with additives, especially for those in recovery, is the potential cumulative effect of all these chemicals. Chemicals that are relatively benign alone or in small amounts can have a synergistic and toxic effect when combined with other chemicals. For millions of people who are chemically sensitive, even minor exposures can have major consequences. Furthermore, those with liver damage from alcoholism or drug addiction are less able to process these chemicals, which can then accumulate in the body.

The problem of additives in processed and prepared foods is compounded by the nutritional effects of refining and processing. With each step of "refinement," crucial nutrients are lost. For example, the whole wheat grain is probably one of the most nutrient-rich foods available (hence the nickname "staff of life"). By the time the grain has been hulled, rolled, scoured, ground, and magnetically separated from the germ and bran, all that is left is a tasteless white powder that contains calories and little else. Gone is more than 80 percent of its cobalt, manganese, magnesium, B_1, B_3, B_6, and biotin; more than 70 percent of its iron, zinc, phosphorus, potassium, folic acid, and vitamin K; and 90 percent of its vitamin E—and this is only a partial list. In their place, we have 7 percent *more* calories! "Enrichment," a process that replaces only four of the more than two dozen nutrients lost in refining, does not even begin to make up the loss. This is why we stress the use of whole-grain flours, breads, and baked goods, which make use of the entire grain, and therefore its nutrients.

While fresh is obviously best, we know that there are times when processed foods—from canned goods to frozen vegetables—are an inevitable part of life. As in all things, there are good choices and bad choices when shopping for such foods. In chapter 15 we will list some of the better sources for prepared foods that use organic ingredients and minimal processing. While it isn't always easy, it is indeed possible to find healthy foods in a can.

Wholefoods are a critical part of the recovery process, for both the nutrients they provide and the chemicals and contaminants they (hopefully) lack. Choosing and preparing wholefoods also puts us more in touch with the nature of food and gives us a creative and emotional satisfaction that simply cannot be had from opening a can and dumping the contents in a pot. In the next several chapters we will introduce you to some specific wholefoods that can become both tools and allies in your recovery.

12 Nutrient-Dense Foods

While all wholefoods are nutritionally superior to processed foods, some can be called more superior than others. These foods provide such a high nutritional return on their caloric investment, and are so tasty, that they should become mainstays of your recovery diet. These "super-foods" are legumes, whole grains, and sea vegetables.

Legumes (Beans)

Beans are probably the best nonanimal source of protein. They are abundant in B vitamins (good for repairing a weakened nervous system), iron (which helps build healthy blood), and fiber (which helps lower cholesterol). They provide minerals such as calcium (necessary if you're cutting down on dairy food), zinc (usually deficient in recovering individuals), magnesium, and copper. And best of all, beans are low in calories, fat, and sodium.

Many people complain of bloating when they eat beans. This can be easily remedied by soaking beans overnight in nine parts water to one part beans. Some B vitamins are lost this way, but after a few weeks your body will adjust and you can reduce the soaking liquid.

Some beans are sold dried and require rehydrating, while others are sold fresh, sometimes in pods. Either way, they are great in chilies, in soups, and pureed for sauces such as an Italian white bean sauce. We can even make breads and baked goods from beans.

Aduki beans (also known as azuki or adzuki), referred to as the king of beans by the Japanese, have been cultivated in Asia for centuries and are now grown commercially in the United States. The reddish-brown bean has a light, nutty flavor, making it a great ingredient in both sweet and savory dishes; it can be simply boiled and eaten with rice or made into candied bean cakes for dessert. An excellent healing food for the kidneys, adukis are an excellent source of carbohydrate, phosphorus, potassium, and iron. They also contain some A and B vitamins.

Black beans, also known as black turtle beans, are native to Mexico, but they are a staple food in South America and the Caribbean. A member of the kidney bean family, the black bean is kidney shaped and shiny black. This hearty but semisweet bean can be eaten boiled, fried, spiced, in a soup, or mixed with rice. Black beans contain high amounts of potassium and phosphorus, and they are also a good source of calcium and iron.

Chick peas (also known as garbanzos in Spain and grams in India) are round beige beans, with a nutty flavor and firm texture. Chick peas can be boiled, fried, roasted, sprouted, or ground into flour. Use them in soups, pâtés, casseroles, stews, and sauces. Perhaps its most popular use is in hummus, a traditional Middle Eastern dish in which chick peas are pureed and mixed with garlic, tahini, olive oil, and lemon juice. Chick pea flour is high in protein and is excellent for wheat gluten-free diets.

Chick peas are considered one of the most nutritious beans; they're high in protein, calcium, and phosphorus, and they have almost double the amount of iron of most other beans.

Black-eyed peas are thought to have originated in China, whence they then traveled the Silk Route into Arab hands, then to Africa, and finally to the Western Hemisphere, brought with slaves.

This medium-size white bean with a "black eye" is traditionally served in the South with collard greens. It is also a great addition to salads or casseroles.

Black-eyed peas are a good source of vitamin A, as well as calcium, magnesium, potassium, and phosphorus. They are lower in fat than other beans.

Lentils were one of the first cultivated crops, originating in southwestern Asia, and are eaten throughout the world as an inexpensive source of protein. They are extremely important in the diets of many underdeveloped countries.

The lentil is shaped like a disk or lens and is usually tan in color. It has a mild flavor, lending itself to use in soups and pâtés. In India, lentils are also used in a dish called dhal—a bean puree seasoned with Indian spices.

There are a variety of different lentils, including brown lentils, green lentils, red lentils, and masoor lentils. No lentils need to be soaked and they all cook much more quickly than other beans. Lentils are richer in protein than other legumes and they are high in calcium, magnesium, sodium, potassium, and phosphorus.

Lima beans are named after the capital of Peru and are otherwise known as butter or sieva beans. These flat, creamy-colored beans come in two species, small and large. One of their more common uses is in a dish called succotash, in which corn and limas are stewed together.

Starchier than other beans and low in fat, limas are also healthy for the liver. They are a good source of B vitamins, iron, calcium, and trace minerals.

<u>Mung beans</u> are most commonly eaten in sprout form in Chinese food, but they actually are native to India. The small, dark green bean is also ground into a flour, which is used to make Chinese noodles referred to as cellophane noodles. Mung beans are high in Vitamin A.

<u>Pinto beans</u> are large tan kidney-shaped beans with brown spots on their skin. They are popular in Mexican and South American dishes. They can be prepared in dishes such as refried beans, chilies, bean burritos, tacos, and tortillas. They are high in calcium, iron, phosphorus, potassium, and B-complex vitamins. They have a high protein content but should be combined with grains, nuts, seeds, or dairy food to provide complete proteins.

<u>Soybeans</u> have been an important ingredient in Chinese cuisine for over 5,000 years. They are grown worldwide. In the United States soybean farming occupies 68 million acres. Much of the crop is used to feed livestock. The beans can be used in casseroles and salads.

Soybeans easily adapt the flavors and textures of many foods, and they are used as meat extenders in many beef and poultry products. Soy milk is a good dairy substitute. The beans are small and creamy white. Soy products now available in the United States include:

<u>Tofu</u> is a cheesy curd used in soups or salads, as a replacement for cream in frostings and icings, and as a substitute for cheese in tofu pies. It also can be marinated and broiled. These days tofu is also making a hit as an imitation ice cream called Tofutti or Icebean.

<u>Miso</u> is a salty fermented soy paste used in soups. The East has long heralded miso for its medicinal properties. It has vitamin B_{12}, a B vitamin found in meat, poultry, and fermented foods such as sauerkraut. A tablespoon of miso in hot water makes a soothing broth.

<u>Tempeh</u>, a fermented soybean cake with a meaty flavor, is also rich in B vitamins. It is available in different flavors, such as garden herb or barbecue. Tempeh can be steamed, sautéed, or roasted and is one of the most digestible forms of whole beans.

<u>Soy sauce</u> is the most familiar soy food. Health food stores carry

the better brands, which are made from fermented soybeans, wheat, and sea salt. Many commercial brands have additives and are not made through fermentation. They are of inferior nutritional quality and are far less tasty than those made through fermentation. One caution: Some soy sauces are preserved with alcohol. Try using shoyu (from whole beans) or tamari (the excess liquid from the miso-making process).

White beans, which include navy beans and great northern beans, are the mature dried bean of a delicate string bean called haricot vert or French bean (see page 118). They are high in protein and carbohydrates, as well as iron, calcium, and the B vitamins. Navy beans are used in the traditional recipe for Boston baked beans.

Grains

Grains are one of the giants of the whole-foods kingdom because they are both high in nutrients and low in cost. They are the main food staple for most of the world's population. Grains are also a primary food source for livestock, which provide us with eggs, meat, and dairy.

Botanically speaking, grains are grasses. To date there are more than 8,000 species of grains. From fields of wispy golden wheat, rye, or barley, to name but a few, come our daily bread, cakes, cookies, muffins, bagels, crackers, matzo, pasta, cereals, and pastries.

Each grain stalk bears many tiny fruit, often called berries. Each berry is covered with a protective hull, which is inedible and must be removed. Just under the hull is the bran layer (containing B vitamins, protein, fats, minerals, and all-important fiber), followed by the starchy endosperm (which is mainly calories and comprises 80 percent of the berry's mass) and, in the center, the nutrient-rich germ. Although the germ comprises only 2.5 percent of the berry's volume, it contains 95 percent of its nutritional value. including the E, A, and B vitamins, protein, and fat.

As we noted in the previous chapter, milling grains into refined flours removes almost all of these nutrients, as well as the grain's fiber content. The growing emphasis on fiber as a cancer preventative and weight-loss aid (since some forms of fiber attract water molecules, expanding to make us feel more full) has led to a renewed popularity of whole-grain products. This healthy trend can be made even better by expanding the types of grains we consume, since there are many wonderful grains besides wheat.

Two of the most common and popular grains—wheat and corn—

are also two of the most common food allergens for people in recovery. It is difficult to find any prepared or processed food that does not contain corn syrup, wheat flour, or both. For persons allergic to these foods, the prospect of finding alternatives to their favorite breads, pastas, snack chips, and the like can seem impossible.

But there are actually many grains and vegetables that can serve as wonderful "starch substitutes" for wheat and corn. Many health food stores now carry wheat-free pastas and breads. The following table lists some of the alternatives.

SUBSTITUTE STARCHES

Amaranth	Chick pea	Quinoa
Arrowroot (thickener)	Lentil flour	Sesame
Artichoke (Jerusalem)	Lima bean	Soybean
Banana/plantain	Lotus root	Spelt
Barley	Malanga	Tapioca (thickener)
Brown rice	Oat	White sweet potato
Buckwheat	Peanut	Yam
Cassava	Potato	

Amaranth was the staple food of the Aztecs, who also used it in religious ceremonies. It was rediscovered in the mid-1970s and continues to gain popularity.

Amaranth is high in lysine, an amino acid that most grains lack. It is up to 18 percent protein, twice that of corn or rice, with respectable amounts of calcium, iron, and vitamin A. It also contains vitamin C, which is uncommon in most grains.

Amaranth can be used to complement other grains, beans, and vegetables. Its sticky, gelatinous quality makes it useful for stuffings in poultry and fish as well as stuffed vegetables. It can also be popped quickly in a pan by dry roasting for use in salads. Amaranth flour makes a sweet crumb crust.

Barley can be traced to the Stone Age, when it was prepared in flat cakes. It originated in North Africa and Southeast Asia and became a staple of the Far East. It was once so popular that it was used to establish standard measures of weight and length (twelve barley kernels equal one inch). As the popularity of wheat increased, barley fell out of favor and became known as the food of the poor.

Barley is low in fiber, which makes it easier to digest than other whole grains. The English still use barley water for stomach upsets. Try to buy the hulled, unpearled barley. Pearled barley is highly processed and contains less than half the original nutrients.

Use barley in soups or stews or as a hot breakfast cereal with fruit. Barley flour cooks up cakelike and sweet and can be used as a substitute for part of the white flour in many recipes.

If you're looking for a coffee substitute, try roasting a few cups of barley in a low pan at 400°F. degrees for 90 minutes. Stir frequently. Just grind and use as you would coffee beans.

When sprouted barley is roasted and the liquid is extracted out of the roasted sprout, the result is a low-cost, high-quality natural sweetener sold in stores as barley malt. Use barley malt in place of white sugar in recipes, but slightly reduce the amount of liquid in the recipe.

__Buckwheat__ is not really a grain, but the seed of an herb plant. Originating in Siberia and northern India, it spread to central Asia and China. Today buckwheat is a staple of Russia, particularly in its roasted unhulled form known as kasha.

Buckwheat has an earthy flavor. It is high in vitamin E and is thought to be a good food for blood building.

Buckwheat seeds are called groats; when they are finely ground, they are known as buckwheat flour. Coarsely cracked groats are called buckwheat grits. Whole groats are best toasted before using. Whole, unhulled buckwheat can be used to make sprouts. The strong-flavored flour makes a fine crumb crust and great pancakes, and when added to breads it will provide a denser, moister loaf.

__Corn__, or maize, was cultivated as far back as 3500 B.C. in Central America and was used by many ancient American cultures, including the Incas of Peru, the Mayas and Aztecs of Central America and Mexico, and North American Indians in the American South and Southwest. Maize is believed to be the only native American cereal grain.

Ancient cultures always processed corn with lime or wood ash to make grits or flour. This effectively released the bound-up niacin in corn. When corn began its migration to other countries, the use of lime or ash was abandoned. This contributed to the development of pellagra (the niacin deficiency disease) in individuals who relied upon corn as a primary dietary staple.

Cornmeal consists of coarsely ground whole kernels. Corn flour is a little sweet, grainy, and tends to be dry. It should be stored in the refrigerator. Cornstarch, which is widely used as a thickener, is very highly processed and should be avoided in a recovery diet.

<u>Millet</u> has been cultivated for more than 6,000 years and can be traced to Africa and possibly Asia.

It is high in B-complex vitamins and contains lecithin (a cholesterol lowerer), calcium, iron, magnesium, phosphorus, and potassium.

Millet is great pan-roasted and then cooked and served like rice. Use it in breads, pastries, or for stuffings. Sprinkle cooked millet on salads for a crunchy, nutritious addition. Millet flour has been described as buttery and a little sweet. It bakes to a dense and crumbly, but not dry, consistency.

<u>Oats</u>, from humble beginnings as a weed in barley and wheat fields, became the staple grain of Ireland, Scotland, and northern England.

Oat groats are cleaned, dried, and toasted to crack the inedible kernel (or hull) surrounding the oat. Hulled oat groats taste more like wheat than the oatmeal we know, and they can be used in soups or breads or cooked like buckwheat.

To make "old-fashioned" rolled oats, the hulled groat is heated and rolled. Steel-cut oats are sliced with thin blades. Quick-cooking rolled oats are heated and sliced an additional time and then prepared as rolled oats. Instant oatmeal comes from precooked oats that are dried and rolled thin.

Oat flour makes a coarse but firm crust with a slightly nutty flavor. It is a good extender for other foods, especially meats.

<u>Quinoa</u> (KEEN-wah) is another rediscovered ancient grain, once known as the "mother grain of the Incas."

It has the most complete protein of any grain and also the highest percentage of protein—between 16 and 22 percent. It supplies methionine and cysteine, vitamin E, several B vitamins, calcium, iron, and phosphorus.

Quinoa has a crunchy, nutty flavor. Use alone or in soups, casseroles, stews, or salads.

<u>Rice</u> is a primary food for more than 50 percent of the planet. The United States, however, consumes less than one-half of 1 percent of the world's rice crop.

There are thousands of varieties of rice. The most common are: long-, medium-, and short-grain brown rice; sweet brown rice (also called sticky rice); basmati rice (popular in Indian cuisine); and wehani (a rich red rice developed in the United States).

Brown rice is the result of removing only the hull of the grain. Milled, unpolished white rice results from an abrasive process that removes the bran and most of the germ. When that rice is further polished with wire brushes, and in some cases with sugar, polished rice is produced. Quick-cooking rice is the most processed and least nutritious rice. Certain nutrients are added back into white rice by spraying them onto the surface of the grain. This is why processed rice should never be washed or rinsed.

Rice is also used to produce a sweet syrup, known as rice yinnie or rice malt syrup, that is a good alternative to sugar or other sweeteners.

Rye originated in central and Southeast Asia and moved west largely as a weed in barley and wheat supplies. Red rye berries are delicious when cooked whole, like rice. Cracked rye or rye flakes are great in granola. Rye flour is one of the few grains other than wheat that is used alone to make bread.

Sorghum is a grain related to millet and similar to corn. The United Nations labeled it the third most important grain in the world after wheat and rye. Africans cook sorghum as a porridge, but in the West we mainly find it processed into a sweetener called sorghum syrup.

Triticale (TRI-ti-kay-lee) is the first man-made grain. It is a laboratory-produced hybrid of wheat (triticum) and rye (secale). It resembles wheat, but is a bit larger, and tastes like both. Early claims about the higher nutritional status have been disproved. Although scientists heralded triticale as the food answer for underdeveloped countries, most of it is used for feed for livestock.

Wheat moved into the West from the Middle East in prehistoric times. Today, wheat is the favorite grain of the western world. We consume 145 pounds per person each year, more than any other grain.

Wheat is classified by its planting season (either spring or winter) and by the composition of the starchy endosperm. The latter classification includes soft wheat (used for pastries and cookies), hard wheat (used in breads), and durum wheat (very hard wheat used to make pasta). Many brands of pasta use a highly processed form of durum wheat called semolina. This variety is less nutritious than whole grain or whole wheat pastas.

The whole wheat kernel is called a berry and can be cooked like rice, used for stuffings or in hot breakfast cereals, or added to soups. Bulgur, or cracked wheat, is partially cooked and often requires only soaking in hot water.

Rolled wheat flakes are processed in the same way as rolled oats. Farina is the most processed form of wheat cereal, made up of the endosperm only.

The most nutrient-rich wheat flour is stone-ground whole wheat flour, followed by whole wheat. Both are coarser and heavier than unbleached white flour and common bleached white flour, which are the most highly processed flours and the lowest in nutritional value. Whole wheat pastry flour makes a sweet, fine crumb for baked goods.

<u>Wild rice</u> is actually a grass that originated in the Great Lakes region of North America. Wild rice is usually fermented for a few weeks and then browned to give it a nutty rich flavor. It is higher in protein than regular rice and is especially rich in lysine, an amino acid that is deficient in most grains.

All of these grains are becoming increasingly available at health food stores and groceries around the country. In appendix M you will find several mail-order houses through which you can buy these grains in bulk.

Sea Vegetables

While most of us are familiar with grains and beans, sea vegetables may seem exotic. Those in urban areas have become casually acquainted with nori, the sea vegetable used to wrap sushi rolls of fish or grains. Most of us have little regard for these foods and refer to them as seaweed.

But until this century, most coastal cultures regularly consumed sea vegetables, and they still are a dietary staple for Alaskans, northeastern Canadians, and many Asians. Sea vegetables are rich in vitamins and minerals but low in calories and fat. The nutrient density of sea vegetables is ten to twenty times that of land vegetables, and since they will not grow in polluted waters they are among the safest of the sea's products. All these facts make sea vegetables one of the best nutritional investments for those in recovery.

Many varieties of sea vegetables now line health food stores, co-ops, and even some of the more progressive or innovative supermarkets. Although they may seem expensive, they expand greatly and only small amounts of these foods are needed daily.

<u>Arame</u> are delicate black strings. The flavor is sweeter and milder than that of most sea vegetables, making it a good choice as an introduction in your diet. Like most sea vegetables, arame is sold dried. Rinse it first, then rehydrate it by soaking it in water for ten minutes before cooking. Remember that it will double in size. Add arame to salads or cooked grains, or serve it as a small side dish. Arame is high in calcium, potassium, iron, and vitamins A, B_1, and B_2.

<u>Agar-Agar</u> is rich in iodine and trace minerals and is used as a vegetarian source of gelatin. To avoid acids and bleaches, which are

sometimes used in processing agar-agar, buy this product in health food stores. When preparing an agar gelatin, remember that acidic foods such as oranges will require a larger quantity of agar-agar than, say, a pear gelatin.

Dulse is a tasty purple leaf vegetable. It is high in potassium and magnesium. When dried, it is a slightly crispy, salty snack. Rinse well before using. Add dulse to soups, salads, casseroles, vegetables, or grains or use in croquettes or as part of a cabbage stuffing.

Hijiki, like arame, is a stringy black cylindrical sea vegetable, but it is wider and has a stronger flavor (the flavor is made milder when hijiki is cooked in shoyu and apple juice). It expands five times while soaking. Serve it with vegetables, soups, beans, or fish. It also cooks well with oil after rehydration—so add it to stir-fries. A one-ounce serving of hijiki has the same amount of calcium as an eight-ounce glass of milk. It also contains protein, vitamins A, B_1, and B_2, and iron.

Kombu comes in dark green, thick strips. It has a wonderful hearty flavor, making it great for stocks. Kombu imparts an almost beefy flavor when added to beans (a 3-ounce piece per pot), and it also makes the beans easier to digest. Kombu is high in iodine, B vitamins, iron, and amino acids.

Nori is one of the most commonly used sea vegetables and it contains one of the highest sources of protein among them. It has substantial amounts of vitamins C, B, and especially A. Its thin green sheets are used to make sushi rolls or can be lightly toasted over an open flame for one or two seconds and eaten as a snack or used as a garnish.

Wakame (kelp) is a brown leafy sea vegetable that has a pleasant, mild flavor. It is rich in calcium and B and C vitamins. Wakame is used in soups, stews, grains, and beans. It can be baked and sprinkled on cooked grains or land vegetables. It is a good sea vegetable for the novice because of its mild flavor. When cooked, wakame turns a lovely green color.

Although some of these foods may seem a tad strange, they should not be allowed to languish in culinary obscurity. Whole grains, legumes, and sea vegetables are some of the most nutrient-dense foods available. As part of a varied diet, these foods can keep scores of diseases at bay, including heart disease, cancer, clinical malnutrition, blood sugar abnormalities, high cholesterol, and anemia. When we include these foods in our regular diet, our recovery process is more assured.

13 Going Shopping: Fruits and Vegetables

How often have you eaten something you didn't really want, just because it was there? Or finished a drink, a snack, or even an entire meal and then asked yourself "Why on earth did I eat that?" This type of impulsive eating is particularly common among those in recovery, since the damage of our addictions and compulsions has dulled our sensitivity to our internal cues. As a result, we all need to become more conscious of what we're eating and when we're eating it.

Whole, natural foods give the body the high-octane fuel it needs to restore and maintain itself. The first step in providing these foods is to actually have them in the house (and on the job, and in the car . . .). And in order to have them in the house, you need to know what foods to choose, how to choose them, and where to find them. This means learning some new shopping skills—particularly how to scout for wholefoods in the modern jungle of the supermarket.

Navigating the Supermarket

The supermarket as we know it is a very new phenomenon. Small specialty shops were the norm until the late 1930s. Although the butcher, the baker, and the farmer's cart with fresh produce are making a slow comeback due to consumer demand, most of us still rely on mammoth markets for our shopping needs.

And super they are. There are currently upwards of 30,000 products on supermarket shelves. Every dollar you spend is also a vote for your food preferences, so if you don't see what you want, ask for it. Although many of these stores are chains (with home offices many states away), they are still eager to please their customers by carrying the foods they request. Remember, in the 1950s yogurt was a crazy "health food" that only a few consumed. Today yogurts of all flavors and sizes fill the dairy case. Consumer demand does have an impact. The prices of some organic produce have already gone down, and as the demand for these products grows, production and supply will increase, reducing prices still further.

You'll probably want to shop for fresh foods at least twice a week and dry bulk items (which can be stored for longer periods of time) once or twice a month. Before heading out to market there are a few things to do in the kitchen.

   *Keep a list of items you run out of during the week on the refrigerator.

   *The evening before shopping, take ten minutes and review some recipes for recovery that you're planning to cook in the next few days. Jot down the ingredients that you don't have on hand.

   *Organize your shopping list into categories to prevent you from running a marathon up and down the aisles. A typical list could be organized into categories such as:
      –Produce (vegetables, fruits, fresh herbs)
      –Meats (poultry, fish, and red meat)
      –Dry goods (whole-grain flours, grains, beans)
      –Baked goods (whole-grain breads, muffins)
      –Specialty foods (Chinese, Mexican)
      –Juices and mineral waters
      –Condiments (mustards, jams)
      –Oils and vinegars
      –Snacks (nuts, seeds, dried fruits)
      –Prepared foods (whole-grain crackers, cereals)
      –Emergency foods such as canned, dried, or frozen foods.

Once your list is completed, and just before you head out to the market, eat something. That's right—eat something. A friend of ours once told us proudly about her recent trip to a health food store, where she had spent almost $75 on "great, healthy foods." She then reeled off a list of organic pecans, almonds, raisins, dates, dried apricots, organic blue corn chips, black bean dip, whole rye bread, eggs, and carrots. While it was true that she had bought whole*foods,* she had bought almost nothing (except the eggs and carrots) that could be used as a base for a whole *meal.* She had shopped hungry and without a list. The result was a bag full of ready-to-eat foods that were great healthy snacks but hardly the ingredients for balanced meals.

You take your chances when you walk into a supermarket when you're hungry. It may not offer such a healthy variety of wholefoods snacks. You may be tempted to eat something full of sugar or refined flour, and in either case you probably won't buy foods that make a whole meal. So we repeat, *Don't shop on an empty stomach!*

When you enter your local market, take another look at it. Check where the wholefoods might be located. Most markets are laid out so that fresh wholefoods are what the customer sees first. The perimeter of the market is where you're likely to find fresh fruits and vegetables, fresh cuts of meat, chicken, fish, baked goods, and dairy products. Note the aisle where dry goods such as packaged or bulk grains and beans are sold. Avoid the aisle where candy, snacks, and soda are displayed —they are not wholefoods. There are many wholefoods choices that offer something sweet, sparkling, crunchy, or gooey. The other inside aisles are variations on the same theme from market to market.

Let's look at choosing fresh produce first. Choose loose unpackaged vegetables and fruit. Precut and wrapped items are difficult to view and may be sprayed with chemicals to keep them from turning brown. This is how some markets sell older produce. Fresh, locally grown vegetables are your best bets for nutritional value, and they may be exactly what your body requires. For example, have you ever noticed that starchy root vegetables are widely available in the colder seasons when the body needs an extra layer on it to keep warm, or that light leafy greens are the first foods in spring when the body needs to slim down?

Remember that, by law, all produce is supposed to be marked if it is waxed or irradiated. In many cases, however, these laws are not enforced, so ask your produce manager to identify items for you and to please mark them. While you're at it, inquire about organically grown fruits and vegetables. (Remember, many individuals in recovery are chemically sensitive.) Many markets are now carrying a wide variety of organic produce because of such requests.

Now let's take a look at some of the specific foods you will be choosing. Review the following sections once in a while before shopping to provide you with shopping ideas and assist you in purchasing the freshest possible foods.

Choosing Vegetables

Artichokes are generally jumbo or baby size. They should feel heavy for their size and the leaves should be compact. Look for bright to olive green leaves and stems (a purple cast is also okay). Avoid yellowing leaves, which indicate an overly mature vegetable. Artichokes store up to a week when refrigerated; make sure to wrap them in a clean, moist towel. Cook artichokes in water with a dash of lemon juice or vinegar (acidulated water) and avoid pots made of aluminum or cast iron, which will turn the artichokes dark brown.

Asparagus is most tender when it's plump. Thin stalks of asparagus tend to be woody. They should be purchased when they are bright green. Look for tight heads that are not slippery. Note the season is fairly short in late spring. If the asparagus begins to wilt, cut the bottoms and stand the stalks in a glass of water and keep in the refrigerator (much the same way we revive wilted celery). Asparagus will last a few days in your refrigerator. Many people prefer to peel the tough outer skin for a smoother look, but this is not necessary.

Arugula is a distinctive peppery-tasting green leaf vegetable also sold as rocket or Italian cress. The leaves are 3 to 4 inches long and scalloped around the edges. Look for bright green leaves without yellow or wilted parts. It will last two to three days in the refrigerator. The leaves get very sandy so be sure to wash it thoroughly before using. Arugula can be used instead of lettuce in a salad. It is a favorite in Italian homes and restaurants.

Avocados come in mainly two varieties. The California avocado, often called the Hass or Hess, is the small dark green one with a warty skin and is the richest in flavor. The Florida avocado is larger and bright green. It has less flavor but it is also less expensive. When selecting an avocado look for a fruit that gives to the pressure of your finger but is firm; brown spots are okay and do not alter flavor. If you feel the pit shaking around inside it is overripe. A hard avocado will need a few days at room temperature to ripen. Once an avocado is cut, the flesh will turn brown quickly at room temperature if not sprinkled with freshly squeezed lemon juice. If you're only using half an avocado, leave the pit in the remaining half; it will keep better.

Green string and yellow wax beans should be free from brown rust spots and should not have bulging seeds. When you break them in half—try this at the store—they should snap crisply and cleanly. String and wax beans will keep for several days in the refrigerator. Haricots verts, often sold as French beans, are delicate little string beans that should not be limp. The color is somewhat darker than regular green beans and haricots verts cook much quicker, too.

Beets are generally red, but yellow beets are making their way to some markets. Both varieties are best when firm, not mushy and soft. Also avoid scales around the top. Remove greens immediately after purchase. (Don't discard them—they are great when sautéed with olive oil and garlic, or steamed.) Beets that are not relatively round will be very strong tasting and tough on the teeth. Smaller beets are sweeter. Although beets sweeten with age, they should be used within a week for optimal nutritional value.

Belgian endive is a tight cluster of white leaves that are shaped like a large closed flower bud. The tips may be light greenish yellow, but avoid brown or torn spots. It is expensive because it is carefully grown by hand in Belgium, wrapped by hand, then shipped to the United States. Belgian endive can be chopped or sliced and added to salads, or braised for an entirely different flavor.

Bok choy, an Asian green, is everywhere these days. It looks like fat white celery stalks with big dark green leaves. It is frequently and incorrectly sold as Chinese cabbage. Look for stalks that are firm with no deep brown cracks, and leaves that are not wilted. Bok choy should have no hole in the bottom (this indicates age and rot). Bok choy will keep under a week in the refrigerator. It is a low-calorie and flavorful addition to stir-fries, or it can be steamed or sautéed by itself.

Broccoli should have tightly packed flowers that are bright green and smell fresh. The larger and more yellow the flower top the older (and less desirable) the broccoli. It can be stored up to 1 1/2 weeks in the coldest part of the refrigerator. The stalk is tasty, so slice it thin and cook it a few minutes longer than the tops (florets). But don't use extra-large stems; they are tough and woody-tasting. Submerge in water to remove any insects.

Broccoli rabe (also called broccoli rape) is a pungent-flavored leafy green vegetable with a few broccoli-like flower buds. The buds are fine when yellow, unlike regular broccoli. Treat broccoli rabe like other leafy greens.

Brussels sprouts look like tiny heads of cabbage. They should be compact, bright green, and free from brown spots or holes. Unfortunately they are usually sold in containers that make viewing anything but the top layer impossible. You can ask the checkout clerk to open the package after it's been rung up to see the lower layers. If they are brown or rotten, ask to exchange them for another package.

Burdock root is a delicious root vegetable. It is a thin (1 inch in diameter) long brown peel root that tastes earthy and nutty. Look for crisp roots. The flesh is white and must be sprinkled with lemon or acidulated water if not served immediately to prevent it from discoloring. It is not necessary to peel it. Don't wash until ready to cook. Wrap it in a damp, clean cloth to store up to two weeks.

Cabbage comes in several varieties. The usual green or red cabbage has crisp outer leaves and no cracks in the head. Check the base to see that it is not dark brown and soft. Also avoid insect holes.

Savoy cabbage has curly leaves but should still be tight in the center.

Napa cabbage has an elongated shape and very light green crinkly leaves.

Cabbage will keep for up to two weeks in the refrigerator. However, if it's cut it should be covered to preserve freshness and prevent the odor from penetrating other foods. Green, red, or Napa cabbage is great raw or cooked, but Savoy is best cooked.

Carrots should be firm and bright orange without green tips or cracks. They are often sold with their leaves, which should be removed immediately after purchasing so carrots do not become bitter. Carrots can be stored for two weeks in refrigeration. Like most root vegetables, they can be kept in cold storage (a cool dark place, covered with sand) for many months.

Cauliflower should be white and firm and should have very tight heads with green leaves. Brown mold spots atop a few flowers can be cut off, but avoid heavily browned heads. Also avoid heads that appear to have been shaved or cut; these are usually very old heads that markets try to keep selling. There are now purple and yellow varieties of cauliflower. All varieties can be stored in the refrigerator for a week.

Celery is naturally a very strong tasting vegetable. Check the base of the stalks for rot and avoid cracked bottoms. Most celery is sprayed with ethylene gas to create a less bitter, light-colored product. Some health food stores and a few markets now sell untreated organically grown celery. The color is a darker green than the light green celery we've been buying for years. However, if you've grown celery in a garden, you've seen the real thing. Celery will keep for one week in the refrigerator and individual stalks can be kept crisp for up to two days when placed standing in a glass of water in the refrigerator.

Celery root or celeriac is more pungent than celery. It is not a root but an enlarged stem bottom. To avoid inside rot, press the top of the celeriac and make sure it's firm. The smallest are the best in taste and texture. Celeriac will store up to a week in the refrigerator and much longer in cold storage. Prepare celeriac as you would any vegetable: Peel, steam, boil, or add it raw to salads.

Chicory is a curly endive that looks nothing like the Belgian endive to which it is closely related. Its leaves are roughly edged and spindly. They are light yellowish green in the center and turn to dark green on the outer leaves. Chicory has a slightly sharp taste and will last for about three days in the refrigerator.

Chilies: (See Peppers)

Chives are seasonally available and sold in small bunches. They look like baby scallions. Their sharp flavor is a favorite with creamy baked potatoes but they are also nice in salads, chopped and added to beans or grains, or tossed on the top of soups. They will keep for a week in the crisper drawer of the refrigerator. (Please note: Most delicate greens should be kept in an airtight drawer, as they will quickly wilt in an open refrigerator.)

Cilantro is a tasty little green that is often sold as Chinese or Mexican parsley. It looks like a bright green, slightly wider leafed parsley. Look for soft clean leaves without slippery decay. The leaves and stems of cilantro can be added to salads to enhance flavor or can be chopped and used to flavor soups and casseroles, much as we use parsley. Cilantro is also a natural with pinto beans. It will store for up to four days in a vegetable drawer, or it can be dried and used as an herb.

Corn is available in many varieties, but sweet corn is the one most of us eat on the cob. Purchase dark green husks with golden silk. Pull a strip of the outer green husk back and press a kernel with your nail; a sugary white substance should squirt out. Store corn in the husks in the coldest part of the refrigerator; it loses 95 percent of its fruit sugar within twenty-four hours if not refrigerated quickly. Grill in the husks or boil without the husks in a large pot of water to prepare. If loose corn is desired, remove it from the cob.

Cucumbers are available in three varieties to most of the nation. The dark green standard cucumber has large seeds and is 8 to 12 inches long. It usually is waxed but is not marked as such. The smaller pickling cucumber has a lighter green skin and, of course, smaller seeds. It is usually not waxed. The very long thin cucumbers often sold as Hollands, Hot House, or Greenhouse are seedless and usually waxed. No matter which variety, look for firm, even shapes. Avoid soft spots or yellow skins, which indicate that the cucumber is overly mature and will taste bitter. Most of the skins are bitter, but to eliminate this problem Evelyn Roehl in her book *Whole Food Facts* recommends "cutting (unpeeled) the cucumber in half [crosswise] and twisting [pressing] the ends together . . . in opposite directions, until foam appears around the edges . . . rinse off the foam and slice."

Dill is often sold fresh. Look for feathery leaves with no sign of slippery rot or flowering. It is a welcome addition to salads for a real fresh flavor. Finely chop it and add it to roasted or boiled beets, carrots, or cauliflower. It will store for only a few days in the crisper drawer, or you can hang it out to dry upside down for a few weeks and then store it in a bottle.

Eggplant (also sold by its French name, aubergine) is available in at least four varieties:

the large standard eggplant—a black pear-shaped vegetable

Italian or baby eggplant—a black, pear-shaped vegetable that is slightly sweeter than the larger standard eggplant

Japanese or Oriental eggplant—long, slender, and more dark brown or purple than black in color

white eggplant—thicker skinned, creamier tasting, and usually less bitter than other varieties.

Look for firm, heavy vegetables without soft or mushy spots. The stems should still be green. Avoid eggplants with wrinkled skin. The skin is edible, but when waxed or not organically grown it should be avoided. All types should be stored in a dark cool place rather than in the refrigerator. Use them within two days. Many cookbooks instruct you to salt the eggplant to get rid of the bitter taste. This is less necessary with organically grown or small sweeter varieties.

Escarole: (See Greens)

Fennel (finocchio in Italian) looks like a white broad-stalked celery with feathery green tops. Its texture is similar as well, but fennel tastes like licorice. Check the base for brown rot or cracks, which are a sign of age. The freshest stalks still have the tops intact. Slice it and steam it, sauté it, add it to tomato sauces, or toss it with salad greens or stir-fries. It has a crunchy, sweet, clean taste. Fennel will keep five days in the refrigerator.

Garlic is sold by the head, which is made up of a cluster of cloves. It should be heavy for its size and the white papery skin should be tight around the cloves. Markets now carry the common small white garlic and the larger pink elephant garlic, which has darker cloves but is much milder in flavor. Infrequently you will find wild garlic, a small red-skinned strong garlic. All garlic should be stored at room temperature in a cool, well-ventilated, dark spot, where it will keep for a few months. Leftover peeled garlic can be stored in a cup with a little olive oil poured over it. The garlic will be well preserved and the oil will have a wonderful garlic flavor after a few days; the oil can be used with or without the garlic itself.

Ginger is a spicy, tan-skinned tuberlike spice. You'll generally find it with imported vegetables even though it's grown in the United States.

Avoid withered, dry, or moldy roots. It is used in small amounts as an aromatic addition to soups, stocks, stir-fries, or sautéed vegetables. To use it, peel the outer skin and chop finely or shred it to extract the juice. A 1 by 1-inch piece is a good amount to add to a stir-fry for four. Store in a cool, dry, airtight place.

<u>Greens</u> (including beet greens, collards, escarole, dandelion, kale, mustard, and Swiss chard) should be selected by looking for firm, unwilted leaves that are not shriveled around the edges. Day-old greens are often on sale carts (great for soup stocks).

<u>Beet greens</u> are often left attached to the tops of beets. Chop and add them to soups, stir-fries, or mixed vegetables. They're even great added to pasta with garlic for a simple dish. Beet greens will keep in the refrigerator for three or four days.

<u>Collards</u> are large, waxy-leafed greens commonly used in Southern cuisine. They require longer cooking time than most other greens. Collard greens can be stored for up to five days in the refrigerator.

<u>Dandelion</u> is making a fanciful comeback in specialty markets and some supermarket shelves. It is slightly bitter when sautéed or steamed and is not the best choice to use in large amounts for stocks. It will store for two days in the refrigerator.

<u>Escarole</u> is one of three members of the chicory family (along with chicory and Belgian endive). Look for bushy, smooth-leafed, 12-inch heads that are crisp. Wash it well because the heads are usually full of sand. To wash, break off leaves and soak them in a bowl full of water, rinse, and repeat. Escarole can be added to salads, but because it is bitter it should be used in small amounts (the inner yellowish leaves are best for salads, but use sparingly). It can also be steamed or braised. It will keep three to four days in the refrigerator.

<u>Kale</u> is appearing not only in its regular, large curly and broad green-leaf forms but also in shorter, more decorative leaf varieties known as purple fancy or white fancy kale. The fancy varieties may be subjected to more spray, but organically grown kale is available in some places. We recommend buying only the organic fancy variety. Although kale is a form of cabbage, it bears little resemblance in flavor. Kale can be tough, so slice it and cook it well. Kale thrives in the cold, so store it in the coldest part of the refrigerator.

<u>Mustard greens</u> are best in the winter and spring. Look for a brilliant shade of green and avoid leaves that are wilted. They

are very pungent. Many prefer to steam the leaves and then sauté them. Plan to use mustard greens quickly, as they will keep for only one day in the refrigerator.

Spinach is commonly seen in two varieties on market shelves: large curly-leaf spinach or the often smaller flat-leaf variety. The delicate flat leaf is our preference for salads, while we tend to cook the crunchy, curly-leaf spinach. Try not to purchase pre-bagged spinach, because it is not as fresh. Avoid slippery, rotten leaves. Remove thick stems and wash quickly but well before serving. Serve raw in salads, steamed, or sautéed. It will keep for a week in the refrigerator.

Swiss chard comes in a red or green variety. Slice the entire leaf, stalklike stem and all, and steam or sauté it. The red is a colorful addition to stir-fries or mixed steamed vegetables. Swiss chard will only survive a few days in the refrigerator (unlike collards and kale).

Horseradish: (See Radishes)

Jerusalem artichoke (often sold as Sunchokes) is not an artichoke at all, but is so named because of its artichoke-like flavor. It resembles the tuber of the sunflower plant found in North America. It looks like a weird-shaped potato with a slightly thinner skin and it is starch-free. The flesh is crisp like that of a water chestnut and sweet. It can be baked, added to stir-fries, served raw in salads, even added to soups. It will last a week in the refrigerator.

Jicama is a root vegetable that is popular in Central America. It looks like a large brown beet or turnip. It's crunchy and slightly sweet. Avoid slippery or soft spots. It can be stored in a cool, dark place or in the refrigerator. The cut root goes bad quickly, so store it for only a day or so. Peel before using. Cook it by steaming or serve raw.

Kohlrabi is often sold as cabbage turnip because it looks and tastes like a combination of both vegetables. The leaves are not edible. Look for green or purple bulbs about the size of a medium tomato; any larger is probably going to be tough. The peel is tough, so it should be cut away with a paring knife, and the inner flesh can be sliced or grated to eat raw or steamed. Kohlrabi will last about seven to eight days in the refrigerator. There's no need to trim the inedible tops from this vegetable before storing it.

Leeks resemble giant scallions; they are long straight-leafed vegetables that are relatives of onions. All but the darkest tough ends can be used. Slice and rinse them well as they generally contain a lot of sand. Use them in soups, stocks, or stews, or finely chop them and use them like onions in other dishes. Store leeks for three to four days in an airtight container or crisper drawer.

Lettuce has come a long way from the days when the only lettuce on the market shelf was boring, tasteless iceberg. Now many varieties are available.

> Romaine or cos has an elongated head with crisp, medium to dark leaves. It has a longer shelf life than most lettuces and can be stored for up to a week in the refrigerator.

> Boston, butter crunch, Bibb, and limestone make up the butterhead varieties—small, round heads of lettuce that are light in weight for their size and have sweet leaves. Boston is cup-shaped with shiny leaves, butter crunch and Bibb are smaller heads, and the limestone is fanlike in shape.

> Green leaf, red leaf, and oak leaf varieties are some of the best-tasting lettuces around (they also have beautiful colors and shapes). Check the base of the lettuce heads for brown spots or cracks, a sign of rot. The leaves should be colorful and free from blemishes, rust spots, or tears.

Lettuce of all kinds is usually used for salads, but it can also be braised or added to stocks and soups. It should be stored at 34 to 38° F. But do not store lettuce near apples, tomatoes, pears, or other vegetables that emit ethylene gas or brown spots will result. Firmer-leafed varieties will last a few days longer than soft-leafed varieties, which will last from two to four days. Do not remove leaves until ready to use or lettuce will wilt quickly. Wash the leaves in large bowls of water before using to remove insects, sand, and at least some of the chemicals if the lettuce is not organically grown.

Mushrooms can be delicious additions to many dishes, and there are many varieties now in the marketplace that range drastically in price. All mushrooms are highly perishable, so use them within a day or two of purchase.

> Button mushrooms are the most common variety. Look for white to tan smooth skin. Avoid black bottoms that are a bit mushy and wet stems. Use within a few days of purchase.

> Shiitake (she-TAK-kee) mushrooms are famous in Japanese and macrobiotic cuisines. They are usually larger than buttons and more capped at the top. They are also darker when dried, which is how they are often sold. Their flavor is rich and

strong. Store fresh shiitakes in airtight containers in the refrigerator for up to one week.

Chanterelles are delicate, trumpet-shaped, and yellow. They should be used the day of purchase. (Both shiitakes and chanterelles are good sautéed in olive oil with a splash of soy sauce.)

Morels are earthy and nutty-tasting. They are spongy, black-topped, cone-shaped mushrooms, a favorite of the French, and they are expensive. Use them within two days of purchase.

Porcini (also called boletes or cèpes) are a meaty-tasting mushroom. Look for blemish-free tops and stems. They must be cooked and should be used within a day or two of purchase. They are wonderful simply sautéed.

Oyster mushrooms are another exotic favorite of gourmets. They are fan-shaped, soft textured, and robustly flavored, and are more expensive at certain times of the year. The tops vary from gray to dark brown. The flavor is more subtle after cooking.

Enoki-daki (en-no-kee-DAH-kee) are thin strands with tiny caps on the top and can be found in Oriental markets. They have a slightly grape flavor and are usually sold prepackaged in plastic or in cans. If you can find them fresh, look for solid white mushrooms with white bottoms that are firm.

Okra is the marvelous seedy green vegetable in gumbo. The young fingerlike pods have a fine, downy, olive-green skin. Avoid brown streaking or rust spots. Steam okra whole or chop and add to soups. The inside of the pods releases a gelatinous liquid that acts to thicken soups or stews. Do not cook in cast iron, aluminum, or copper or the okra will turn black.

Onions are members of the lily family, which also includes garlic, leeks, and scallions. Numerous varieties are currently found in the marketplace.

Globe onions are the strong-flavored, common yellow or white cooking onion.

Spanish onions are yellow skinned. They are larger and sweeter than the globe.

Bermuda onions are mild, sweet onions popular on sandwiches. They come in red and white varieties.

Red onions come in round Italian and elongated varieties.

Boiling onions are mild white onions, about 1 inch in diameter.

Pearl onions are tiny, white bulbs that are used in pickling or served sautéed or boiled.

Vidalia onions (named after the town of Vidalia, Georgia) are sweet and juicy with a very short season.

Walla Walla onions (named for Walla Walla, Washington) are delicious onions with a short season.

Maui onions (from Hawaii) are as mild and sweet as a piece of fruit and, like fruit, can be eaten raw out of hand.

Shallots are the prize ingredients of many cooks. The shallot is a wonderful-tasting member of the onion family with a distinctive flavor that some describe as a cross between a clove of garlic and an onion. The bulb has a pale brown to gray skin with a large double clove. Look for firm bulbs. Store in a cool, dark place up to one month. Fresh green shallots should be refrigerated.

Look for firm onions with papery tight skins intact. Avoid brown spots, very green onions, and those that are beginning to sprout. Onions can be stored in a cool, dry location for three months. Refrigeration is not necessary.

Parsley is a subtle-tasting herb that belongs to the carrot family. It is sold fresh in bunches at most markets. Two varieties are commonly available, the strong-flavored, broad-leaf Italian type and the tight curly-leaf form. Cilantro is also sold as Mexican or Chinese parsley (see Cilantro above). Infrequently, parsley root or Hamburg parsley is available. Its flavor is similar to that of celeriac. Look for bright green bunches. Avoid wilted, yellow, or slippery leaves and stems. Rinse all varieties well before using. Stems can be chopped and used. If you wish to dry parsley, hang it upside down for a week and then store it in a jar.

Parsnips look like white carrots and have a distinctive sweet, earthy flavor. Look for firm, blemish-free roots. Add parsnips to soups, stews, or roasted or steamed vegetables, or cook as a companion to sautéed carrots. Store them in an airtight container in the refrigerator. They will keep for two weeks.

Peas can rarely be found fresh anymore, which is sad because canned or frozen peas will cook up soft but not crisp. If you have the opportunity to shop at a farmer's market you have a better chance of finding fresh peas. Look for velvety pods that are crisp but not bulging. Older pods are wilted and often yellow. Keep peas cold until ready to use. Shell them by pulling the connective string that runs from one end to the other along the side. The peas will pop out. Steam them quickly or add them to soups, stews, or pasta dishes.

Snow peas are more frequently available, but they are often expensive and they still require de-stringing. They have a nutty taste and an edible shell and are quick-cooking.

Sugar snaps also have an edible pod, and the strings must be removed.

All varieties can be stored for two to three days in the refrigerator.

Peppers can be purchased in numerous sweet or hot varieties. The most common sweet peppers are the green or red bell pepper. They are 2 to 3 inches in diameter and bell shaped. There is also a tricolored bell pepper and a bell-shaped orange pepper called a banana pepper. Look for smooth skin without wrinkles or soft spots.

Chili peppers come in all shapes, sizes, and intensities of hotness. Hot peppers act as a coolant for the body by causing the body to sweat (hence their popularity in warmer climates).

—The Anaheim grows up to 8 inches long. It is a brilliant green color and has a milder flavor.

—Jalapeño peppers are a very hot little pepper usually sold and consumed in green form; they turn red if left to ripen. They are between 1 and 3 inches long. Select smooth, shiny skins.

—Serrano chilies are tiny too, between 1 and 2 inches long and 1 inch wide. They are green and orange and extremely hot.

—Poblano chilies are dark green, 5 inches long, and similar in shape to bell peppers but a little narrower. They are a milder chili.

—The habañero is a red lantern-shaped chili that is powerfully hot.

Remember to wear gloves when preparing chili peppers and to avoid contact with the inner flesh and seeds. Rinse the gloves after use before removing. Many a careless cook has for hours felt the pain of burning hands, eyes, and nose when gloves were not worn.

Potatoes, ever popular, can be roasted, fried, mashed, baked whole, or boiled. They come in as many varieties as there are ways to cook them. Denser varieties such as the russet are the best baking potatoes; creamier potatoes like the red bliss and new potatoes are lovely boiled.

New potatoes have thin red or tan skins and are creamy rich. They are quick-cooking and store only one to two weeks.

Red bliss potatoes are often dyed (ask your produce manager to avoid these dyed varieties as there are no sure ways to tell, by sight, if they have been dyed), but they are favored by many gourmets for their flavor. They are especially nice tossed in olive oil with rosemary and roasted.

Idaho potatoes are all-purpose round or long white potatoes that are used in salads or stews or as french fries.

Western russets have a scaly, thick, brown skin. Their density makes them the perfect choice for baking.

Yellow Finns are a delicious treat if you can find them; they usually sell out quickly. They have a pale yellowish-tan skin and a delicate flavor, and they are good baked or boiled.

Avoid potatoes that are green or have green spots; they are not underripe but have been exposed to sunlight and contain a toxin called solanine. Also avoid moldy potatoes or those with too many eyes or cracks. Purchase smooth-surfaced potatoes. Also note that many potatoes are waxed, so peel them before eating or purchase unwaxed organically grown potatoes.

Pumpkin: (See Squash)

Radicchio (rah-DEEK-ee-oh), also sold as red chicory, is a red-and-white-veined leaf lettuce with a slightly bitter taste. Look for crisp leaves and white bottoms. Avoid brown spots or cracks at the base. Add to salads or sauté with olive oil, garlic, and mushrooms and toss with pasta. A few leaves make a lovely edible bed for grains or beans. Store for up to one week in the refrigerator.

Radishes are a relative of the mustard family. The pungent or hot taste of raw radishes is changed to a sweet, sometimes earthy flavor when cooked.

Red radishes should be about the size of a cherry tomato, firm with leaves attached. Avoid prepackaged whenever possible. They are great in salads.

Daikon radishes are long and white. They start about the size of a large carrot but can be found five times that size. The daikon has been popular for centuries with the Japanese, who claim it helps to break down fats in the body. Always peel it, then shred it, and serve it raw with fish or slice it and add it to soups, stews, or steamed vegetables.

Black radishes look like small black beets and should be peeled. The flesh is very hot and pungent.

Horseradish, the magically hot ingredient found in cocktail sauces, is a long knobby root. Look for firm radishes; softness indicates age and lack of crispness. Peel the radish and grate slivers to serve alongside tempeh sandwiches, fish, beans, and rice.

Radishes can be stored in the refrigerator for up to one week.

Rutabagas are not giant turnips (as they are often sold), but they are a relative of the turnip. Look for heavy rutabagas in relation to their size. Most of them are sprayed with a heavy wax, so the yellowish tan skin should be peeled. Serve raw or quickly cook rutabaga for ten minutes for a sweeter flavor. It will store in the refrigerator up to one month.

Sprouts are a nutritious food derived from the germinating and sprouting of seeds from various plants. Look for firm sprouts with white bottoms, as yellow or brown bottoms indicate age and decay. They are a tasty addition to any meal—soups, salads, stir-fries, and sandwiches. Use sprouts within one week of purchase and store in the refrigerator. Sprinkle or rinse in water once a day to keep sprouts fresh.

Alfalfa sprouts are the delicate ones with tiny, dark green leaves that we see at salad bars everywhere.

Mung bean sprouts, also known as "bean sprouts," are long, white, crunchy sprouts often seen in Chinese dishes and soups.

Mixed sprouts are made up from radishes, cabbage, garlic, onions, and clover, or from bean sprout combinations such as pea, lentil, and chick pea.

Sunflower sprouts are a new addition to this group. This is a lovely 3-inch-high sprout with a large double-leaf top. It's a beautiful edible garnish and a crunchy addition to salads.

Seeds for sprouting can be purchased and easily grown in a few days on a sunny windowsill in a glass jar.

Squash is available year round in one variety or another. Look for a firm squash that is heavy for its size. The skin should be soft, but avoid soft spots.

Summer squashes are more delicate and can only be stored for a few days in the crisper of the refrigerator.

Zucchinis come in green and gold varieties. They can be eaten cooked or raw.

Yellow crooknecks (also known as yellow summer squash) can
be steamed, sautéed, or eaten raw in salads.

Pattypan squash is yellow or light green and shaped like a flying
saucer. It is also available in a baby variety. It is delicious cut
in half or quarters and just steamed.

Bitter melon or Chinese bitter melon is a summer squash shaped
like an Anaheim pepper. It's an interesting addition to stews
and roasted vegetables.

Spaghetti squash is, technically, not a squash at all, but a gourd.
It is a large yellow elongated vegetable with a sweet strandlike
flesh that appears after cooking. Bake spaghetti squash for an
hour and a half, then slice open lengthwise, remove the seeds,
and scoop out the strands of squash. Toss in olive oil with
herbs, cover with a tomato sauce, or serve as a side dish.

Avoid winter squashes and pumpkins with black stems or soft spots.
The winter squashes are usually harder skinned and can be stored for
longer periods of time.

Acorn squash (named for its distinctive shape) is dark green or
orange and ribbed. Its flesh is sweet and fibrous. Slice in half,
scoop out the seeds, and bake facedown with a small amount
of water in a baking pan until the skin can be easily pierced
with a fork.

Banana squash looks more like a pod than a squash. It is pale
pink and very large, and it can weigh up to thirty pounds.

Buttercup squash has an orange flesh that's creamy and sweet.
It has a green skin and a turbanlike top. It weighs about
5 pounds.

Butternut squash is a large, tan, pear-shaped squash, also with
sweet, creamy, orange flesh. It weighs up to 4 pounds.

Delicata squash is a scrumptious winter squash with green stripes
running lengthwise along its cream-colored, elongated body.
It weighs up to 3 pounds. Its taste has been described as a
cross between sweet potatoes, corn, and butternut squash.

Pumpkin is a close cousin of the squash and thus is included
here. Pumpkins vary in size from a few ounces to a few hundred pounds. Some varieties are better for baking than others.
If you're buying directly from a farmer, which many do in the
late fall, ask which type is better for carving jack-o'-lanterns
and which is better for baking. Once again, fresh is superior
in flavor to anything canned. Try making pumpkin pies at
least once from fresh pumpkin. Pumpkins will keep for several weeks in a cool, dark location.

Kabocha squash is the sweetest squash, with a corresponding high natural sugar content. There are two varieties, one with a bright orange skin, the other greenish blue. It's a native American known by a Japanese name.

Winter squashes may be stored in a well-aerated, cool, dry environment for several months.

Sweet potatoes are bright orange, sweet root vegetables that are often sold as yams. True yams have a yellow flesh, not orange, and are generally not sold in our supermarkets. However, they *can* be found in many Latin American markets. When choosing sweet potatoes, avoid moldy soft spots, and store in a cool, dry location for a week or two. They do not last as long as other varieties of potatoes.

Taro root or dasheen is a tuber that appears in markets on both coasts. It is a hairy brown-skinned tuber with pale pink flesh. Look for firm tubers without mold or soft spots. It is popular in Oriental and North African dishes and is a staple in Polynesian, Central American, and South American cuisines. Prepare it by peeling and always cooking it. Use taro in steamed vegetable dishes (it takes longer than most to cook, so start it first) or stir-fries.

Tomatillos (toe-mah-TEE-yohs) or green tomatoes are often sold as Chinese Lanterns. Look for very firm tomatillos with a brown papery skin that is very close fitting (the skin should be peeled before using). A pungent, slightly sweet green sauce can be made by sautéing tomatillos with onions and garlic. They will keep for a few weeks in refrigeration.

Tomatoes are really only worth eating fresh when in season locally. It's sad to think that many children have never tasted anything but the mealy pink, tasteless flesh of non–vine-ripened tomatoes. Generally tomatoes are picked green, shipped, then sprayed with ethylene gas to ripen. Look for firm, sweet-smelling, bright-colored tomatoes without soft spots, but avoid great-looking, very firm hothouse tomatoes, as these have little flavor and fewer nutrients. Tomatoes should be heavy for their size. If they are slightly underripe, place upside down in front of a sunny window for a day or so. Choose among the many varieties: tiny cherry tomatoes, tiny pear-shaped yellow or red tomatoes, flat Italian or plum tomatoes, juicy round beefsteak tomatoes, or the new yellow or orange low-acid variety. Canned whole tomatoes are fine for sauces, but these sauces are even better when fresh, sweet, local vine-ripened tomatoes are used. Store ripe tomatoes at room temperature for 2 or 3 days.

Turnips are round, white roots with purple tops and a nutty flavor. Look for firm, 2- to 3-inch roots rather than larger, tougher ones. They are also available in a baby variety the size of a cherry tomato. The green fresh leaves are also edible. Turnips are great roasted or steamed. Refrigerate them up to one week.

Watercress is a peppery-tasting green with a thick stem and small, round leaves. Look for unwilted, undamaged leaves. It can be steamed, sautéed, and added raw to salads. Watercress will keep for a few days only in the refrigerator.

Yams: (See Sweet Potatoes)

Choosing Fresh Fruits

Fresh fruits are by far the most nutritious way to satisfy a sweet tooth. While some fruits may be out of season, remember to choose at least two to three servings of fruit per day. It is sometimes difficult to tell if fruit has been waxed (and impossible to tell if it has been irradiated). By law, these products should be labeled, but the law is rarely followed or enforced. Some waxed fruits will have a very shiny, or white, flaky appearance, but the best way to determine if food has been waxed or irradiated—and where it has come from—is to ask your produce manager. When buying wrapped products (such as berries), open the container before you leave the checkout counter and check the lower layers of fruit for mold and leakage. If the fruit is damaged, you can make an exchange before leaving the store. Use the following list to make up your shopping list beforehand.

Apples grow in the wild and have been cultivated in more than 7,000 varieties, but fewer than 22 of the more marketable varieties are available in the United States. Apples are graded according to appearance, not flavor or nutritional value, so growers have been forced to produce attractive but often tasteless and unhealthy fruit. Despite this, there are still some notable varieties available.

Red or golden Delicious apples are sweet and crisp. The goldens are super for apple butter.

Cortlands, both red and green, are tart and tasty.

Newtown Pippins are light green, tart, and firm.

McIntosh apples come in red and green varieties and are very juicy.

Rome apples are red, semi-firm, and slightly tart.

Stayman apples are red and green, tart, and crisp.

Granny Smiths are another popular tart green apple.

Gravensteins are tart, green, and very juicy.

Lady Apples are tiny yellow or bright red fruits that are sweet and tart.

Cortland, Granny Smith, McIntosh, Newtown Pippin, and Rome apples are all good for baking.

Apples are available much of the year, since they store well in a cool, dark (but not dry) environment or in the refrigerator. Apples are often waxed in supermarkets, so peel before eating or purchase unwaxed, organically grown apples and enjoy the fiber.

Apricots, Nectarines, and Peaches are relatives that must ripen on the branch or they will never become sweet. While it is true that these fruits will get *softer* when off the branch, they will not truly ripen or get sweeter. When choosing these fruits, avoid brown spots, which may indicate internal damage.

Apricots are so fragile that they bruise easily when ripe. Once overripe, they lose their flavor and texture. They should be stored in the refrigerator and eaten within three or four days of purchase.

Peaches have a fuzzy skin, which is often shaved before they reach the market. There are two varieties of peaches, the firmer cling (whose flesh "clings" to its pit) and the freestone (whose flesh doesn't). Choose the cling for poaching. Ripe peaches will last two weeks. Peaches should be kept in the refrigerator.

Nectarines, like peaches, are yellow with rosy red patches. But unlike peaches, their skins are smooth. Ripe nectarines can be stored for four days and should be refrigerated.

Bananas are unusual in that they are picked green and sweeten off the tree. Although they are not locally grown, they are one of the commonly consumed tropical vegetables. Purchase green bananas; they have not been gassed with ethylene to hasten the ripening process. Avoid gray or discolored bananas—they will never ripen. Store at room temperature until ripe and yellow with light brown spots, then refrigerate. This will not hurt the flavor.

Blackberries (also sold as brambleberries) and **Raspberries**, their close relative, should be purchased plump and unbroken. Avoid berries that stick together. Keep them in the refrigerator for only a day; they're highly perishable. Before using blackberries or raspberries, gently rinse. Unlike blackberries, raspberries separate from their hull (each tiny bump on these berries is actually an individual fruit).

<u>Blueberries</u> are sometimes called huckleberries. Ripe berries should be plump and have a pawdry bloom on the skins. Store up to six days in the refrigerator.

<u>Cantaloupe:</u> (See Melons)

<u>Cherries</u> are the sweetest in June, when they are dark red to black. (These are the Bing cherries.) Watch out for rotted stems and waxed cherries. The former are overripe and the latter impossible to peel. Ask your produce or grocery manager if the cherries are waxed. When baking, simply slice the cherry in half and take out the pit. Two other varieties of cherries are:

<blockquote><u>Royal Anns,</u> which are yellow or red.</blockquote>

<blockquote><u>Sour cherries,</u> which are generally used in pies and are rarely sold fresh, are small and light red.</blockquote>

<u>Cranberries</u> should be red, firm, and full. They are usually sold in bags that weigh between 12 ounces and a pound. Avoid wrinkled skin and any moldy berries. The mold can be highly toxic. Rinse well prior to using. Store in the refrigerator for up to two weeks. Freeze for off-season use.

<u>Coconuts</u> are actually the largest seed in the world. They are also one of the few nonanimal sources of saturated fat, so we use them sparingly. A fresh coconut looks like a brown hard-skin fruit about the size of a grapefruit. Its surface is fibrous and hairy. Some dried coconut contains sugar and additives, so try to use fresh whenever possible. To open a coconut, pierce one of the three "eyes" at one end with a nut pick or other sharp object. Turn the coconut upside down and drain the coconut milk into a bowl. (The milk can be used for thickening soups or added to frozen fresh fruit drinks.) To crack open the coconut, strike it with a hammer on a hard surface. Cut out the hard white flesh. The thin brown skin that sticks to the flesh is edible. Fresh coconut must be refrigerated and used within a few days. Unopened coconuts can be kept at room temperature for a few months.

<u>Dates</u> have been consumed for more than 5,000 years. It's easy to understand their popularity if you've ever eaten plump fresh dates. They are unbeatable for a sweet tooth. Fresh dates are unripe when green. Most dates are sold dried, but these are often fumigated with methyl bromide and then treated with sulfur dioxide. Whenever possible buy fresh or look for unsulfured, organically grown dates.

<blockquote><u>Deglet Noor</u> is the largest-selling variety, comprising 85 percent of the market.</blockquote>

Medjool is the largest and richest-tasting date.

Barhi dates and the early-season Khadrawi dates are commonly available fresh (although pressed).

Holawi dates have an unusual flavor.

Zahidi dates are somewhat less sweet than the other varieties.

Fresh dates should be stored airtight and eaten within two weeks, but dried dates will last for six months at room temperature and up to a year if refrigerated.

Figs are another fruit that is usually sold dried and prepackaged, but more and more we're finding this succulent treat fresh. (Dried figs are often treated with potassium sorbate, which is considered one of the safer additives.) Figs sold fresh are deep purple or tan. Avoid cracked or sour-smelling figs. Eat fresh figs immediately. Dried figs will keep for three or four months. Store both fresh and dry figs in the refrigerator in an airtight container.

Mission figs are dark purple and very sweet.

Adriatic figs are tan-skinned and less sweet.

Climyrna figs are large with a yellowish or green skin.

Kadota figs are small and white-skinned.

Grapefruits are available in two varieties, white or ruby.

White grapefruits have light yellow flesh, a yellow skin, and are fairly small.

Ruby or pink grapefruits have a pink glow to the skin and a dark pink or red flesh. They are larger than white grapefruits. A seedless variety is also available.

Look for a thin-skinned, heavy grapefruit—it will be the juiciest. Store at room temperature for a day or two, then refrigerate in the vegetable or fruit drawer for as long as two weeks.

Grapes are a luscious, thirst-quenching cluster fruit that originated in Asia. They can be eaten out of hand, as many prefer, or used in salads or cereals. One of America's favorite varieties is the pale green Thompson seedless grape. Some other preferred grapes are the plump, blue-black Concord and the plump, black, mildly sweet Ribert. Other types are the warmly sweet Red Flame seedless and the bright red "cherrylike" Emperor. Try small white Perlettes, pale green Calmeria, or the Tokay or Cardinal, which is red with gray blushes. All grapes stop ripening after they are picked. Look for plump grapes that are firmly attached to the stem. The dark varieties should have no hint of green and should be deeply colored. The lighter green or white grapes should have a yellow blush to them, which indicates ripeness. Do not wash grapes until ready to use. Wash thoroughly, because grapes are one of the most heavily sprayed fruits. Or better yet, purchase organically grown grapes. Grapes will keep in the refrigerator up to one week.

Guavas originated in the American tropics and there are more than 100 varieties. They are currently grown in California, Florida, and Hawaii. Though guavas vary in size, they are usually 2 inches in diameter. The musky odor is deceiving as the pink flesh is quite sweet. Guavas ripen if they are kept at room temperature until they yield slightly when pressed. When fully ripe they should be stored in the refrigerator.

Kiwifruit is a small soft, furry brown-skinned fruit about the size of an egg. Inside is a bright green flesh with tiny black seeds that are edible. The inedible skin should be peeled away before cutting. Ripe fruit will yield slightly when pressed. Kiwis can be used in salads or desserts or can be sliced and served plain. Ripe kiwis can be stored for three weeks but keep them separate from other fruit.

Kumquats are a dry, bitter citrus fruit. They resemble very small flat oranges about the size of a date. They should be heavy for their size as well as firm. The skin is edible and spicy, but make sure to wash it well. Kumquats are delicious when used for chutneys. (Rinse them, slice, and remove the seeds, then finely chop. Heat 10 to 12 of them with ½ cup of fruit juice and a touch of honey. Simmer 20 minutes and serve along with chicken or turkey dishes.) Kumquats are also used in preserves and sauces. Kumquats will keep for a week in the refrigerator.

Lemons should have a deep yellow color. The lighter the fruit, the more tart it will be. The juiciest lemons have the smoothest skin. Good lemons will be firm and plump. A few brown spots won't affect the flavor. Always wash them before using, since most lemons are sprayed. There are two common varieties: the Eureka, a very round lemon, and the Lisbon, which is rather elongated. If using the skin of the lemon (as in zest, thin strips of skin), the lemon zest should be blanched for thirty seconds. This will remove any sharp acidity. Also, lemon juice can be substituted for wine vinegars in many recipes. Use fresh lemon juice for recipes that require lemon juice; the bottled stuff bears no comparison in flavor or nutrition. Fresh lemons will store in the refrigerator in an airtight container up to two weeks.

Limes are bright green, lemon-shaped citrus fruits. They come in two varieties: the Persian and the Key lime (made famous by the pie of the same name). The Persian is larger than the Key lime and more common. The Key lime has a lighter skin and rounder shape. Both are less tart than lemons. Look for heavy, smooth-skinned fruit. Store airtight in the refrigerator for ten days.

Loquats are often sold as a Japanese plum. They are currently cultivated in California and Florida. The light yellow, small, pear-shaped fruit should be crisp but juicy. Handle with care as they bruise easily. Ripen at room temperature, then store airtight in the refrigerator for a few days.

Mangoes are a highly aromatic, succulent fruit. They have smooth, yellow skins with a blush of red. Avoid mushy, overly soft or black-spotted fruit. Green mangoes will ripen if left at room temperature for a few days. Mangoes must be peeled and pitted before eating. Begin by making a cut in the peel and pulling it back—if the mango is not ripe it will be extremely difficult to remove the peel. Wash your hands immediately after peeling to prevent a rash. Mangoes grown outside the United States are sprayed with chemicals banned for their cancer-causing results, so purchase only those that are domestically grown or those labeled "organically grown." Use mangoes in salads, chutneys, fresh fruit drinks, or alone. Store ripe mangoes in an airtight container for three to four days.

Melons actually belong to the gourd family (as do their cousins, pumpkins and squash). There are four classifications of melons: canta-loupes, muskmelons, winter melons, and watermelons. When picking any of the following melons, avoid those with mold on them and search for ones with even color. Melons do not become sweeter after picking, but they do get softer. Store hard melons a few days at room temperature. Refrigerate after cutting and use within two days.

Cantaloupe melons found in the marketplace are really muskmelons (true cantaloupes are grown and sold only in Europe). These tan or beige melons have a raised netlike surface and creamy orange flesh. It is ripe when it smells sweet and when the blossom end (the side with a small indented circle) yields to gentle pressure.

Honeydew melon is probably the biggest-selling muskmelon. It is a bowling ball–size melon with a pale yellow-green rind and it weighs between 4 and 8 pounds. When ripe the honeydew is sweet and juicy and has a very fine little wrinkle on the surface of the rind.

Casaba melon has a yellow to light green rind with deep crevices and an ivory flesh. It is very juicy. The flavor is often described as resembling that of cucumbers. It is odorless when ripe.

Cranshaw melon, sometimes called Crenshaw, is a spicy-sweet, very juicy melon that weighs between 5 and 9 pounds. The rind is yellowish green and the flesh is a deep orange coral color. It becomes yellow as it ripens. Once again the sweet aroma is a sign of ripeness. The spot or circle at one end should not be too soft or the melon is overripe.

Persian melons look like very large cantaloupes. They have a green rind with raised netting and coral-colored flesh. They weigh upwards of 5 pounds and are ripe when they yield to gentle pressure.

Winter melons have a silvery green rind and are quite large, up to 30 pounds. They look like giant honeydews and taste like summer squash. The white flesh is briefly cooked before eating.

Watermelons are actually members of the cucumber family. Like cucumbers, they have green skins and an oblong shape, but on a much larger scale. If you've always wondered why people thump their watermelons, it's because a ripe watermelon will resonate when tapped. The sweetest watermelons will be light yellow to light green on the bottom side of the melon. This indicates that it ripened on the vine. Watermelons will keep for five to six days in the refrigerator.

Charleston Gray is the largest member of the watermelon family.

Miyako and Crimson Sweet both average about 30 pounds each.

Sugar Babies are small and sweet and average 8 pounds.

Oranges have been cultivated for 4,000 years. There are juicing and eating varieties. Search for firm oranges that are heavy for their size. Many are waxed and dyed, so appearance has little or nothing to do with flavor or ripeness. Unfortunately the Florida varieties are most often dyed, so avoid these if you're planning to serve the skin in any fashion, such as in zest or compotes. Although 80 percent of the U.S. crop is used for juice, more and more Latin American oranges are being used. To date, produce from other countries is not subject to the same laws regarding use of cancer-causing pesticides, so avoid imported oranges if possible and make your orange juice from fresh oranges.

Juicing oranges—such as Parson Browns, Hamlins, Pineapple oranges, and the queen of the juicers, the Valencia—primarily come from Florida. These oranges are thin-skinned and vary in size.

Temple oranges are good for both juicing and eating right out of the hand.

Navel oranges from California are thick-skinned, plump, and the best for eating. They turn bitter when exposed to the air, so they're not good for juice.

Mandarin oranges are very sweet and are great for salads because the sections separate easily and cleanly.

Blood oranges have bright red flesh with a unique sweet-tart taste. In Italy blood orange juice is popular served over crushed ice.

Seville oranges are quite tart and are great in chutneys or marmalades.

Tangerines, clementines, pomelos, and tangelos are cousins of oranges. All varieties will store for a few weeks in the refrigerator and a few days at room temperature.

Tangerines are a loose-skinned orange fruit that tastes like a cross between a mandarin and an orange. Tangerines always feel flabby. They will store for a few weeks in the refrigerator or a few days at room temperature.

Clementines are a cross between a tangerine and an orange (considered a variety of tangerines).

Pomelos are actually related to grapefruit, but they are not as moist. They have thick skin.

Tangelos are a thin-skinned cross between a tangerine and a pomelo. They should feel heavy.

Papayas are large, yellow avocado-shaped fruit grown domestically in Florida and Hawaii. They have black edible seeds. The taste is sweet but spicy, a bit like pepper. Search for a firm papaya without soft spots. The Spanish used to tenderize meat with papaya juice when the fruit was green because of the presence of papain, a tenderizing enzyme that helps digest proteins and is still used today commercially. Wear gloves when peeling a papaya because many people experience an allergic reaction to the papaya skin. Papaya will ripen in a day or two at room temperature, then can be refrigerated for up to two days

Pears come in thousands of varieties. Pears should be purchased when firm, not rock hard. They are usually picked early and allowed to ripen after they have been picked. To ripen at home, keep pears at room temperature in a dark, humid location.

Anjou pears come individually wrapped and have a spicy-sweet flavor. They have short necks and yellowish-green or red skin.

Comice pears have a short top or neck and are similar to the Anjou in shape. They have a yellowish-red to solid red skin and are quite moist.

Bartlett pears are very juicy, yellow-skinned pears. They are also available in solid red varieties.

Bosc pears are crisp, long-necked, and have dark yellow to brown skin. They are perfect for poaching.

Forell pears have reddish-gold skin.

Seckel pears have a grainy texture and a reddish-green skin. They are small and juicy.

Winter Nellis have a brownish-green skin.

Asian pears are sold in several varieties. They are moist, crisp, round, and less sweet than the more common varieties.

Persimmons are cultivated in the Gulf areas and California, and they grow wild in the Southeast. They are also imported from the Orient. The American variety is a smooth orange-skinned fruit that resembles a tomato; the imported type has a pointy end. The American variety has many times the iron, potassium, and vitamin C of the imported. The softer the persimmon, the sweeter. Search for fruit with green stems and solid skins. Handle with care. Remove the seeds and peel, and slice to eat out of hand or in salads. Persimmons will keep at room temperature for several days.

Pineapples are picked mature but hard. They will soften if left at room temperature for a few days. It's debatable whether easy removal of the inner leaves is a sign of ripeness, but a ripe pineapple will have a fragrant scent. Search for fruit that has yellow to reddish-brown skin tones under the "eyes." They should be heavy for their size. Pineapples contain bromeline, a digestive enzyme also used as a meat tenderizer. Most dried pineapple contains a huge amount of sugar (used to preserve it), so it's best to eat unsweetened or domestically grown organic pineapple. Sliced pineapple will last a few days in an airtight container in the refrigerator.

Plantains look like oversized, often overbrowned bananas, and they taste less sweet than regular bananas. They are ripe when the skins are spotted brown. Unlike bananas, though, plantains must be cooked before eating. In South American cuisine they are often sliced and either dried or fried. A healthy preparation of plantains would be to sauté them in a little oil. Like potatoes, plantains are high in starch. Leave unripe fruit at room temperature for a few days.

Plums are available in more than 150 varieties. When ripe, store them in the refrigerator.

> Damson plums are small and oval. They have an almost blackish blue skin and dark flesh. They are the favored plums for preserves as they are quite tart.
>
> Empress plums are also dark-skinned and oval but are more purple than blue.
>
> El Dorado and President plums are large with maroon skins.
>
> Friar plums are another dark red plum, but they are smaller than the El Dorado or President.
>
> Greengage Kelsey plums are yellowish green and midsize with yellow flesh.
>
> Umeboshi plums are pickled plums used in Japanese and macrobiotic cooking. They are often used to add a salty flavor to dishes.

Prickly pears are also sold as Indian figs. They are the plum-size fruit of the Opuntia cactus. Choose pears that are plump. Their flesh is bright red and very seedy. The skin must be removed before eating. Serve raw by peeling and slicing, or puree it for its colorful juice. Prickly pears can be stored for one week in the refrigerator.

Quinces look like a green or gold oddly shaped pear. Choose firm, gold, unblemished, smooth fruit. The peel is edible, but the seeds are not. Once popular in preserves or jellies, quinces are now served braised, baked, or in soups (particularly Mulligatawny). Most quinces will store up to a month in the refrigerator.

Raspberries (See blackberries)

Rhubarb is a vegetable but we use it like a fruit. Choose red firm stalks. The tart red stalks that resemble celery are used in pies and preserves, but the leaves are poisonous so make sure you remove them. Rhubarb requires cooking and sweetening. Store at room temperature for a day or so and then refrigerate up to three weeks.

Strawberries are best when they're small, and locally grown strawberries are the sweetest because they're often riper when picked. Look for firm bright red berries with stems attached. Wash them immediately before using. They will store only a few days in the refrigerator.

Choosing Dried Fruits and Vegetables

Some fruits and vegetables are sold dried (with only their moisture removed), prepackaged or in bulk. Dried fruits are lightweight, quick-energy snacks that fit easily into briefcases, backpacks, or purses. Dried vegetables make a good part of a healthy "brown bag" lunch, either as is or rehydrated with hot water.

Dried foods store well for long periods of time. Dried fruit will last months at room temperature and as long as a year in the refrigerator. The white powdery buildup you'll notice is only the fruit sugars and not mold. Dried vegetables are prepackaged with expiration dates. They can be stored at room temperature until opened.

Purchase organically grown or at the least sugar-free and unsulfured produce. Some dried fruits are preserved in a heavy sugar solution, and both fruit and vegetables may be preserved with sulfites (sulfur dioxide). Sulfites are one of the most dangerous food additives and have been conclusively linked with several deaths over the last decade. In some individuals, sulfites can prompt allergic reactions such as headaches, chest pains, runny nose, difficulty breathing, tightening in the throat, nausea, diarrhea, and even anaphylactic shock and death. A recent ban on sulfites only restricts their use on *fresh* fruits and vegetables, so be wary when buying dried produce.

Buying in Bulk

Many foods are available in bulk form, including seeds, nuts, herbs, spices, pastas, flours, dried fruits and vegetables, grains, and beans. Many major supermarkets have become very aware of the American public's concern for healthful foods and have responded by offering a greater selection of bulk foods, in either help-yourself bins or prepackaged form. Buying foods in bulk can be much less expensive than purchasing small quantities, so if you haven't tried bulk shopping you may want to start. Refer to the list of mail-order sources in appendix M for places in your area.

Bulk grains may look like commercial bird food, but they remain one of the best nutritional investments around. From amaranth to wehani rice, grains are a hearty dietary staple. As we saw in chapter 12, there are many grains available, most of which can be purchased in bulk either at the market or by mail.

Bulk grains should be stored in airtight glass jars to prevent spoilage or insect infestation. The more colorful grains are really quite lovely to look at as well, so leave jarred grains (and beans) in view to serve as inspiration. If you know you will not be using the grain for a while, keep it in a cool, dry place or the refrigerator.

Dried beans are another visually and nutritionally pleasing bulk food option. Beans will keep many months; just remember that the older they are, the longer they often take to cook. See chapters 12 and 17 for information on specific beans and how to cook them.

Flours can be as varied as the grains and beans from which they are derived—which is quite a boon for those who are sensitive to wheat or cannot tolerate gluten. We have included several recipes that make use of nonwheat flours, and we recommend that you experiment with a variety of flours as you get into recovery cooking.

The beneficial oils in whole grains make flours more susceptible to spoilage, so store whole-grain flours in airtight containers and keep them refrigerated.

Seeds and nuts may well be the most widely available bulk foods, and they are terrific to have around as quick, high-nutrition snacks. Choose raw, unroasted products. Roasted nuts are frequently salted and rancid. Nuts are best if purchased in the shell, as shelled nuts are often dipped in a caustic solution to remove the skins. And please avoid the red-dyed pistachios even if they're in their shell. Store nuts and seeds in the refrigerator in airtight containers.

Now that we have reviewed some of the best sources of complex carbohydrates, vitamins, and minerals that the store has to offer, let's move on to the primary protein sources: fish, poultry, eggs, meats, and dairy products.

14 *Fish, Poultry, Eggs, Meats, and Dairy*

Fish, poultry, eggs, meat, and dairy products are excellent sources of protein, iron, and many other nutrients. They can also be sources of various chemicals, drugs, and disease-causing bacteria that upset our chemical balance and compromise our immune systems. The trick to making these foods part of your balanced recovery program is to learn what to look for when buying these products, and to take the time to choose your purchases carefully.

Choosing Fresh Seafood

Fish and other seafoods are a terrific source of the high-quality protein and essential fatty acids that are important to a healthy recovery. But seafoods (from the fastest tuna to the most stationary mussel) that develop in polluted waters inevitably absorb the toxins from their environment, and fresh fish that are improperly stored or handled during transport can become infected with disease-causing bacteria. These toxins and contaminants are a serious health threat to humans, recovering or otherwise.

Certain waterways and ocean areas are notoriously polluted, and fish taken from these waters are likely to be heavily contaminated. Fatty fish, in particular, store chemical contaminants within their fat cells, and large, older fish tend to have greater concentrations of toxins than their small, youthful peers. So bigger is not necessarily better when choosing fresh, whole fish.

Table 14.1 lists the safety levels of several kinds of seafood, regardless of where it has been caught or harvested. Green-light items have the smallest concentration of toxins and pollutants and can be eaten often as part of your recovery program. Yellow-light items tend to have moderate concentrations of pollutants and should be eaten only occasionally. Red-light items are those that have been found to have high concentrations of toxins and pollutants and should be avoided.

The best way to be certain that you are buying the freshest fish available is to develop a relationship with a reputable fishmonger. He or she can tell you when the fish came in to port and where it was caught.

When purchasing an entire fish, choose fish with clear, bulging eyes. Check behind the gills; they should be bright red, not brown. The skin should be shiny and should not have a strong odor. Many fresh fish smell like cucumbers.

Also check for a fresh smell when buying fish steaks or fillets. The flesh should feel firm and moist and spring back when compressed. Avoid fish that is hard, dark-colored, or crusty around the edges.

If your supermarket packages fish in plastic, always ask what day the fish was delivered, and when they get seafood deliveries in general. (Most markets don't get fresh deliveries on weekends, so don't buy fish on Sunday night.)

Fish should be kept refrigerated in airtight containers and should be cooked within two days of purchase. When freezing fresh fish, clean it first, then wrap it tightly and mark the date it was put into the freezer. Most fish will store well when frozen for six months but will be less moist and firm when cooked.

Shrimp should always be purchased in the shell. Whenever possible, cook shrimp in the shell as well—it will preserve the shrimp's moisture and flavor. Small shrimp average fifty-five shrimp to the pound. Medium shrimp have about thirty shrimp per pound, large anywhere from eight to twelve. Store shrimp in the coldest part of the refrigerator. Ideally, shrimp should always be cooked on the same day it is purchased.

Scallops are available in two varieties: the large sea scallop and the tender tiny bay or cape scallop. Either can be used in most recipes that call for scallops. The larger scallops often need to be cut into smaller bite-size pieces.

Clams, mussels, and oysters (mollusks) should be chosen with care. Fresh shellfish of this type should be bought while still living. Look for those with closed shells or with slightly open shells that close when touched. The shells will open when cooked (any that don't should be discarded). Steer away from eating raw shellfish, which are a high risk for bacterial contamination.

Fresh clams, mussels, or oysters will keep for twenty-four hours when covered with a damp cloth and refrigerated. Wash the shells well prior to cooking.

To shuck mollusks, run a small, strong knife along the top and bottom half of the shell to cut the muscle that holds the shell closed. Remove the flesh and cook immediately.

Lobsters should be purchased live, with their claws fastened closed. Prior to cooking, place live lobsters in the freezer for two hours

14.1 BUYING SAFE SEAFOOD

GREEN LIGHT

Abalone	Grouper	Orange	Spiny lobster
Arctic char	Haddock	roughy	Squid
Crawfish	Halibut	Pacific salmon	Talapia
Dover sole	Imitation crab	Red snapper	Tuna
English sole	(surimi)	Scallops	Wahoo
Dungeness	Mahimahi	Sea bass	Whiting
crab	Marlin	Sea urchin roe	Yellowtail
Fish sticks	Monkfish	Shrimp	
Flounder	Octopus	Sole	

YELLOW LIGHT

Belt fish	Norwegian	Pacific	Sea trout
Bonito	salmon	mackerel	Smelt
Bream	Ocean perch	Porgy	Spot
Butterfish	Pacific	Rock cod	Thresher
Drum	barracuda	Rockfish	shark

RED LIGHT

Bass	Croaker	Sablefish	Weakfish
(freshwater)	Dace	Sea herring	White bass
Black cod	Eel	Shark	White croaker
Bluefish	Great Lakes	Sheepshead	Whitefish
Buffalo fish	salmon	Striped bass	(freshwater)
Carp	Lake trout	Sturgeon	White perch
Catfish	Lobster	Swordfish	Yellow eel
Caviar	Mackerel	Trout	Yellow perch
Chub	Mullet	Walleye	
Cod	Northern pike		

Source: David Steinman, *Diet for a Poisoned Planet* (New York: Harmony Books, 1990), 120. Used with permission.

(this will cause them to gradually lose consciousness and die). After two or more hours, remove them from the freezer and place them head-first into a gallon of boiling water per lobster.

Choosing Poultry

When selecting poultry, particularly chicken and turkey, the premier choices are organically raised free-range birds. These birds taste sweet and tender, with no chemical flavor. They have not been fed hormones or growth enhancers, dyes, antibiotics, or other chemical additives. They're raised in barnyards rather than tiny cages. Many markets now carry these products, so if yours doesn't, ask. There are many small local farms throughout the country that produce drug-free poultry, so inquire at your supermarket, butcher, or farmer's market for a source.

When free-range or organically grown poultry is not available, look for labels that say "all natural, no additives, no preservatives, and antibiotic free." This will also help you avoid other additives such as coconut oil, partially hydrogenated vegetable oil, and sodium-based phosphates, which are supposed to add juiciness. Table 14.2 lists some of the major companies that are producing relatively drug- and chemical-free poultry.

14.2 PURER POULTRY

Chicken	Turkey
Foster Farms	Foster Farms
Holly Farms	Norbest
D'Artagnan	Louis Rich
	Swift-Eckrich

When selecting poultry, always check the expiration date on the package or ask about the delivery date. Many markets leave birds on the shelves several days past their expiration for consumption date, increasing the risk of contamination with salmonella bacteria.

Fresh poultry should be stored in the refrigerator (at 40° F. or below) for a day or two at most before it is cooked. When freezing fresh poultry, remove it from the original package, rewrap it well, and mark the date on the package before freezing. Frozen poultry can be stored for up to six months. Always defrost frozen poultry (and other meats) *in the refrigerator.* Thawing food at room temperature encourages the growth of harmful bacteria.

Always clean your hands and work surfaces well before and after working with raw poultry. The U.S. Department of Agriculture recommends washing the hands with hot soapy water for at least twenty seconds. To prevent cross-contamination, never let the juices of raw poultry come in contact with other foods. Wash hands, utensils, and work surfaces with hot soapy water after working with poultry as well.

If you are fond of chicken liver, remember to use only the livers of organically raised birds, since the liver is the organ that processes (and therefore may contain) toxins.

Choosing Eggs

Although eggs are generally found in or near the dairy section (since they are stored at similar temperatures), they are most certainly not dairy products. Indeed, the egg has been called one of nature's perfect foods—high in complete protein and all the vitamins and minerals except vitamin C.

Concern over the dangers of cholesterol has led many health practitioners to advise against eating eggs. But eggs are rich not only in cholesterol but in lecithin—which acts to break down fats and which may balance out eggs' cholesterol equation. In fact, the relationship between eggs in the diet and high cholesterol in the blood has not been well established, and there is some evidence that eggs have no effect on blood cholesterol whatsoever.

This doesn't mean that you should start eating three eggs with every meal. But eggs have exceptional nutritional value and should be included in your balanced recovery diet. Eggs can be used as the protein centerpiece for meals in place of fish, meat, poultry, or grain and bean combinations.

When purchasing eggs, check the expiration date and purchase the best quality available. Look for eggs from free-range (and/or organically raised) hens. They're freer from drugs and are superior in taste. The difference in taste is astounding. After eating a few free-range eggs you'll find it hard to be satisfied with commercially produced eggs.

For all their benefits, eggs are also a potential source of salmonella poisoning and should be treated with care. Eggs should be refrigerated immediately and used within one week of purchase. They should *not* be eaten raw (even if mixed in a beverage), and cracked eggs should always be discarded. Egg substitutes, dried eggs, and liquid egg mixtures are poor nutritional alternates and should be avoided.

Choosing Fresh Meats

As we noted in chapter 11, much of conventionally raised meat is contaminated with antibiotics, hormones, pesticides, and a variety of other chemicals. Fortunately, there are an increasing number of non-toxic options for meat lovers in recovery.

Several companies are responding to consumer demands for cleaner meat. They have signed agreements with the Department of Agriculture to raise their cattle with a strict eye on eliminating drugs and pesticide residues from their feed and water as well as to avoid antibiotics and hormones. Table 14.3 lists some of these companies. Several major supermarket chains are now carrying these products, so if your local market doesn't have organic meat, make sure to ask for it.

Purchase leaner cuts of meat and remove as much fat as possible. This means avoiding fatty, "marbled" cuts of meat, which are very high in saturated fats. Always check the label for consumption and/or expiration dates. In general, try to limit your intake of red meat in favor of other low-fat forms of whole protein (such as poultry or fish).

14.3 ORGANIC MEATS

Bradley 3R (Texas)
Coleman Natural Beef (Colorado)
Harris Ranch (California)
Hitch Enterprises (Oklahoma)
Kohler Farms (Wisconsin)
Larsen Beef
Laura's Lean Beef
Lean & Free (Iowa)
Maverick Ranch Lite Beef
Nebraska Beef (Nebraska)
Organic Cattle Co. (New York)
Quality Steaks

Choosing Dairy Products

Dairy products are milk-based products that include milk, buttermilk, hard and soft cheeses, yogurt, butter, margarine, kefir, goat milk, and goat and sheep cheeses. Some dairy products—most notably cream, sour cream, evaporated milk, and crème fraîche—are low in nutritional value and extremely high in fat, while others, such as ice cream and sweetened condensed milk, are high in both sugar and fat. Products such as evaporated milk or evaporated skim milk are highly processed.

In general, dairy products are excellent sources of protein, but they can pose significant problems for those with:

*Lactose intolerance—an inherited inability to digest lactose (or milk sugar). This condition affects up to 15 percent of the general population but is even more common (as high as 80 percent to 90 percent) among blacks and Asians.

*Adverse reactions to milk protein—a condition that is particularly prevalent among people in recovery (see chapter 8).

*Atherosclerotic disease, high cholesterol, or disordered lipid metabolisms—since many dairy products are high in saturated fat.

Those who are lactose intolerant can now take enzyme formulations that will help them digest proteins, while individuals who are limiting fat can choose some of the dairy products (such as skim milk) that are low in saturated fat. If you have adverse reactions to milk products, however, it is important to limit and rotate dairy foods in your diet. In these cases, it is important to eat other foods that provide dietary calcium and protein.

Many milk-allergic individuals become almost panicked about calcium deficiency when they hear they have to limit their milk intake. But calcium is found in many foods other than milk. After all, cows make milk out of grass! So cutting back on dairy products does not mean automatic osteoporosis. It just means being aware of the many other food products—particularly green leafy vegetables—that are also rich in calcium.

Bones are an excellent source of calcium when boiled for stock, soups, or stews. Some fish are good sources of calcium, particularly those that are eaten whole, such as sardines, herring, and kippers. Table 14.4 lists particularly good alternative sources of calcium for people in recovery.

When you do choose dairy products, there are two crucial facts to keep in mind. First, dairy products that come from commercially bred dairy cows can contain residues of the hormones, pesticides, antibiotics, and other chemicals used in raising these animals. Second, the removal of fat from milk products (to make skim or low-fat milks) is a double-edged sword. While it lowers the concentration of saturated fat and cholesterol, it also reduces the milk's nutrient value. Fat is crucial to the absorption of calcium, and removing fat from milk also removes

14.4 NON-DAIRY SOURCES OF CALCIUM

Almonds	Filberts
Avocados	Fish
Barley	Greens
Beet greens	Kelp
Beans (of all kinds)	Kohlrabi
Bran	Lentils
Brazil nuts	Millet
Broccoli	Oats
Brussels sprouts	Onions
Buckwheat	Parsnips
Cabbage	Prunes
Carrots	Rice (brown)
Cauliflower	Rye
Coconut	Sesame seeds
Dandelion greens	Soy milk
Dulse	Walnuts
Egg yolk	Watercress
Figs	Wheat (whole)

the fat-soluble vitamins A, D, E, and K. When whole milk is processed into skim or low-fat forms, vitamins A and D are usually the only ones restored.

Therefore, although we recognize that some health authorities are advising the public to use dairy products sparingly, we want to add a caveat. Limit consumption, and when you do use dairy products, go for those that are as whole and organically produced as possible rather than skim or low-fat versions. In this way, you can get the most nutritional benefit from dairy products, while avoiding some of their pitfalls.

Dairy products of all kinds should be among the last items you pick up when shopping, so that they stay refrigerated as long as possible. Milk is sold in glass, plastic, and cardboard containers. Some nutritional experts have found that light can degrade vitamins A and B_1, and they recommend that milk be purchased in opaque cardboard containers. Others have found that cardboard milk cartons contain a toxin that may be passed to milk in the cartons. Given the contradictory evidence, we recommend purchasing milk in quart-size glass containers and using the milk within a week of its purchase. Never buy milk past its labeled last date of sale.

Milk should be kept at 40°F. or cooler at all times to prevent bacterial growth. The exception is when making a fermented milk product such as buttermilk, yogurt, or kefir—when the growth of bacteria is encouraged to alter and enhance flavor and nutritional value.

<u>Whole milk</u> is 86 percent water. The remainder is protein; some B vitamins; the fat-soluble vitamins A, D, E, and K; 3 to 4 percent fat (65 percent of which is saturated); and lactose (milk sugar).

Milk goes through several processes, which typically are noted on its label. Pasteurization is a process of heating milk or cream to destroy contaminants. Ultra-pasteurization is a variation of the same process using higher temperatures. Although pasteurization has made our milk supply immeasurably safer, both processes also destroy or inactivate enzymes and some vitamins. As a result, most pasteurized milk products need to be enriched or fortified with synthetic vitamins A and D.

Whole milk is also usually homogenized—a process that prevents the heavy fat globules of cream from separating from the rest of the milk. To achieve this, whole milk is sprayed at high pressure against a hard surface, breaking up the fat molecules and dispersing them throughout the milk. Ironically, this actually makes milk more bland tasting and also more susceptible to spoilage (making pasteurization even more necessary).

<u>Low-fat milks</u> (1% and 2% milks, etc.) are made by combining milk solids with water. While it is true that these products contain a lower percentage of fat *by weight* than whole milk, they are not really low in fat. As you shall see in the next chapter, the central issue of nutritional content is not the *amount* of a specific dietary component, but its contribution to the overall caloric load of the product. For example, 2% milk is made up of 10 percent milk solids and 90 percent water. Take away the water and you are left with a product that is 20 percent fat by weight. In a single 8-ounce glass of 2% milk, which contains 130 calories, fully 45 percent of the calories are derived from fat. When looked at from this perspective, these "low-fat" milk products are still fairly high in fat.

<u>Skim milk,</u> on the other hand, is made by literally skimming cream off the top of nonhomogenized whole milk. Skim milk products have had all or most of their fat removed and thus are the real low-fat alternatives for those who want to avoid saturated fat and cholesterol.

<u>Raw milk</u> is neither pasteurized nor homogenized. By law, raw milk cannot be transported across state lines, but it is available in more than half of all states. Raw milk is subjected to very strict standards

and testing. It has a rich, unadulterated flavor and is highly nutritious. It is labeled "certified raw milk." There are a growing number of raw milk products, cheeses, and yogurts available in health food stores and supermarkets.

Goat's and sheep's milk and milk products are becoming increasingly popular in health food stores and some larger markets. They have distinctly different tastes from cow's milk and can sometimes be tolerated by those who have difficulties with cow's milk.

Cheese is high in calcium, protein, and some vitamins, but it may also be high in fat, cholesterol, and sodium. Cheeses may contain dyes without notice to consumers on the label.

> Natural cheeses generally use unhomogenized milk. Many brands (European in particular) use raw milk and allow a slow, natural aging process to kill harmful bacteria.

> Soft cheeses (such as cottage cheese) are made from skim milk with the addition of pasteurized cream. Soft cheeses should be refrigerated immediately and used within a few days. They are highly perishable even with preservatives.

> Hard cheeses should be wrapped airtight and refrigerated. Storage time will vary according to the type; most will keep for at least a few weeks.

> Processed cheese foods (such as so-called American cheese) have no place in a diet based on whole foods. Processed cheese foods contain bleaches, dyes, preservatives, animal rennet, and other additives.

Yogurt is a fermented milk product that can be made with any kind of milk. Yogurt is often easier to digest than other dairy products. The bacterial cultures that cause yogurt to thicken and give it its distinctive tart flavor are nutritionally valuable. Pasteurization kills these cultures, so look for products that contain "active yogurt cultures."

Many commercial brands of yogurt contain artificial additives in the form of food starches, thickeners, artificial flavors, colors, and sugar—all of which can add up to 150 calories per serving. Look for yogurt flavored with natural fruit, or buy plain yogurt and add your own fresh fruit. Not only is it better for you, it is often less expensive.

Kefir is a fermented or cultured milk drink. This pleasant thick shake has been enjoyed for thousands of years. It is high in B vitamins. Like yogurt, kefir is good for the immune system in that it replaces intestinal flora that is destroyed in many cases through the use of antibiotics.

<u>Ice cream</u> as we know it today can contain up to sixty additives and derives up to 75 percent of its calories from saturated fat. So-called low-calorie brands basically have more air whipped into them and more additives to keep it together.

Since ice cream, by definition, is a product that contains scores of additives, it really isn't a whole food. Although some health food stores carry fresh whole-milk ice cream sweetened with real fruit, there is no guarantee it is additive-free. Good over-the-counter options for those who love sweet cold things are increasingly popular fresh fruit sorbets. Better still, however, is to make your own frozen desserts using fresh fruits, yogurt, ice, and fresh juices. See the dessert recipe section for some ideas.

This brings us to the end of our many wholefoods choices and to the beginning of the prepared foods quagmire. Finding healthy, additive-free prepared foods is one of the great adventures of recovery shopping, and the quest opens up a whole new literary universe: that of the product label. Prepare to be amazed.

15 Healthy Prepared Foods

All prepared foods are not created equal. Many (if not most) contain additives such as salt, sugar, fats, preservatives, colors, and other unpleasant chemicals, and offer few nutritional benefits to balance the equation. Prepared foods—from the simplest can of peas to the most elaborate frozen pie—never come close to the taste and quality of products made fresh from wholefoods. Once you get used to the superior tastes and textures of fresh, wholefoods cooking, it will be hard to go back.

However, we all know that there are times when making a complete meal simply isn't possible and when chewing on granola simply isn't enough. Learning to eat well in recovery is a process, with many pitfalls along the way. In the early days of recovery the prospect of cooking a complete meal may seem very daunting. On these occasions, you may want nothing more than to open a can and pour something, anything, into a pot. But that doesn't mean you have to settle for the type of high-calorie, high-additive, low-nutrient prepared foods that line most grocery shelves. A growing number of companies are making prepared foods that are low in (or free of) chemical additives and preservatives, and that use whole or organically grown ingredients. By keeping the larder stocked with these healthy forms of canned, frozen, and otherwise prepared food products, you can make your life much easier and still provide your body with above-average nutrition when time doesn't allow you to cook.

Avoiding the Worst

Generally speaking, the problem with prepared foods is both what they lack (the nutritional value of wholefoods) and what they contain (an inordinate amount of additives). The process of choosing healthy prepared foods is often a matter of avoiding those with excessive additives.

The easiest way to avoid unhealthy prepared foods is to *read the label*. This sounds easier than it is. Product labeling can be confusing, misleading, and at times downright untrue. To be a truly smart shopper you need to read between the lines and find out what the label is *really* telling you.

156

Food labels contain several key pieces of information: the name of the product, the manufacturer and its address, the quantity of the food (in weight or volume), the number of servings in the package, and—last but not least—its nutritional information.

It is the nutritional information portion of most food labels that is problematic for consumers. Most manufacturers list the number of calories; grams of fat, protein, and carbohydrates; and specific vitamins found in *each serving* of the food product. The typical bag of potato chips, for example, contains two servings (when was the last time you ate only half a bag?). The unwary consumer who reads a potato chip label and sees "150 calories per serving" may blithely finish the whole bag without realizing that he or she has just eaten 300 calories worth of chips.

An even more confusing aspect of food labels is the relationship of grams to calories and their real meaning in the world of nutrition. Many products call themselves low-fat on the basis of the number of grams of fat they contain. In many cases the validity of these claims is dubious.

Let's look at the ingredients listed on the label of a popular cereal. Per 1-ounce serving, this product contains:

*119 calories

*5 grams of protein

*9 grams of carbohydrates

*7 grams of fat

On the surface, this would seem to be a relatively low-fat product. But let's look at it again.

Each gram of protein or carbohydrate contains 4 calories. Each gram of fat contains 9 calories. (See pages 17–18 for a discussion of calories.) When evaluating the nutritional content of a food, we want to know *what percentage* of its total calories come from fat, carbohydrates, and protein. In this case:

*5 grams of protein × 4 calories per gram = 20 calories

*9 grams of carbohydrate × 4 calories per gram = 36 calories

*7 grams of fat × 9 calories = 63 calories

When these caloric breakdowns are compared with the food's total caloric value, we find that fully 53 percent of each serving's calories come from fat. Far from being low-fat, this product is more than half fat! Since we recommend that fat make up less than 15 percent of the diet, it is clear that this particular cereal is not a great nutritional choice.

Another problem with most food labels is that they do not specify the *form* of carbohydrates the food contains. As we have seen, highly refined carbohydrates such as sugar and white flour are definite no-nos for recovering people. Complex carbohydrates such as whole wheat, brown rice, and other whole grains are far preferable. A food that contains 9 grams of carbohydrate in the form of sugar or corn syrup is much different from one that contains 9 grams of carbohydrate in the form of whole ground oats.

For this reason, it is important to cross-reference the nutritional information list with the list of ingredients. Specific ingredients are listed in descending order of volume, from greatest to least. If you calculate from the nutritional label that the food is 45 percent carbohydrates, but sugar, refined bleached white flour, and corn syrup top the ingredients list, it's time to look at another product.

There are several common additives/ingredients that should be strictly avoided by those in recovery (a longer list can be found in appendix N). Keep an eye out for these items when reviewing ingredients lists, and avoid products that contain them:

  * Artificial flavorings

  * Artificial colors (usually indicated by a number, i.e. "Blue number 1")

  * BHA (butylated hydroxyanisole) or BHT (butylated hydroxytoluene)

  * Highly refined sweeteners: corn syrup, dextrose, dextrins, invert sugar, lactose, mannitol, sorbitol, sucrose, turbinado sugar

  * Highly processed fats and oils: brominated vegetable oil, hydrogenated or partially hydrogenated vegetable oil, palm oil, coconut oil

  * Hydrolyzed vegetable protein

  * MSG (monosodium glutamate)

  * Nitrite (or sodium nitrite)

  * Phosphates

  * Phosphoric acid

*Propyl gallate

*Refined, bleached, white, or "enriched" flours

*Sulfites (sulfur dioxide, sodium bisulfite)

*TBHQ (tertiary butylhydroquinone)

Although analyzing labels may seem complex at first, once you get into the habit of reading labels you will find that it is easy to spot the most common nutritional pitfalls. And, of course, never buy a product that requires an advanced degree in chemistry to read the ingredients list!

Choosing the Best

Once you have mastered the art of label reading, you are well on your way to becoming a master shopper. But smart shopping is not just a matter of avoiding the wrong foods, it's also choosing the right ones. Table 15.2 lists some of the most common prepared foods and companies that make healthful, additive-free alternatives to the major commercial brands. Keep in mind, however, that even these companies are not perfect; make sure to read labels of individual products before buying.

If you cannot find products by these companies in your local market, don't despair. Many of the larger food companies are beginning to pay attention to consumer interest in healthy foods, so check labels and purchase the best foods available. You can also investigate health food stores and food co-ops in your area (see page 166), or make use of some of the mail-order sources of wholefoods products (see appendix M). The important thing is to purchase the best-quality foods that are available and to *start eating them.*

When buying baked goods (breads, muffins, cakes), there are several rules of thumb. Always look for breads made with whole-grain flour: wheat, rye, barley, oat, rice, millet, multigrain, and so forth. Refined, bleached, and even enriched flours can't hold a nutritional candle to whole-grain products. Whole-grain baked goods are often labeled as "only stone-ground whole-grain flour, water, and salt," to assure the consumer that no preservatives or additives were used in making the product.

Avoid white breads, which can contain more than 100 food additives that need not be listed on the label—many of which have known adverse health effects. Dark, hearty breads are a much better option, but even these should be chosen carefully. Pumpernickel, for example, is a dark bread that generally contains bleached white flour and uses coffee and/or chocolate to achieve its dark color. Do not rely on appearance alone when making your choices; always check ingredients.

Choosing fresh whole-grain breads and other baked goods is easy if the expiration date or baked date is on the package. If your market has a bakery on the premises and does not mark its baked goods, ask the department manager when these products are baked or delivered, and buy your breads on or close to these days. Don't squeeze these goods to test for freshness, since the squeeze test doesn't work for hearty, whole-grain goods. You should store baked goods in the refrigerator to avoid molds and rancidity—although they will become harder when refrigerated.

Canned vegetables, fruits, soups, and other foods are never as tasty as their fresh homemade counterparts, but they can be a real help when time is pressing (canned beans are particularly useful). If you are going to keep canned goods in your larder, make sure to choose them carefully. Avoid cans that have been soldered with lead (lead-free cans are usually labeled as such), and never store open canned goods in their original can. Transfer unused canned foods to glass or plastic containers instead.

Many canned foods are packed in liquids that can contain chemical additives, preservatives, and colorings, excess salt, and various forms of sugar (most notably corn syrup). Although the brands listed in table 15.2 tend to be relatively free of such additives, always check the label. Look for products that are packed in water or their own juices (or, in the case of fruit, natural fruit juice).

When looking for oils to use in cooking or salad dressing, it's a good bet to avoid most brand-name commercially processed oils. They have been overly processed and stripped of their nutritional value. Processed oils, when rancid, can increase the level of LDL (or bad) cholesterol in the blood.

Get acquainted with some of the many delicious nut and vegetable oils that are now available (see table 15.1). Look for oils that have been cold pressed or expelled. The best olive oils are labeled "extra virgin" or "first pressing." Oils should be kept refrigerated in airtight, preferably opaque containers. Light and oxygen can cause natural oils to go rancid.

15.1 HEALTHY ALTERNATIVE OILS
cold-pressed varieties: keep refrigerated

Almond	Pumpkin
Apricot kernel	Safflower*
Avocado	Sesame
Canola*	Soy
Olive (extra virgin)*	Sunflower
	Walnut

* highly recommended

15.2 PREPARED FOODS: HEALTHY ALTERNATIVES

Food Type	What To Look For	Brand Names
Batters (pancake)	Whole grain	Arrowhead Mills, David's Goodbatter, Granny's Buttermilk Pancake and Waffle Mix, Fearn
Beans (canned)	Packed in water. No added sugar.	Eden, Goya (some), Hain, Health Valley, Old El Paso
Breads/baked goods	Whole grain, stone-ground flour. Low salt. Natural sweeteners.	The Baker, Baldwin Hill Corp. (organic), Bread Alone (organic), Food for Life, Lifestream Natural Foods (organic), Manna Breads/Nature's Path (organic), Matthew's, Nature's Garden, Shiloh Farms, Walnut Acres
Butters, fruit (also sauces)	No added sugar. Sweetened with fruit juice.	Eden, Organic Farms, Santa Cruz Natural, Sonoma Gold, Tree of Life, Walnut Acres

Food Type	What To Look For	Brand Names
Butters, nut	No added sugar. No added salt. (Oil on top of product can be skimmed off or stirred back in.)	Arrowhead Mills, Hain, Walnut Acres
Cereals (breakfast)	Whole grain. No added sugar. No additives.	Alpenzell, American Prairie, Arrowhead Mills, Back to Nature, Barbara's, Con Agra (cream of rye), Country Life Natural Foods, Eden, Erewhon, Familia, Golden Harvest, Grainfields, Health Valley, Kashi Company, Kellogg's (some), Kolln, Little Bear Trading Co., Lundberg Family Farms, Manna/ Nature's Path, Mother's, Muesli, Nectar Sweet Granola, New Morning, Oro Wheat, Pacific Rice, Pocono, Quaker (not instant), Safeway, Shurfine, Stone Buhr, Stow Mills, Tree of Life, Walnut Acres, Wheatena
Condiments (dressings, sauces, etc.)	No added sugar. Low salt. Additive-free. No hydrogenated oil. No tropical oils.	Chalif, Cardini Natural, Cuisine Perel, Marie's, Nasoya, Paul Newman's, Premier Japan, San-J, Walnut Acres
Crackers	Whole grain. No salt. No sugar.	AK Mak, Edward & Sons, GG, Hain, Ryvita, San-J, Washa
Desserts (frozen)		Cascadian Farms, Gone Bananas, Nouvelle, Rice Dream

Food Type	What To Look For	Brand Names
Fish (frozen)		Medallions, Natural Sea
Frozen foods (general)		Anyo, Amara's, Boil-a-Bag, Cascadian Farms, Coleman Meats, Eden, Empress, Fumaro, Health Is Wealth, Health Valley, Jaclyn's, Legume Densi, Mitohu, Natural Touch, Premier Japan, Shelton, Shiloh, Simply Natural, Sohen, Taj, Wholesome 6 Hearty Foods, Worthington
Frozen foods (meals)		Healthy Choice Dinners, Stouffer's Right Course
Fruit (canned)	No added sugar. No added salt. Packed in water or own juice.	Alpha Beta Natural, Coop, Country Pure, Del Monte Lite, Diamond, Diet Delight, Dole (pineapple), Eden, Featherweight, Finest, Food Club Natural Style, Gathering Winds All Natural, Golden Harvest, Kroger Lite, Libby (pineapple), Lucky Leaf No Sugar Added, Motts Natural, Mrs. Gooch's Natural, New England Organic, Nutradiet, Pathmark Unsweetened, Ralph's Unsweetened, S & W Unsweetened, Shiloh Farms, Thrifty Maid Natural, Very Fine Unsweetened, Waldbaum's Natural Unsweetened

Food Type	What To Look For	Brand Names
Fruit (frozen)	Unsweetened. Additive-free.	Big Valley, Cascadian Farms, C & W, Flavorland, Kroger, Snow Kist, Stillwell
Grains and beans (dried and flours)	Organically grown	Arrowhead Mills, Country Grown, Eden, Erewhon, Fantastic, Grainaissance Inc., Health Valley, Little Bear Trading Co., Lundberg Family Farms, Natural Way Mills, Quinoa, Shiloh Farms, Westbrae
Grain dishes (dry mixes)	Whole grain. No additives. No colorings.	Ancient Harvest, Casbah, Country Grown, Grainaissance Inc., Little Bear Trading Co., Natural Way Mills, Quinoa, The Original Near East
Jams and jellies	No added sugar.	Berry Best Farms, Fruitfully, Cascadian Farms, R. W. Knudsen, Polaner, Sorrell Ridge, Walnut Acres
Juices (fruit and vegetable)	100 percent juice No added sugar. Low salt.	After the Fall, Knudsen & Sons, Lakewood, Santa Cruz Natural
Margarines	Soy brands	Willow Run
Meats (canned)		La Loma, Worthington
Oils (vegetable)	Cold pressed. Extra virgin. First press. Preferably in opaque glass containers. Keep refrigerated.	Arrowhead Mills Co. (organic), Greek Gourmet, Hain, Loriva, Supreme Foods, Omega Nutrition, Spectrum Naturals, Spruce Foods, Tree of Life

Food Type	What To Look For	Brand Names
Salads (deli)		Abrahams, Brightsong, Nasoya, Simply Natural Foods, Spring Creek, Soy Shop, 21st Century Foods, Watkins
Sauces (spaghetti)	Sugar-free. Corn syrup-free.	Ci' Bella, Eden (organic), Enrico, Pritikin, Tree of Life
Snacks/ Cookies	Low or sea salt. Fruit sugar.	Barbara's, Bearitos (organic), Garden of Eatin', Health Valley, Little Bear Trading Co., Maine Sea Vegetables, Nanak's Gourmet Cookies, Nature's Warehouse, Pacific Gardens, R. W. Frookie, Tree of Life, Walnut Acres, Westbrae
Soups (canned)	Additive-free. Low fat. Low salt. Sugar-free.	Eden, Erewhon, Fearn, Hain, Health Valley, Nile Spice, Premier Japan, Lundberg Family Farms, Pritikin, Sohen, Walnut Acres, Westbrae
Sweeteners (natural)		barley malt, honey, pure maple syrup, molasses (unsulfured), rice yinnie
Vegetables (canned)	Sugar-free. Low salt, or no salt added.	Bertolli (tomato), Big Star, Contadina No Salt Added, Coop Unsalted, Country Pure, Del Monte, Diet Delight, Eden (organic tomato), Edward's Finest, Featherweight, Finest, Giant Foods, Grand Union, Green Giant, Food Club No Salt Added,

Food Type	What To Look For	Brand Names
Vegetables (dried)	Sulfite-free. Avoid potatoes.	Hunt's, Kroger, Libby's Natural Pack, Libby's Solid Pack, Nutradiet, Natural, Pathmark, Parade, Pritikin, Ralph's, Staff, Stokeley's 100% Natural, Von's Eden, Marine Coast Sea Vegetables, McCormick's Freeze Dried, Premier Japan Seaweeds, Tree of Life, Wel Pac

For a comprehensive overview of the contaminants in our food supply and how to avoid them, read David Steinman's excellent book, *Diet for a Poisoned Planet* (New York: Harmony Books, 1990). Beautifully written, researched, and referenced, this is an essential reference for everyone who cares about the quality of the food supply.

Health Food Stores and Food Cooperatives

If your local supermarket doesn't have a decent selection of healthy prepared foods, don't give up. First try to interest the manager in stocking some of the larger "health food" brands (Erewhon, Hain, Eden, Health Valley, etc.). Then scope out your neighborhood for some of the best shopping alternatives to supermarkets: health food stores (also known as organic markets or wholefoods stores) and food cooperatives.

Health food stores are usually smaller, better staffed, and somewhat less structured than big supermarkets. In fact, one of the reasons these markets seem to thrive is because of their ever-present and knowledgeable staffs. Take the time to get to know your health food market and feel free to ask questions of the staff. Most markets also have a book section, and many hold cooking classes to help educate the community about more healthful ways to prepare food.

Health food markets have greater independence in food choices, since major food companies do not rent space in these small markets as they do in larger chains. Some of the larger health food markets

(Bread and Circus in New England, Earth's Harvest and Perelandra in New York, and Quinn's in Los Angeles) offer an amazing variety of wholefoods and fresh organic fruits, vegetables, meats, and cheeses. If you can't find a particular product, a health food market is more likely to special order that item for you. One warning, however: Not everything in a health food store is a wholefood, so remember to still read the labels before buying.

Establishing a food cooperative (or co-op) is one way in which health-conscious consumers can ensure that they are getting healthy, wholefoods products. In the United States today more than 2,000 food cooperatives are already established, so check around for co-ops in your area. Another money-saving idea is to look for a local farmer's market and ask who sells organic produce. Prices are usually much cheaper when you purchase direct from the farmer.

Food co-ops take advantage of the old axiom that everything is cheaper in bulk. Food producers, warehouses, and distributors have minimum orders that are usually too large for any family but are perfect for an enterprising band of consumers. Co-ops are usually not-for-profit markets where organic wholefoods are sold at close to cost—a 40 to 50 percent savings off retail prices. Those who wish to purchase foods through a co-op must become members, usually by paying a small fee and volunteering a few hours a month to help run the market. Volunteering offers a great opportunity to learn more about wholefoods and find support for healthful eating. Some co-ops offer nonworking memberships as well. These members receive a smaller discount on purchases.

Any group can form a food co-op—a group of parents, artists, people in recovery, or just neighbors. Co-ops offer a full variety of wholefoods, from sugar-free condiments to nuts, grains, beans, meats, dairy products, cereals, breads, and healthy snacks. Many now offer environmentally safe home and beauty products. Many co-ops also offer fresh organic fruits and vegetables by contacting local organic farmers, who are usually very happy to find a sure market for their produce.

Food co-ops are a wonderful way to work with others and save big on the best-quality foods, and also to learn more about nutrition and the use of wholefoods. For more information about starting a co-op, write:

Blooming Prairie
2340 Heinz Road
Iowa City, IA 62240
(319) 337-6448

Or read the following books:

The Blooming Prairie Buying Club Manual
The Blooming Prairie Manual on Bookkeeping for Buying Clubs
The Catalogue of Healthy Foods. John Lepper Marlin, Ph.D., and
   Dominick Bertelli (Bantam Books, 1990).

Dining Out

For people in recovery, dining out can prompt both pleasure and anxiety. Those in recovery from eating disorders must deal with their new relationship with food, while those in recovery from alcoholism must learn how to dine without drinking alcohol. And every recovering person must apply his or her new awareness of nutrition to the food choices made in restaurants.

Whether you're looking for new places to "do lunch" or visiting the old favorites, here are some tips to make eating out a more recovery-supportive event.

1. Don't go out to eat when you're starving. Brain functions get cloudy, leading to poor food choices. If you're headed to a restaurant after another activity, to help you avoid overeating try to munch on a high-protein or complex carbohydrate snack—such as a whole-grain muffin—before you sit down for a meal. It's always a good idea to stabilize your blood sugar. Healthy snacks keep us out of the HALT (Hungry, Angry, Lonely, and Tired) stage.

2. Think ahead. Whether you're invited out or you make the plans, call ahead and ask about the menu. Make sure there are foods you can eat. Avoid dishes with rich sauces, which often contain alcohol. Alcohol is equally hazardous for those in drug and eating disorder recovery. It clouds perception, weakens willpower, and can create cross-addictions.

    While it's true that much of the alcohol is cooked out of most foods that contain it, some does remain. Liquors in dessert frostings or uncooked fruit desserts do not vanish. In either situation, the taste of the alcohol lingers and may be restimulating for recovering individuals.

    Restaurants use a lot of other unnecessary and occasionally unhealthy tricks to raise the flavor of foods. For example, sugar is added to fresh vegetables such as carrots, butter to grilled chicken, MSG to stir-fries. Salad bars are fine if the contents are not sprayed with preservatives, but not all salad bars are properly labeled. So call ahead and ask about specific practices. The same rule holds true when flying. Gourmet foods on planes are high in spirits these days. Request an alcohol-free or vegetarian meal. Vegetarian meals typically will not contain alcohol.

3. Arrive early. Check out the environment and get as comfortable as possible. Notice the music; check out the temperature near your table. Relax and get ready to enjoy the evening. Those with eating disorders know how debilitating fear can be when it comes to eating.

4. Set your limits. For example, if you are accustomed to rich desserts and you're trying to eliminate them, look for fresh fruit on the menu or plan to have your dessert of fresh fruit later at home. This is especially important if you're in alcohol or drug recovery and it's an anxiety-producing business lunch or dinner, or if you're in eating disorder recovery and it's a family gathering.

5. Maximize the nutrient value of your food. Request undercooked vegetables. Select steamed or roasted foods rather than high-fat, high-calorie fried food. When in doubt about salad dressings (some have sherry, wine, or liquors), request oil and vinegar. Since many pasta dishes also include liquor, choose simple tomato sauces or pasta tossed in olive oil with herbs and vegetables.

In a word, never be afraid to ask about the ingredients in a dish. If your family or friends roll their eyes, recognize that that's their problem—you're appropriately dealing with yours.

Part Three

16 Recovery Cooking: Getting Started

Most of us spend thousands of dollars (and hours) each year on maintaining our appearance and keeping ourselves entertained, but few of us devote any real time to choosing and preparing the foods that nourish every aspect of our lives. Yet cooking—for yourself or for others—is one of the most self-affirming things you can do in recovery. Few activities provide more simple pleasure or lasting benefit.

Unfortunately, few modern-day Americans feel sufficiently at home in their kitchens to fully appreciate the pleasures of cooking for themselves. Whether it is the impact of addiction, the pressures of day-to-day life, a lack of knowledge, or simple inertia that is the cause, the end effect is the same: millions of people who do not know how to cook more than a few basic foods, and who rely on Mrs. Smith, Mrs. Paul, Sara Lee, or the Swansons to do their cooking for them.

The most common excuse for not cooking must be "I haven't got the time." This may be true if you want to cook a six-course dinner, but the fact is there are many simple, quick, tasty, and nutritious meals that you can make from scratch without spending hours in the kitchen. If you are in recovery, you can't afford *not* to take the time to nourish yourself properly. And who knows, once you get started you may find that preparing meals is relaxing and creative, not an odious chore. Most people learn to enjoy cooking once they learn to shop, store, and cook a large enough variety of wholefoods. The important thing is to start.

Getting Organized

Many people feel uncomfortable in their kitchens because their kitchens *are* uncomfortable. It's difficult to enjoy cooking if you are constantly searching for the right tool or ingredient, or running to and fro around your kitchen to get them. If you are going to make a commitment to cooking, you need to make your kitchen user-friendly.

First, take stock of your kitchen. What does it need to make it more comfortable, inviting, and workable? Don't worry about major remodeling, just look at what you have and how it can be adjusted to make cooking easier. For example, is the lighting adequate? Can you easily see what you are doing at all locations throughout the kitchen, or do you need an extra bulb or lamp somewhere? What about your cooking utensils and pots? Are they in easy reach for when you are working at the stove? Do you have a good cutting board for slicing vegetables, meats, and other ingredients? Are your pot holders close to the stove? Do you have enough accessible storage space?

When assessing your kitchen, consider how you like to work. Do you prefer cutting vegetables while sitting at the table or while standing at the counter or near the sink? Your preference will determine where you want to keep your knives and cutting board. Similarly, you will probably want to keep large spoons and other cooking utensils fairly close to the stove so that you can reach for them easily while working at the stove. Spices should also be relatively close at hand, but not too near the stove, since heat will destroy their freshness. Always remember that this is your work space—it should meet your individual work needs.

Once you've figured out what you need, it's time to do some reorganizing and modifying. Don't worry about creating a *House Beautiful* kitchen. The point is to make it functional. Your kitchen's beauty will come from the foods that emerge from it. For example, if you are short on counter space, an over-the-sink cutting board can give you needed space at a relatively low cost. Do you need more storage space? Open metal shelves are a snap to install; stacked plastic cartons work, too. Try not to store heavy pots and pans on top of each other, because they'll be hard to reach when you most need them. Try hanging pots and pans overhead, or on large hooks or grids near the stove.

Storing Your Ingredients

When storing foods—particularly bulk grains, beans, pastas, and frozen and other prepared goods—keep fresher items behind older ones, and use the oldest products first. When freezing foods, remember to label packages with the name of the item and the date it was frozen. There are few things more disconcerting than finding a package of "mystery meat" in the bottom of your freezer bin.

Oils, whole grains, and whole flours will go rancid unless refrigerated. Store grains like millet, oats, quinoa, spelt, kasha, and amaranth in separate jars in the refrigerator. Rice, wild rice, wehani rice, dried beans, and pastas can be stored in jars at room temperature. Natural sweeteners (rice yinnie, barley malt, fruit juices) also need to be refrigerated after opening. Honey does not.

Choosing Your Tools

Don't put off cooking because you don't have the latest and most perfect cooking tools. Get started with the equipment you have, even if it is a bit old and battered, and upgrade as you go along. You'll have a much better idea of what you really need after you've become a little more experienced at cooking. Table 16.1 lists the basic tools needed in a "start-up" kitchen, as well as a few more advanced items.

If you do need to buy new cookware, we suggest that you use either cast-iron or stainless steel cookware with copper bottoms (copper conducts heat well). Glass or enamel-clad metal (in that order) are good alternative choices. Nonstick pans are not good choices; some are made of coated aluminum, and the aluminum will be exposed if the nonstick surface is scratched. There is still some debate about the use of aluminum cookware. Although aluminum is an excellent heat conductor, many authorities believe that the toxic metal can leach into food during cooking. Aluminum is also known to react with acidic foods and alter the color and flavor of certain dishes. We therefore suggest that you avoid using aluminum unless it's sandwiched between layers of stainless steel.

One of the best first investments you can make is a good knife. A good knife is one that feels comfortable in your hand. It should be balanced, which means it should rest horizontally in your open hand (your index finger under the end of blade at the handle). Prior to the introduction of stainless steel, all knives were made of carbon steel. Carbon steel lasts longer and stays sharper than stainless and is the preferred choice for food preparation.

A standard kitchen knife set usually consists of a saw-edged knife, a chopping knife, one all-purpose knife, a carving knife, a thin knife for filleting fish, and a parer for peeling vegetables. A good chef's knife—heavy with a wide blade—can be used for many kitchen tasks such as chopping, slicing, shredding, and carving, thereby eliminating the need for a large set of knives. A good French chef's knife works well for many, but some prefer a large Chinese cleaver or a square-bladed Japanese knife. Always clean your knife immediately after use and try to keep it well sharpened.

16.1 OUTFITTING YOUR KITCHEN

Pots and pans

saucepan
2-handled saucepan
(1 to 3 quarts)
5- to 7-inch skillet
9- to 12-inch skillet
large sauce pot (4 quarts)
sauté pan (10 to 14 inches)
steamer basket
stainless steel colander
smaller sieve
broiling pan with a rack
muffin pan
baking sheet (12 by 18)
pie pan
round baking dish
(preferably glass)
loaf pan

Utensils

chef's knife
paring knife
potato peeler
can opener
measuring spoons
large slotted spoon
large solid spoon
(wood or stainless
steel)
long-handled fork
cutting board
grater
rolling pin
kitchen scissors
tongs
oven thermometer
vegetable brush

Miscellaneous

measuring cups (liquid
and dry)
mixing bowls
airtight containers
pot holder and/or towels

Small appliances

blender
food processor
toaster oven
pressure cooker

Cooking Techniques

Most of the recipes in this book describe the processes needed to prepare them, but there are several common cooking techniques and basic cooking rules that all cooks should know. Understanding these concepts will broaden your ability to use other cookbooks and try different recipes for whole foods.

Cooking in Liquids

Blanching: the brief immersion of a food in boiling water followed by immersion in a bath of cold water or ice. It is used to soften food, enrich the color, remove skins (tomatoes), or

16.2 BASIC MEASUREMENTS

Liquid measurements

Pinch = $\frac{1}{16}$ teaspoon
Dash = $\frac{1}{8}$ teaspoon
1 teaspoon (tsp.) = $\frac{1}{3}$ tablespoon (tbsp.)
3 teaspoons = 1 tablespoon
1 fluid ounce (fl. oz.) = 2 tablespoons
$\frac{1}{4}$ cup = 4 tablespoons or 2 ounces
$\frac{1}{3}$ cup = $5\frac{1}{3}$ tablespoons
$\frac{1}{2}$ cup = 8 tablespoons or 4 ounces
1 cup (c.) = 16 tablespoons, 8 ounces, $\frac{1}{2}$ pint
1 pint (pt.) = 2 cups or 16 ounces
1 quart (qt.) = 4 cups, 32 ounces, 2 pints
1 liter (ltr.) = 35 ounces
1 gallon (gal.) = 4 quarts

Dry measurements

1 quart = 2 pints
8 quarts = 1 peck
4 pecks = 1 bushel

remove the bitter flavor of acidic foods such as citrus fruit zest. Blanch harder vegetables before adding them to stir-fries or pasta dishes. (Also known as *parboiling* or *scalding*.)

Boiling: bringing a liquid to 100° Celsius or 212° Fahrenheit. There are varying degrees of boiling, such as a low boil, which is a gentle boil, and rapid or rolling boil, which is a vigorous boil. Since boiled food loses many of its nutrients to the liquid it's boiled in, boiling is one of the least nutritious ways to prepare a food unless the liquid is also consumed.

Steaming: cooking food above a few inches of boiling water in a steamer basket or colander. The food does not touch the boiling water or liquid but is cooked by the steam. This extremely healthful cooking method preserves water-soluble vitamins.

Simmering: cooking food in liquid below the boiling point. This technique is often used for soups and long-cooking sauces.

Stewing: slowly cooking food in a small amount of liquid in a covered pan or container over low heat. This process makes food more tender and also blends flavors.

Poaching: cooking in simmering (see above) water, stock, or other liquid. The food is usually completely covered with the liquid. This process is used for fish, chicken, fruit, or vegetables. For chicken or fish the liquid will often contain aromatic vegetables or herbs. It is a way of cooking without oils or fats.

Pressure cooking: a quick method of cooking food at extremely high temperatures. It is done in a covered special pot called a *pressure cooker*. An attachment at the top of the pot jiggles as it cooks and releases steam to prevent the pot from exploding. Never open the lid while the attachment is still jiggling. Instead, run the pot under water until cool and then open the cooker. It is used for beans, grains, vegetables, and stews.

Braising: a method using both oil and liquid. The food is usually lightly browned in a small amount of oil (or *seared,* see below), then immersed in water or stock and simmered in a covered pan. The liquid usually turns a rich golden or brown color and only a tiny amount may be left in the pan. Also known as *pot roasting.*

Cooking with Oil

Sautéing: quickly cooking food in a small amount of oil over a high heat. It is done in a skillet or sauté pan. It is used for vegetables, lightly floured fish, and chicken cutlets. This process is sometimes called *pan frying.*

Searing: cooking food over high heat in order to brown the exterior of the food. Also known as *browning.*

Frying: completely immersing a food in very hot oil. Potatoes (french fries), breaded mushrooms, zucchini, and even fish can be prepared this way. Tempura is a method of deep-frying batter-dipped foods in a wok very quickly so that very little oil is absorbed. The batter can be made from whole-grain flour and ice water. This is about the only time we deep-fry foods for those in recovery.

Stir-frying: sautéing in a wok (a pan shaped like a large bowl, usually with two handles on either side or one long handle). A small amount of oil is heated in the wok and foods are added and quickly sautéed. Add the longest-cooking foods first. As foods are cooked they can be pushed up the sides of the wok where the temperature is lower, so that they will not overcook. The idea is to cook foods only until their color is bright and they are still crispy and crunchy. Remember to season a new wok before using.

Sweating: cooking vegetables in a small amount of fat (oil) over low heat to allow the natural moisture to come out of the food. The foods do not brown. In many recipes aromatic vegetables are sweated as the first step to making a sauce or soup.

Dry Cooking

Baking: cooking with dry heat, usually in an oven.

Broiling: cooking under high heat, with the heat source from above. Broiling is fast and helps rid certain foods of excess fat, which drips away while cooking. Use a broiling pan that is 1 to 2 inches deep with a rack on top to allow the fat to drip through. Cover the rack with foil or use a solid pan for fillets, as the fish tend to fall through the rack. Fish fillets are best cooked 1 to 2 inches from the broiler, whereas poultry on the bone, shellfish, whole fish, and vegetables should be cooked farther away from the flame, about 3 to 5 inches. This type of cooking does not make foods more tender, and many foods require marinating beforehand and/or basting (a process of brushing liquids onto the food while it cooks) to retain moisture.

Grilling: cooking with high heat, with a heat source from below. Use a bit of oil in the pan or on the grill rack to prevent sticking. Whole fish with the skin on are usually fine cooked on the grill.

Roasting: oven-cooking fish, chicken, vegetables, and tender cuts of meat in an uncovered pan, creating a crispy brown exterior and moist interior. A rack can be used to cook the food evenly on all sides. Often the food is basted with a marinade or with fat from the bottom of the roasting pan. Many recommend cooking a turkey or chicken with a thermometer in the breast until it is approximately 165° F., then letting the bird sit for ten to fifteen minutes at room temperature. Another "doneness test" is to shake the legs; if they are flexible and loose the bird is done. A third test is to puncture the thigh; if the juices run clear, the bird is done. Organic birds seem to take a little longer to cook, so watch them carefully toward the end of the process. Stuffed birds and fish take longer to cook.

Toasting: subjecting a food to high heat from above and below to brown the exterior while minimally affecting the interior. This can be done on a rack (as in toasting bread) or a pan. It is a lovely way to bring out the flavor in foods such as grains and spices.

If this all seems a little overwhelming, don't worry. You probably know a lot more than you think. Try the simpler methods (such as steaming or roasting) first. Try to use one new method per week until you're comfortable with five or six. The more cooking methods you know, the less likely you are to become bored with cooking and the more confidence you'll have.

Other Odds and Ends Now that you're a bit more familiar with some of the basic cooking techniques, here's a quick glossary of other terms you're likely to encounter while learning to cook, followed by a final word about the secret ingredients in recovery cooking.

Acidulated water: Water with vinegar, lime juice, or lemon juice added to help prevent the discoloration of foods. Used for cooking and soaking.

Al dente: An Italian term meaning "to the tooth." It describes food cooked to the point of firmness (usually applied to pastas).

Aromatics: Vegetables such as onions, leeks, carrots, parsnips, and celery, and herbs and spices used in cooking for the flavorful scents they impart to other foods.

Bind: To hold together or stir ingredients to cause something to thicken.

Blend: To mix together two or more ingredients.

Bruise: To crush the leaves of herbs to release their flavor before using them in cooking.

Bouquet garni: Several herbs, including parsley, thyme, bay leaf, and others, tied up in a piece of cloth and used to flavor dishes. It is removed after cooking and before serving.

Caramelization: A method of releasing the natural sugars in food to turn the food a golden brown and add natural sweetness to the food. Usually achieved by lightly sautéing (see below).

Chop: To cut pieces of food coarsely.

Coat: To cover a food with another ingredient such as bread crumbs, a sauce, or eggs.

Coddle: Cooking foods (usually eggs) by placing them in a special pan with individual sections, immersing the pan in water, and cooking for a long period of time on very low heat.

Condiment: An accompaniment to dishes. It is usually very high in flavor: piquant, tart, sweet, or salty. Some condiments for the recovery recipes are soy sauce, umeboshi vinegar, gama-shio, curry chutneys, and salsa.

Cut in: A term (usually used in pastry cooking) to describe the way a fat is mixed with dry ingredients. Butter is cut into flour by using a fork, two knives, or a pastry cutter. The fat (butter) is cut and mixed with the dry ingredients until the mixture forms tiny balls.

Deglaze: To heat a stock or other liquid together with the juices and residue left in a pan after roasting or sautéing. A small amount of liquid is poured into the pan and stirred over medium heat until the residue is incorporated and the liquid reduces, becoming darker and thicker.

Degrease: To remove the excess fat from a stock, soup, or sauce. This is best achieved by chilling the liquid until the fat solidifies on the surface, then skimming it off. A special degreasing cup (the spout of which comes from the bottom) is handy for degreasing hot liquids.

Dice: To cut foods into ⅛-inch to ¼-inch cubes.

Dilute: To reduce the intensity of a mixture by adding liquids.

Dissolve: To mix dry ingredients with a liquid until the dry is fully incorporated into the liquid.

Drain: To strain the liquids away from a food (for example, draining cooked pasta).

Dredge: Dipping foods in dry ingredients such as bread crumbs, flour, or cornmeal, then shaking off any of the extra crumbs, etc. This process is often used for sautéing or pan-frying thin, delicate fish fillets, pressed chicken cutlets, or thinly sliced vegetables.

Dress: To add dressing to a salad. Also to clean and trim fish or poultry.

Drizzle: To pour a sauce or other liquid over a food, usually in a thin stream.

Dust: To lightly cover a food with flour or another dry ingredient.

Emincer: To cut food into very thin pieces for even cooking.

Entrée: In America, the main course. In most of Europe, the first course of a meal.

Floret: The separate, small flowers of broccoli or cauliflower.

Flour: To lightly coat a pan or food with flour to prevent sticking.

Fold: A process of combining lighter foods with heavier ones by placing the light foods in the bowl on top of the heavy foods, then blending the two by bringing a rubber spatula through the mixture with a folding motion. Continue until the foods are gently combined. An example of this process is when whipped egg whites are folded into a batter.

French cut: A cut made to food at a 45-degree angle.

Garnish: To add a decoration, such as a sprig of parsley or slice of orange, to a dish before serving. In recovery cooking we try to use edible parts of food as garnishes, which enhance nutritional value as well as ornamentation.

Glaze: To coat food with a thin, shiny mixture.

Grate: Shredding food (into various sizes) by rubbing it up and down the sides of a grater (or by using a rotary grater).

Infusion: Adding aromatic foods or seasonings (spices, herbs, pepper, fruit, garlic, tea, etc.) to a liquid such as hot water, oil, or vinegar in order to "infuse" the liquid with flavor.

Jardiniere: A preparation style that uses vegetables for garnish.

Julienne: A cut made to foods that is ⅛ by ⅛ inch thick and 2½ inches long. Also referred to as a *matchstick* cut.

Marinade: A seasoned liquid mixture, usually with lemon juice or vinegar, in which food is soaked to heighten flavor or tenderize.

Marinate: The process of soaking food in a marinade.

Matchstick: See Julienne

Mince: To cut food into very tiny pieces.

Mirepoix (mere-PWAH): A mixture of vegetables and herbs used to flavor soups, sauces, and fish or chicken. The common mirepoix ingredients are carrots, celery, onions, and herbs.

Pare or peel: To remove the outer layer of a fruit or vegetable.

Proof: A process of "proving" that yeast is active before using it to bake with. The yeast is placed in water with a sweetener for ten minutes and if it bubbles it's still good to use.

Puree: A food that is mashed until smooth; the process of blending or mashing and straining foods until soft.

Reduce: To cook a liquid until it reduces in volume and its flavors are concentrated.

Refresh: To sprinkle cold water over foods.

Roux: A cooked mixture of flour and fat used to thicken soups and sauces.

Sauce: A flavored liquid served with foods to enhance their flavor.

Scale: A process of removing fish scales by scraping them off.

Scallop: Slicing vegetables thinly. The term also refers to thinly sliced pieces of meat and to a pretty edge on pie crusts.

Score: To thinly pierce or cut the skin of a fish or the surface of a piece of chicken so that it will not curl while cooking and will be better able to absorb a marinade. The pattern of the cut is parallel lines in two directions, creating a diamond shape.

Shock: To add cold water to certain foods while they cook.

<u>Shred:</u> To cut foods narrowly with a knife, grater, or processor.

<u>Steep:</u> To soak food in liquid so that the liquid picks up the flavor of the food (for steeping tea). Steeping is also used to rehydrate dry foods such as dried mushrooms.

<u>Truss:</u> To tie up food (usually poultry) to maintain its shape.

<u>Whisk:</u> A wire tool used to beat or whip foods.

<u>Whip:</u> To beat food to increase its volume by incorporating air into it. Used especially for egg whites and cream.

<u>Zest:</u> The outermost layer of skin of an orange, lemon, or lime. The white portion, or pith, of the skin is not used for zest.

Seasoning Traditionally, foods are flavored with salt, sugar, and cream or butter. The recovery recipes use herbs and spices to heighten flavor, maximize good dietary habits, and maintain nutrient density. The following chart lists some popular spice combinations.

In the early stage of recovery, milder spices such as bay leaves, thyme, or rosemary work wonders in stimulating a desensitized palate or appetite. More robust spices, such as those used in curries or peppers, can be enjoyed during the later months of recovery, when damaged digestive tracts have become stronger. Experiment with various combinations of spices from each group. Try using two spices in a group and then experiment with adding others. These combinations will work well with vegetables, grains, beans, fish, poultry, or meats.

16.3 HERB AND SPICE COMBINATIONS

PARSLEY	BASIL	GARLIC
THYME	OREGANO	OREGANO
ROSEMARY	THYME	CUMIN
SAGE	PARSLEY	PAPRIKA
BAY LEAF	CHILIES	
ALLSPICE	DILL	CORIANDER
CINNAMON	CARAWAY	GARLIC
CLOVES	CHIVES	ONION
NUTMEG	CUMIN	CELERY SEEDS
GINGER		
PARSLEY	TURMERIC	CUMIN
TARRAGON	CORIANDER	CARDAMOM
SAVORY	FENNEL SEEDS	THYME
LEMON RIND	CAYENNE	ROSEMARY
MARJORAM	ALLSPICE	PARSLEY
CHIVES	PARSLEY	BASIL
CHERVIL		

17 *The Recipes*

Fresh wholefoods are the centerpiece of a good recovery program, but few of us take the time to enjoy their benefits, for a variety of reasons. We may think it will take too long to prepare wholefoods, or that we don't have the skills needed to cook for ourselves. Or our palates may have been dulled by the effects of alcohol, drugs, and a diet that is overloaded with sugar, salt, fat, and the other additives found in processed foods. But wholefoods cooking does not have to be difficult or time consuming, and deadened taste buds will perk up remarkably fast when they are exposed to new and interesting flavors and sensations.

The single most important step in maintaining long-term recovery and vigorous and long-term health is learning to choose and prepare wholefoods. We've already reviewed the basics of how to shop for healthy whole and (occasionally) processed foods. Now is the time to learn how to make these good foods into equally good meals.

The following recovery recipes rely on satisfying, healthy foods that will leave you rejuvenated and energized instead of stuffed and sluggish. However, not every food is appropriate for every recovering person. In addition, different stages of recovery are marked by different nutritional needs and biochemical abilities. In the early days of recovery most people are malnourished and plagued by gastrointestinal problems, disrupted carbohydrate metabolism, and cravings for sugar and other unhealthy foods. The same is true of those in long-term recovery who have not paid attention to the biochemical connection in their recovery.

The order of these recipes corresponds with various stages of recovery. Foods that are easier to prepare and/or digest are at the beginning of each section; spicier dishes, or those that may take more time to prepare, are at the back. The recipes also include alternatives for those with food sensitivities or other disorders that restrict food choices.

All the recipes are nutritionally dense while low in calories, cholesterol, and saturated fats. They are flavored without the use of refined sugar, salt, heavy creams, high-fat cheeses, gravies, or alcohol. Each recipe includes a brief description of some of the nutrients it contains (for a full listing of the major nutrients, their sources, and their effects, see pages 33–36).

We've tried to anticipate the questions and needs of novice cooks by making the preparation instructions clear and complete. Read through all the recipes at least once, and note the ones that appeal most to you. If a recipe calls for cooked grains or beans, refer to the cooking charts (pages 241 and 248) for amounts of liquid, cooking methods, and cooking times. Remember to peel all fruits and vegetables that are not organically grown. Although peels can be rich in nutrients, they can also be rich in pesticides and other chemicals. If you're using organic produce, simply wash away any sand or dirt and prepare according to the recipe. When a recipe calls for olive oil, use cold-pressed extra virgin olive oil. When a recipe calls for vegetable oil any cold-pressed oil will do, such as canola, safflower, or soy.

When deciding what foods to prepare when, keep in mind that menu planning can be as individual and eclectic as you wish. Don't limit yourself to an egg dish or cereal for breakfast or soup and sandwiches for lunch. After all, in many Oriental nations, noodles and fish are a breakfast staple. Omelettes can make a delicious light dinner. And you should never underestimate the pleasures of rice and beans for breakfast. Every wholefoods dish can provide a healthy collage of nutrients, no matter when you eat it.

If you have medical or dietary limitations or unique requirements—such as food sensitivities or a need for more protein—you will of course need to plan your meals accordingly. But a good rule of thumb is to keep an open mind about what to eat when, and to create as much variety in your diet as possible.

Challenge yourself with a few new recipes a week. Within a year you will have more than 100 recipes and most basic cooking techniques under your belt. Cooking is like dancing: It gets easier as you learn the steps. You'll eventually reach a point where you won't need the recipes, you'll just get inspired by fresh ingredients and start creating your own dishes! So start the fires burning—the riches of recovery await you.

Breakfast

Breakfast is a vitally important meal for people in recovery. It can set the tone and temperament of your body and brain for the entire day. High-protein foods tend to wake us up and the complex carbohydrate of whole grains tends to help keep us calm and regular. A combination of the two makes for a good start to the day.

The traditional hearty American breakfast of eggs with all the trimmings has come under attack from every corner in the last decade and with good reason. More often than not it is high in saturated fats, salt, and sugar, and remarkably low in nutrient value. A breakfast of whole grains, hot or cold breakfast cereals, or whole-grain breads, muffins, or pancakes is the best way to maintain energy through the day and build resilience to stress.

We have a lot of preconceived notions about what constitutes a breakfast food. Many cultures start the day with fish or beans and corn bread. A tuna salad on whole-grain toast would make an excellent breakfast and yet most of us classify this as lunch or dinner fare. So keep in mind that many recipes outside the breakfast section make for a super breakfast and last night's leftovers are often great morning foods.

Len's Parsley Scramble

This high-protein recipe is for the first stages of recovery, although it can be enjoyed any time—not just in the morning. Blanching the parsley makes it less bitter and easier to digest. Basil or cilantro can be substituted for the parsley.

Serves 4

> 1 bunch parsley, finely chopped (about ¾ cup)
> ¼ teaspoon salt
> Dash freshly ground black pepper
> 8 eggs, beaten
> 2 tablespoons olive oil

1. Bring a medium pot of water to boil over high heat. Add the parsley and blanch: Cook 1 minute, then drain and rinse under cold water.

2. Add the parsley, salt, and pepper to the bowl of beaten eggs. Whisk to combine.

3. Warm a heavy skillet, preferably cast-iron, over medium heat. Add the oil and, when hot, pour in the eggs. Stirring constantly, cook for about 2½ minutes, or until the eggs are firm and not runny.

Zucchini, Tomato, and Onion Frittata

The frittata is the Italian version of the omelette. It can be enjoyed hot or cold.

Serves 4

2 tablespoons olive oil
1 medium onion, sliced
2 large garlic cloves, minced
1 medium zucchini, washed and julienned
3 plum tomatoes, chopped
1 tablespoon finely chopped fresh parsley, or 1½ teaspoons
  dried
1 teaspoon dried oregano
8 eggs, lightly beaten
Dash freshly ground black pepper

1. Preheat the broiler.

2. Warm the oil over medium heat in a medium frying pan with an ovenproof handle. Add the onion and cook until lightly browned. Add the garlic, cook 1 minute, then add the zucchini, tomatoes, parsley, and oregano. Cook for about 3 minutes, or until the zucchini is soft. Remove from the heat and pour the eggs over the vegetables. Sprinkle with pepper.

3. Place the pan under the broiler and cook about 4 minutes, or until the top of the frittata is golden. Remove from the broiler. Run a knife around the sides, place a plate over the pan, and turn the plate and pan over. Slice into 4 pieces and serve warm, or chill and serve later.

Red Pepper and Olive Frittata

Here's another tasty variation of the frittata. Red peppers are a good source of vitamin C, and olives are high in monounsaturated fatty acids. Let your imagination run wild and add your favorite vegetables. Try fennel and olive, or parsley and garlic.

Serves 4

2 tablespoons olive oil
1 medium onion, sliced
2 garlic cloves, minced
1 medium zucchini, julienned
3 plum tomatoes, chopped
1 red bell pepper, seeded and diced
⅓ cup finely chopped black olives
1 teaspoon dried oregano
½ teaspoon finely chopped fresh parsley
½ teaspoon salt
¼ teaspoon freshly ground black pepper
8 eggs, lightly beaten

1. Preheat the broiler.

2. Warm the oil in a large ovenproof skillet over medium heat. Add the onion and cook until lightly browned. Add the garlic, zucchini, tomatoes, red pepper, olives, oregano, parsley, salt, and pepper. Cook about 3 minutes, or until the zucchini is soft. Remove from heat, pour in the eggs, and place the pan under the broiler. Cook about 3 to 4 minutes, or until the frittata is firm and golden brown on top.

Whole Wheat Pancakes with Strawberry Syrup

Pancakes made from whole-grain flours have a richer flavor and are more filling. Here, their nutrient density is augmented by the topping. In addition to being high in vitamin C, the sauce has fewer calories than commercial maple syrup. Other fresh fruit—such as blueberries, blackberries, raspberries, or peaches—can be substituted. This breakfast is high in B vitamins, manganese, calcium, protein, complex carbohydrates, and phosphorus.

Makes 8 4-inch pancakes

Sauce

> 1 cup chopped strawberries
> ½ cup water
> 2–3 tablespoons maple syrup, rice yinnie (page 112), or
>   honey

Pancakes

> 1½ cups whole wheat pastry flour
> 2 teaspoons baking powder
> 1 egg
> 2 tablespoons vegetable oil, plus more for greasing pan
> 1½ cups soy milk, milk, or buttermilk
> 1 tablespoon maple syrup or barley malt (page 110)
> 2 teaspoons molasses
> ½ cup chopped walnuts
> ½ cup chopped strawberries (optional)

1. In a small pot, combine the strawberries, water, and maple syrup. Bring to a boil over high heat, then reduce heat to a simmer and cook until the mixture becomes thick and syrupy, about 20 minutes. Keep the mixture warm while preparing the pancakes.

2. In a large bowl, combine the flour and baking powder. In a smaller bowl, whisk the egg. Add the oil, milk, maple syrup, and molasses. Stir well, then add the wet ingredients to the dry. Stir a few times to mix. There may be some lumps in the batter but that's okay. Gently add the walnuts and strawberries, if using.

3. Preheat the oven to 200° F.

4. Oil a cast-iron skillet and warm it over medium heat until a few drops of water sprinkled in the pan skip across the surface. Pour about ⅓ cup of the batter into the pan. The first pancake is always a tester. Cook until bubbles form on the surface, then flip it over. The second side will cook faster than the first, but it will look as attractive as the first side. Place cooked pancakes on a baking sheet in the oven to keep them warm while you are making the rest. Don't stack the pancakes until ready to serve, then top with the sauce.

Vanilla French Toast with Slivered Almonds

Melt-in-your-mouth French toast combines high protein and complex carbohydrates in the same meal. Almonds add crunch and nutrients like iron and vitamin B$_2$ (also known as riboflavin). The vanilla used in baking is generally high in alcohol, so read the label and purchase only alcohol-free vanilla extract. (Check your local health food store.)

Serves 4

> 1 cup slivered almonds
> ½ cup apple juice
> 2 tablespoons honey
> 1½ teaspoons alcohol-free vanilla extract
> 2 eggs
> 2 egg whites
> 2 teaspoons vegetable oil
> 8 slices whole-grain bread

1. Preheat the oven to 325° F. Place the nuts on a baking tray and toast in the oven until golden brown, about 10 minutes. Remove and set aside.

2. In a small saucepan, bring the apple juice to a boil over high heat. Reduce to a simmer and add the honey. Stir to melt. Add the vanilla extract and remove from heat. Cool to room temperature.

3. In a large bowl, whisk together the eggs and egg whites. Add the apple-honey mixture and whisk to combine.

4. Warm a large skillet, preferably cast iron, over medium heat. Add 1 teaspoon of the oil and when hot, dip a slice of bread into the egg mixture and drop it into the pan. Add enough slices to fill the skillet with one layer. Cook for about 4 minutes per side, or until golden brown, being careful that the pan does not get too hot, or the toast will burn. Repeat with each slice of bread, adding oil as needed. Remove the toast to a baking pan and cook 6 minutes in the oven, or until the toast looks puffy. Top with toasted almonds, and serve with maple syrup, fruit sauce, or Fresh Fruit Compote (page 305).

Cornmeal Griddle Cakes

Griddle cakes are an old-fashioned breakfast. The cornmeal provides minerals such as calcium, magnesium, phosphorus, potassium, iron, and zinc as well as vitamin A, protein, and plenty of fiber. Serve these with your choice of protein food such as baked fish, beans, eggs, or dairy food.

Makes 6 medium cakes

3/4 cup water
2 teaspoons honey or rice yinnie (page 112)
1 cup cornmeal
1 egg
1/2 teaspoon salt
2 tablespoons vegetable oil

1. Preheat the oven to 200° F.

2. In a small saucepan, bring the water to a boil over medium heat. Add the honey and stir until melted. Remove from heat and add cornmeal. Allow to cool.

3. In a small bowl, whisk the egg with the salt. Add to the cornmeal mixture and stir well.

4. Warm a medium skillet (preferably cast iron) over medium heat. Add the oil and when it is hot drop 1/4 cup of the batter onto the skillet. Cook 4 minutes per side, or until golden brown and cooked through. Place each cake on a baking sheet and keep warm in the oven until the others are cooked.

Potato Basil Crisp

This recipe gives you the satisfaction of crispy potatoes without the fat of deep-frying and for fewer than 200 calories per serving. Serve with eggs for breakfast or as a side dish at dinner, lunch, or brunch.

Serves 4

> 1 medium onion, finely chopped
> 4 cups shredded or grated peeled potatoes (about
>   6 potatoes)
> 2 tablespoons finely chopped fresh basil or parsley
> ½ teaspoon salt
> Dash of freshly ground white pepper
> 2 tablespoons canola or olive oil

1. In a large bowl, combine the onion, potatoes, basil, salt, and pepper. Mix well.

2. In a large skillet, warm 1 tablespoon of the oil. When the oil is hot, place half of the potato mixture into the skillet. Press down with a spatula to flatten and shape to the bottom of the pan. Cook about 15 minutes, or until the bottom is browned evenly. Run a knife around the sides of the pan, then place a large plate over the pan. Using oven mitts, grip both sides of the pan with your hands and flip the crisp over onto the plate. Then gently slide the crisp's uncooked side into the skillet. Cook 10 to 15 minutes more, then remove and repeat the procedure with the remaining potato mixture and oil.

Granola

A great breakfast cereal that's full of fiber, protein, and many vitamins and minerals, granola is also a crunchy snack, a good topping on yogurt or fruit compote, and a great stuffing for baked apples or pears.

Makes 5 cups

> 3 cups rolled oats
> ½ cup rye or soy grits
> 1 cup nuts: walnuts, almonds, hazelnuts, or cashews
> ⅓ cup raisins

¼ cup sunflower seeds or pumpkin seeds
¼ cup sesame seeds
¼ cup chopped dried fruit (optional)
¼ cup vegetable oil, such as corn, safflower, or canola
⅓ cup barley malt or molasses

1. Preheat the oven to 350° F. In a large bowl, mix the oats, grits, nuts, raisins, seeds, and fruit.

2. In a small bowl, mix the oil and malt and then add to the large bowl. Stir well to coat the oat mixture.

3. Spread on a large baking sheet and bake 20 minutes, or until crispy brown.

Bulgur Muffins

Bulgur is a nutty-tasting form of wheat made by parboiling and cracking wheat berries. Since it is already parboiled it cooks quickly. Bulgur is a rich source of fiber, protein, and B vitamins.

Makes 8 muffins

½ cup water
¼ cup bulgur
1 cup soy milk or buttermilk
2 tablespoons oil, plus more for greasing muffin pan
2 tablespoons honey, barley malt (page 110), or rice yinnie
  (page 112)
1½ cups whole wheat flour, plus more for dusting muffin
  pan
1½ teaspoons baking powder
⅛ teaspoon salt

1. Preheat the oven to 350° F. Lightly grease and flour 8 muffin cups.

2. In a small pot, bring the water to boil over high heat. Add the bulgur, remove from heat, cover, and let sit for 15 minutes.

3. In a large bowl, whisk together the soy milk, oil, and honey. In another bowl, combine the flour, baking powder, and salt. Pour the dry ingredients into the wet, stir well, then add the cooked bulgur. Stir to mix. Spoon the batter into the muffin cups and bake 45 minutes, until golden brown.

Blue and Yellow Corn Muffins

Here's a sweet quick bread made from whole ground cornmeal. It provides ample carbohydrates, vitamin A, and calcium. This muffin has one-third the calories of a plain bagel. Spread a hot piece with one tablespoon of tahini and add even more calcium and fewer than 90 calories.

Makes 8 medium-large muffins

> 1 tablespoon vegetable oil, plus more for greasing pan
> 1¼ cups blue cornmeal
> 1 teaspoon baking powder, divided in half
> 1 teaspoon baking soda, divided in half
> 1¼ cups yellow cornmeal
> 1½ cups soy milk, buttermilk, or milk
> 3 tablespoons honey

1. Preheat the oven to 425° F. Oil the muffin tin.

2. In a large bowl, mix the blue cornmeal with ½ teaspoon each of the baking powder and baking soda. In another bowl, mix the yellow cornmeal with the remaining ½ teaspoon each of baking powder and baking soda. In a third bowl, combine the milk, honey, and oil. Mix well, then split the wet ingredients between the 2 bowls of cornmeal.

3. Fill the muffin molds halfway by pouring the yellow cornmeal mixture except for 1 cup into the tin, then fill the molds with the blue cornmeal mixture. Swirl 1 to 2 tablespoons of the reserved yellow cornmeal on top of each muffin. Bake 20 to 25 minutes, or until a tester comes out clean. (You can also bake the mixture in a greased 8 x 8-inch pan.)

Scones

These scones are humdingers! Serve them warm from the oven with jam. A favorite of recovery cooking students, this recipe is donated from Mary Estella's Natural Foods Cookbook. Naturally sweetened and yeast-free, these scones are full of whole-grain goodness. They provide lots of vitamin C, E, and B-complex as well as calcium, magnesium, phosphorus, selenium, and zinc.

Makes 16 scones

⅓ cup currants (use raisins if currants are unavailable)
⅓ cup apple juice
2 ½ cups whole wheat pastry flour
Pinch of salt
1 teaspoon baking soda
1½ teaspoons baking powder
¼ cup corn oil
¼ block tofu (4 ounces)
Juice and zest of 1 lemon
2–3 tablespoons grade A maple syrup (see Note) or rice yinnie (page 112)

1. Preheat the oven to 350° F. Soak the currants in the apple juice.

2. In a large bowl, stir together the flour, salt, baking soda, and baking powder.

3. In a blender, puree the corn oil, tofu, lemon juice and zest, and syrup until smooth. Pour the liquid ingredients into the dry. Add the currants and the apple juice and gently mix together. The dough should hold together; if it doesn't, add more liquid.

4. Place the dough on a floured surface and roll out ½ to ¾ inch thick. Using a glass or cookie cutter, cut 2-inch circles and place on a lightly oiled baking sheet. Leave a little room for them to expand as they begin cooking. Bake 12 minutes, or until golden on top. Serve warm.

Note: Maple syrup should be grade A or better; most commercial brands contain additives.

Almond Milk

This is a nutritious milk substitute for those who are lactose intolerant but love cereal with milk. Almonds are a good source of iron as well as many other minerals.

Makes 2 cups

> 1 cup raw almonds
> 4 cups water
> ¼ cup pitted dates, roughly chopped

1. Place the almonds in a bowl and cover with 2 cups of water. Soak 8 hours or overnight.

2. Drain and rinse the almonds. Place them in a blender with the additional 2 cups of water and puree.

3. Place a strainer over a large bowl and press the liquid out of the almond puree. Discard the solids. Return the almond liquid to the blender and add the dates. Puree completely and refrigerate until ready to use.

Fruit Smoothies

Smoothies are great for breakfast as well as dessert. Invent your own by trying different combinations of fruits in season. For all smoothies, simply blend all of the ingredients in a blender until creamy and smooth.

Peach Smoothie

This creamy and filling smoothie contains fewer than 90 calories per serving.

Serves 2

> 4 peaches, peeled and pitted
> 1 banana, peeled
> ½ cup crushed ice
> ¼ teaspoon alcohol-free vanilla
> Dash of ground nutmeg

Blueberry Smoothie

We could call this a manganese-potassium smoothie. Blueberries are one of the best sources of manganese and bananas are a good source of potassium.

Serves 2

1 cup blueberries
2 bananas, peeled
½ cup apple juice
½ teaspoon maple syrup
½ cup crushed ice

Soups and Stocks

Soup is a great food for the early part of recovery, when the body's fluid balance may be depleted and the gastrointestinal tract is often impaired. Soups, be they hot or cold, are an easy way to obtain needed nutrients without stressing the digestive tract or spending lots of time in the kitchen. (If you are using organic vegetables, you will get maximum nutritional benefit if you don't peel them.)

Stocks, broths made by simmering vegetables and/or leftover bones, are the basis for most soups. While not always essential, they add a depth of flavor and nutrients that water can't supply on its own.

Making a stock can be as simple as throwing some greens and bones into a pot or as complex as spending hours roasting and sautéing individual stock ingredients. Prepared stocks are often high in sodium and additives and relatively low in nutrients, so take the time to make your own. We recommend making large batches of stock and keeping it on hand in several containers in the freezer.

The best stocks start with leftovers—the trimmings of raw organic vegetables, leftover cooked vegetables, and the bones of fish, chicken, or meats. Almost any vegetable will work in stock, with the exception of cabbage and broccoli, since their strong flavors can overwhelm the stock and soup made with it. Bones and cooked vegetables can be stored in the freezer until you're ready to make stock, while raw vegetable trimmings will keep for up to a week in a plastic bag in the refrigerator. We also recommend adding a piece of sea vegetable such as kombu or wakame to stocks to boost their mineral content.

The following recipes will get you started, but remember, some of the best soups are created from a few leftover vegetables, an herb or two, and a bit of water or stock.

Quick Super Stock

*This soothing soup stock has been a favorite medicinal prepara-
tion for the Japanese for thousands of years. Alone it's perfect for
the early stages of recovery when simple broths are gentle to the
digestive system.*

*The resulting broth is a clear stock called a dashi. Add tofu
squares, scallions, thinly sliced carrots, and daikon radish for a
light soothing soup. A small amount of alcohol-free soy sauce
can be used instead of salt to flavor the broth.*

Makes 1½ quarts

> 2 medium dried shiitake mushrooms
> 1½ quarts water
> 1 3-inch piece kombu or kelp (page 114)

1. Rinse the mushrooms and cover with the water in a small
bowl for 4 minutes. Remove the mushrooms and cut off the
stems. Slice the mushroom tops and return to the water.

2. Remove any sand from the kombu by brushing it off. Do
not rinse, as the white powder on the surface, which is high
in minerals, would be rinsed away.

3. Combine the water, mushrooms, and kombu in a medium
pot. Bring the water to a boil, then lower the heat and cook
for 10 minutes. Serve hot.

Vegetable Stock

Vegetable stock is the queen of stocks. Cooks worldwide use stocks to enrich the flavor of soups and sauces. Moreover, this vegetable stock increases the nutritional value of any dish it's added to. Try using this stock to cook grains in as well.

Makes about 1½ quarts

1 tablespoon vegetable oil, preferably canola or olive
1 onion, chopped
2 carrots, chopped
2 celery stalks, chopped
3 cups raw vegetables (do not use broccoli or cabbage)
3 sprigs parsley or 2 tablespoons dried parsley
1 bay leaf
1 tablespoon fresh thyme or 1 teaspoon dried
2 whole cloves
2 garlic cloves (optional)
2 quarts water
1 3-inch piece kombu (page 114)

1. Rinse and peel all nonorganic vegetables. Rinse the organic produce.

2. In a large pot, heat the oil. Quickly add the onion and cook until light brown, stirring occasionally. Add the remainder of the ingredients except the kombu and cover. Cook 10 minutes on low heat.

3. Cover with the 2 quarts of water, add the kombu, bring to a boil, reduce heat, and simmer 1½ hours. Strain the stock and use immediately or refrigerate for future use. If a more intense flavor is desired, return strained stock to stove and reduce the liquid by half.

Chicken or Turkey Stock

Chicken or turkey stock is the base for many soups and sauces. It can also be served with brown rice for a soothing simple soup. Use all leftover parts of a chicken or turkey except the skin, which is high in fat.

Makes about 1¹/₂ quarts

> 1 chicken or turkey carcass (or 3–4 pounds chicken pieces)
> 1 large onion, quartered
> 2 carrots, coarsely chopped
> 2 celery stalks, coarsely chopped
> 2 sprigs fresh parsley
> 1 bay leaf
> 1 tablespoon fresh thyme or 1 teaspoon dried
> 2 whole cloves
> 2 fresh peppercorns or a pinch of freshly ground black pepper
> 1 tablespoon fresh lemon juice or vinegar (see Note)
> 2 garlic cloves (optional)
> 2 quarts water

1. Put all the ingredients in a large pot. Cover with the 2 quarts of cold water.

2. Bring to a boil, reduce heat to a simmer, and simmer 2 hours. Strain and use immediately or refrigerate. When using refrigerated stock, spoon off any waxy (fat) top layer before proceeding.

Note: The lemon juice or vinegar helps to extract more calcium from the chicken or turkey bones.

Broccoli Soup

This low-fat, cream-free broccoli soup contains only 24 calories per cup. It is high in vitamin K. Broccoli is a member of the cruciferous family, which has strong anti-cancer properties.

Serves 6

> 2 tablespoons vegetable oil
> 1 onion, peeled and finely chopped
> 3 garlic cloves, peeled and chopped
> 1 tablespoon fresh marjoram or 1 teaspoon dried
> 1 tablespoon fresh thyme or 1 teaspoon dried
> ⅛ teaspoon nutmeg
> 2 celery stalks, finely chopped
> 2 scallions, trimmed and coarsely chopped
> 1 medium potato, peeled and chopped
> 1½ pounds broccoli, washed, separated into florets (tops) and stems
> 6 cups vegetable stock (page 199) or water
> 2 tablespoons minced fresh dill, plus a few sprigs for garnish
> Salt
> Freshly ground black pepper

1. Warm the oil in a large stockpot over medium heat. Do not ever let the oil smoke. If oil does smoke, your heat is too high; let the pan cool, drain, then wash and begin over. Add the onion and cook until it is translucent, then add the garlic, marjoram, thyme, and nutmeg. Sauté 3 minutes. Add the celery, scallions, and potato and cook 5 minutes. Add the broccoli stems and the stock and cook, covered, 30 minutes.

2. Add the broccoli florets and cook 2 minutes. Remove from heat and blend in a food processor or blender, adding the dill as it's blending. Season with salt and pepper and serve.

Pop's Thick Pea Soup

Split peas are high in fiber, and fiber helps control blood sugar levels and may also lower blood pressure. Fiber in peas is soluble (unlike the fiber in whole grains) and thus it helps to reduce LDL cholesterol.

Serves 8 to 10

2 tablespoons olive oil
1 large onion, finely chopped
3 medium carrots, finely chopped
2 celery stalks, finely chopped
2 garlic cloves, minced
1 bay leaf
1 tablespoon thyme
2 teaspoons dried marjoram or oregano
2 teaspoons ground cumin
1 teaspoon sage
4 cups green split peas
10 cups vegetable stock (page 199) or water
1 teaspoon salt
½ teaspoon freshly ground black pepper

1. Warm the oil in a large stockpot over medium heat. Add the onion and cook until golden, then add the carrots, celery, garlic, bay leaf, thyme, marjoram, cumin, and sage and cook on low heat for 10 minutes.

2. Add peas and stock and bring to a boil. Reduce heat and simmer 1½ hours, covered (uncover for the last 10 minutes). Season with salt and pepper and serve.

Beet Soup with Fresh Dill

Beet soup can be served hot or cold with a cooked potato or tomato and topped with tofu or sour cream. Beets are high in calcium, phosphorus, sodium, potassium, iron, and magnesium.

Serves 6

2 teaspoons vegetable oil, such as canola
1 medium onion, finely chopped
4 medium beets, peeled and shredded
6 cups stock (pages 198–200) or water
4 tablespoons minced fresh dill
2 scallions, finely chopped
2 tablespoons vinegar
1–2 tablespoons freshly squeezed lemon juice
1 tablespoon honey
Salt
Freshly ground black pepper

1. In a large stockpot, warm the oil over medium heat. Add the onion and sauté until light golden; do not brown. Add the beets, cover the pot, and cook 5 minutes.

2. Add the stock and bring to a boil. Reduce heat and simmer for 25 minutes, then add the dill, scallions, vinegar, lemon juice, honey, salt, and pepper. Simmer 5 minutes more and serve hot, or remove from heat, cool to room temperature, and chill.

Root Soup

Root soup is soothing and easy to digest. There are no heavy spices in this soup but it's strong in flavor. Root vegetables offer good amounts of vitamin A (in the form of beta carotene), folic acid, and minerals such as iron, magnesium, and potassium.

Serves 4

4 medium yellow onions
3 small beets
2 carrots
2 parsnips
1 medium daikon radish
4 small red potatoes
1 large turnip
1 small rutabaga, peeled, or 1 large sweet potato (optional)
10 cups water

1. Peel the onions. Wash all the vegetables and peel them if they are not organically grown. The beets can be quartered, the carrots, parsnips, and daikon can be cut into 2-inch pieces, and the potatoes, turnip, and rutabaga can be cut into 2-inch chunks.

2. Fill a large stockpot with the 10 cups of water. Add the vegetables, cover, and bring to a boil. Reduce heat to a simmer and cook for 30 minutes. Serve with warm whole-grain bread.

Tomato Cabbage Soup

Cabbage has traditionally been considered a "blood purifier," and recent research has confirmed its beneficial health effects. To date, it is believed that cabbage can help prevent cancers, stimulate the immune system, and, when eaten raw, prevent and heal ulcers. The simple ingredients belie the rich taste of this soup.

Serves 6

- 1 tablespoon vegetable oil
- 1 medium onion, chopped
- 1 teaspoon dried tarragon
- 1 teaspoon dried dill
- 1 teaspoon dill seed
- 3 cups green cabbage, cut into ¼-inch by 2-inch strips or shredded
- ½ cup chopped kale
- 6 cups stock (pages 198–200)
- 4 ripe tomatoes, peeled, seeded, and chopped (see page 269 for directions) (any juice reserved)
- 1 tablespoon finely chopped fresh parsley
- 1 tablespoon finely chopped fresh dill
- 1 tablespoon honey
- Salt
- Freshly ground black pepper

1. In a large stockpot, heat the oil over low heat. Add the onion and cook until golden brown.

2. Add the tarragon, dried dill, and dill seed. Cook 3 minutes and add the cabbage. Cover and cook until tender, about 10 to 15 minutes.

3. Add the kale, stock, tomatoes, and juice. Simmer 30 minutes.

4. Add the parsley, fresh dill, honey, and salt and pepper to taste. Simmer 2 minutes and serve.

Chicken or Turkey Soup

Delicious, nutritious, and so soothing, this soup contains all the major vitamins and minerals as well as complete protein, fiber, and carbohydrates.

Serves 6 to 8

1 tablespoon vegetable oil
1 medium onion, finely chopped
2 garlic cloves, finely chopped
2 cups finely chopped carrots
2 cups finely chopped celery stalks
2 cups finely chopped parsnips
1½ cups chopped mixed vegetables, such as greens, corn, rutabaga, green or yellow beans, mushrooms, or tomatoes
2 teaspoons dried thyme
2 teaspoons finely chopped fresh parsley
½ teaspoon dried marjoram
½ teaspoon dried sage
⅛ teaspoon freshly ground black pepper
1½ quarts chicken or turkey stock (page 200)
1½ cups cooked chicken or turkey, chopped
1 cup cooked brown rice or millet
1 tablespoon alcohol-free soy sauce or shoyu (if allergic to soy products, use 1½ teaspoons salt)

1. Heat the oil in a large stockpot. Add the onion and cook until golden brown. Add the garlic, carrots, celery, parsnips, mixed vegetables, and herbs. Cover and cook over medium-low heat for 8 minutes. Add the stock and chicken or turkey and simmer for 1 hour.

2. Add the cooked brown rice and soy sauce and cook a few minutes more to rewarm the rice.

Quick Vegetable Herb Soup

Serve piping hot with warm whole-grain bread. Loaded with vitamins and minerals, a bowl of this soup is a great way to get lots of vegetables.

Serves 4

1 tablespoon vegetable oil
1 medium onion, diced
1 carrot, washed and diced
1 celery stalk, finely chopped
1 potato, washed and diced
2½ cups mixed vegetables, diced (use any of the following: cabbage, corn, green or yellow string beans, kale, peas, parsnips, turnips, tomatoes, sweet potatoes, squash, zucchini)
1 bay leaf
1 teaspoon dried thyme
½ teaspoon dried rosemary
½ teaspoon dried dill
¼ teaspoon dried sage
1 tablespoon finely chopped fresh parsley or 1 teaspoon dried
5 cups stock (pages 198–200) or water (if using water, include tomato among the mixed vegetables)
½ teaspoon salt, or more to taste
¼ teaspoon freshly ground black pepper, or more to taste

1. In a large stockpot, warm the oil over medium-high heat. Add the onion and cook until translucent, about 5 minutes.

2. Add the carrot, celery, potato, and mixed vegetables, except string beans, which will cook quickly at the end. Add the bay leaf, thyme, rosemary, dill, and sage. Cook 3 minutes, stirring to combine all the vegetables and herbs.

3. Add the stock, cover, and bring to a boil. Reduce heat and simmer 20 minutes. Add any remaining vegetables and cook 5 more minutes. Season to taste and serve.

Ginger Carrot Soup

Carrots contain beta carotene, a precursor of vitamin A. Pureeing cooked carrots actually makes the vitamin A more available to the body. Other sources are yellow fruits and vegetables, dark green fruits and vegetables, eggs, liver, and whole milk products.

Serves 4 to 6

> 2 teaspoons dark sesame oil (if unavailable, use vegetable oil)
> 1 medium onion, minced
> 1 garlic clove, minced
> 1 teaspoon minced ginger root
> 8 carrots, peeled and finely chopped
> 2 sweet potatoes, peeled and finely chopped
> 1/4 teaspoon allspice
> 6 cups stock (pages 198–200) or water
> Salt
> Freshly ground black pepper
> 1 tablespoon lime zest for garnish

1. In a stockpot, warm the oil over low heat. Add the onion, garlic, and ginger and cook 3 minutes.

2. Add the carrots, sweet potatoes, and allspice. Stir and cook 3 minutes.

3. Add the stock and cook 35 minutes, or until the vegetables are soft.

4. Puree in small batches in a blender or food processor. Season to taste, garnish with lime zest, and serve.

Butternut Squash Soup

This soup is buttery but dairy-free. Squash soup has been popular for generations in South America. It's a great source of vitamin A and potassium, as well as vitamin C, calcium, and fiber.

Serves 6 to 8

2 tablespoons olive oil
1 medium onion, diced
2 garlic cloves, minced
1 bay leaf
2 teaspoons ground cumin
1 teaspoon dried oregano
2 large carrots, diced
2 medium potatoes, peeled and diced
3 pounds butternut squash, peeled, seeded, and diced
1 teaspoon salt
½ teaspoon freshly ground black pepper
6 to 8 cups stock (pages 198–200) or water
2 red bell peppers, seeded and minced

1. In a large stockpot, warm the oil over medium heat. Add the onion and sauté until golden. Add the garlic and cook 2 minutes, then add the bay leaf, cumin, and oregano and stir to combine flavors. Add the carrots, potatoes, squash, salt, and pepper. Cook 5 minutes, then add the stock. Bring to a boil, then reduce heat to a simmer and cook, covered, 1 hour.

2. Remove the bay leaf and puree the soup in small batches in a food processor or blender. Sprinkle the top with minced red peppers and serve.

Fresh Fruit Soup

Soup doesn't always have to be hot. This light summer soup is high in vitamins C and A and contains good amounts of manganese from the blueberries.

Serves 4

½ cup freshly squeezed orange juice, strained (about
    2 medium oranges)
2 tablespoons freshly squeezed lime juice, strained (about
    1½ limes
½ cup cold water
1–2 tablespoons honey or rice yinnie (page 112)
¼ teaspoon salt
3 cups very ripe cantaloupe, peeled and diced (about
    1½ small cantaloupes)
½ cup fresh blueberries
4 sprigs fresh mint

1. In a large bowl, combine the orange and lime juices, water, honey, and salt. Stir until completely blended.

2. Puree the melon in a blender or food processor. While the machine is running, pour the juice mixture into the fruit through the feed tube at the top of the processor or blender. Chill for 2 to 3 hours and garnish with blueberries and mint.

Blender Gazpacho

This refreshing cold soup provides us with vitamins A, B, and C, calcium, iron, magnesium, manganese, phosphorus, and potassium.

Serves 6 to 8

1½ pounds (6 to 7) ripe tomatoes, peeled (see page 269 for
    directions)
1–2 garlic cloves, peeled (or more to taste)
½ medium onion, chopped
1 carrot, coarsely chopped
1 small cucumber, peeled and coarsely chopped
1 green pepper, seeded and coarsely chopped
2 parsley sprigs, chopped

3–4 tablespoons chopped fresh basil (to taste)
Juice of 1 to 2 lemons (to taste)
Salt
Freshly ground black pepper
3–4 cups tomato juice

1. Blend together all the ingredients in a blender until smooth.

2. Chill several hours if possible. Adjust seasonings. The soup will keep in the refrigerator for 2 or 3 days.

Persian Red Bean and Carrot Soup

This traditional Persian soup is rich but low in calories and fat. The kidney beans have ample amounts of fiber and copper, a trace mineral found in all body tissues.

Serves 6 to 8

2 tablespoons vegetable oil
2 onions, finely chopped
3 garlic cloves, minced
1 medium eggplant, peeled and diced
2 tablespoons chopped fresh parsley
8 carrots, peeled and diced
1 celery stalk, diced
2 potatoes, peeled and diced
2 cups cooked kidney beans
7 cups stock (pages 198–200) or water
1 teaspoon salt
2 teaspoons freshly ground black pepper
Mint sprigs

1. In a large stockpot, warm the oil over medium heat. Add the onions and cook until translucent. Add the garlic and cook 1 minute. Add the eggplant, parsley, carrots, celery, and potatoes and stir to combine. Cook 15 minutes over low heat.

2. Add the beans, stock, salt, and pepper and cook 20 minutes. Remove from heat and puree in batches in a blender or food processor. Return to heat and simmer 5 minutes, or until soup is hot. Garnish with mint and serve.

Red Lentil Soup

This is a quick-cooking bean soup because unlike most beans, lentils need no soaking. Lentils contain protein, iron, thiamine, riboflavin, and niacin. This soup is meaty-tasting and very low in fat. Green lentils work just as well here. Cumin is a South American spice that gives this soup its characteristic flavor.

Serves 6 to 8

2 teaspoons extra virgin olive oil
3 shallots or 1 medium onion, minced
1 garlic clove, minced
1 carrot, finely chopped
1 parsnip, peeled and finely chopped
1 celery stalk, finely chopped
2 teaspoons ground cumin
1 bay leaf
2 cups red lentils, rinsed and picked over
7 cups vegetable stock (page 199)
1 tablespoon finely chopped fresh parsley or 1 teaspoon
    dried
1 tablespoon freshly squeezed lemon juice
2 tablespoons chopped scallions
½ teaspoon salt
¼ teaspoon freshly ground black pepper

1. In a large stockpot, heat the oil over medium heat. Add the shallots and cook until golden, about 7 minutes. Add the garlic and cook 2 minutes.

2. Add the carrot, parsnip, celery, and cumin. Cook 5 minutes.

3. Add the bay leaf, lentils, and stock. Cook 30 minutes.

4. Add the parsley, lemon juice, scallions, salt, and pepper. Cook 1 minute longer and serve.

Mushroom Barley Soup

The British have long used barley soup for tummy aches. This soothing soup is great for cold winter nights. Barley helps prevent dietary fats and cholesterol from being absorbed in the intestines.

Serves 6 to 8

1 tablespoon vegetable oil
1 medium onion, coarsely chopped
10 ounces mushrooms, sliced
1 garlic clove, minced
2 carrots, finely chopped
1 celery stalk, finely chopped
1 parsnip, peeled and finely chopped
1 turnip, peeled and finely chopped
1 sweet potato, peeled and finely chopped (optional),
   or 1 cup chopped white potato
1 cup corn kernels, fresh or frozen (optional), or 1 cup
   peas
2 bay leaves
1 tablespoon finely chopped fresh parsley
1 teaspoon dried thyme
1/2 teaspoon dried marjoram
1/2 teaspoon dried dill
1 cup barley
8 cups vegetable stock (page 199) or water
1 1/2 teaspoons salt
1/4 teaspoon freshly ground black pepper

1. In a large stockpot, warm the oil over medium heat. Add the onion and cook until light golden brown, about 6 minutes. Add the mushrooms and cook 7 minutes, until softened and lightly browned. Add the garlic and cook 2 minutes, stirring frequently. Add the remaining vegetables and herbs and cook 5 minutes. Add the barley, 6 cups of the stock, salt, and pepper, reduce heat to simmer, and cook 30 minutes.

2. Add the remaining 2 cups stock and cook 15 minutes more. Adjust seasonings and serve.

Salads

Salads are the cornucopias of wholefoods: hot or cold bouquets of vegetables, fruits, herbs, legumes, grains, pasta, chicken, fish, or meat. They can be given additional texture by adding crunchy seeds, nuts, or grains.

Dressings, like the salads they top, ought to be fresh. Extra-virgin olive oil with a dash of freshly squeezed lemon juice, a clove of garlic, and a pinch of herbs such as basil, oregano, chervil, or parsley is not only suitable for many salads but is the savory best choice. Add a bit of mustard for more zing or try orange juice as a sweetener. Here too, the limitless possibilities are inspiring. Use brown rice, apple cider, or balsamic vinegar instead of red or white wine vinegars, which contain alcohol. Many herb vinegars also contain alcohol, so read the label.

Sweet Potato Salad

Here's a welcome change from standard potato salad. Sweet potatoes are a super source of vitamin A, and this is super easy to make.

Serves 6

3 large sweet potatoes, rinsed and cut into 1-inch pieces
¼ cup olive oil
1 tablespoon balsamic vinegar (see Note)
3 garlic cloves, minced
2 tablespoons dried rosemary
½ teaspoon salt
⅛ teaspoon freshly ground black pepper
3 scallions, thinly cut on the diagonal

1. Fill a medium pot with water. Add the potatoes and bring the water to a boil. Cover and simmer until a fork can pierce the potatoes halfway, about 15 minutes. Drain the water from the pan. Quickly return the hot pan with the potatoes in it to the stove. Turn off the heat, cover the pan, and let the potatoes sit for 5 minutes. The potatoes will finish cooking but will not turn mushy. Remove the potatoes from the pan, place in a bowl, and chill slightly.

2. In a large bowl, combine the oil, vinegar, garlic, rosemary,

salt, and pepper. Add the scallions and chilled potatoes, toss, and serve.

Note: Lemon juice can be substituted for those who have a problem with the naturally occurring sulfites in balsamic vinegar.

Seasonal Veggie Salad with Crispy Tempeh Croutons

Tempeh is a fermented food made from whole soybeans. It's a great way to get the nutritional goodness of beans without the gas. The salad contains B vitamins including B_{12}, beta carotene, vitamin C, iron, potassium, phosphorus, protein, carbohydrates, and fiber.

Serves 4

Tempeh Croutons

    ¼ cup olive oil
    1 tablespoon soy sauce
    2 teaspoons toasted sesame oil
    ¼ teaspoon ground ginger
    4 ounces tempeh (page 107), sliced into 1-inch cubes

Salad

    1 head butter lettuce, cored, rinsed, and separated into
        leaves
    2 carrots, peeled and grated
    1 red onion, sliced
    1 green pepper, seeded and julienned
    1 yellow squash, sliced thin

1. In a medium bowl, combine the olive oil, soy sauce, sesame oil, and ginger. Add the tempeh, toss to coat, and set aside to marinate 10 minutes.

2. In the meantime, arrange the lettuce leaves on a flat platter. Arrange the remaining vegetables over the lettuce.

3. Warm a skillet over medium heat and with a slotted spoon add the tempeh, reserving the marinade. Brown on all sides, then remove with the slotted spoon to the platter and drizzle the remaining marinade over the salad.

Grilled Chicken Salad

This is by far the favorite recovery salad. Crispy grilled chicken with red potatoes, greens, and other vegetables is complemented by a lightly herbal garlic dressing. It's a meal in itself.

Serves 4

2 boneless, skinless chicken breasts, halved

Marinade

¼ cup olive oil
1 bay leaf
½ teaspoon dried rosemary
½ teaspoon dried thyme
1 garlic clove, minced
¼ teaspoon salt
Dash of freshly ground black pepper

Salad

2 medium red potatoes, rinsed and diced
½ cup green beans, rinsed, trimmed, and cut in half
1 carrot, peeled and grated
½ cup mixed vegetables, such as broccoli florets,
    cauliflower florets, snow peas, diced yellow squash, or
    zucchini
1 head green leaf lettuce, rinsed, cored, and cut into thin
    strips
2 medium tomatoes, cut into quarters
1 red pepper, cored, seeded, and julienned

Dressing

¼ cup extra virgin olive oil
¼ cup canola or safflower oil
3 tablespoons vinegar
1 tablespoon minced garlic
1 teaspoon dried parsley
½ teaspoon dried thyme
½ teaspoon paprika
Salt
Freshly ground black pepper

1. Slice the chicken breasts in half lengthwise. In a bowl, combine the olive oil, bay leaf, rosemary, thyme, garlic, salt, and pepper. Add the chicken and marinate at least 15 minutes.

2. Fill a small pot with water and bring to a boil. Add the potatoes and cook for 14 minutes, or until a fork easily pierces the potato. Drain and rinse in cold water.

3. Fill a medium pot with water. Bring to a boil and add the green beans, carrot, and mixed vegetables. Cook 2 minutes, then immediately drain, reserving ½ cup of the cooking water, and rinse with cold water.

4. Prepare a grill or preheat a broiler. Remove the chicken from the marinade and discard the marinade. Place the chicken on the grill or under the broiler for 4 minutes per side. Cooking time will vary depending on the thickness of the breast. After 8 minutes, check the chicken by piercing with a sharp knife. The juices should run clear when done. Remove from heat, let cool 2 to 3 minutes, and then slice into thin strips.

5. In a small bowl, whisk together the dressing ingredients with the reserved vegetable cooking liquid.

6. In a large bowl, toss the lettuce, tomatoes, and red pepper. Add the beans, carrot, and mixed vegetables. Add the chicken strips and dressing and toss again. Serve on chilled salad plates.

Soba Noodle Salad

Soba noodles are flat buckwheat noodles that are egg-free. They make a meal in themselves when paired with vegetables and Tahini Dressing. Tahini is a creamy paste made from sesame seeds. This nutritional salad has protein, complex carbohydrates, and many vitamins, minerals, and enzymes.

Serves 4

8 ounces buckwheat soba noodles or udon noodles
1 tablespoon toasted sesame oil
1 cup thin-sliced red cabbage
1 head green leaf lettuce, washed, drained, and sliced thin
½ cup broccoli florets
½ cup cauliflower florets
A few snow peas

Tahini Dressing

½ cup tahini
½ cup water
2 teaspoons brown rice vinegar or freshly squeezed
   lemon juice

2 medium daikon radishes, shredded
2 medium carrots, shredded
1 scallion, thinly sliced

1. In a large pot, bring 2 quarts of water to a boil. Add the soba noodles and cook 6 to 8 minutes. Remove the noodles and rinse them under cold water. Set the noodles aside and sprinkle with the toasted sesame oil.

2. Combine the cabbage and lettuce and divide among 4 bowls. Top with the noodles and surround the noodles with the broccoli, cauliflower, and snow peas.

3. In a medium bowl, combine the dressing ingredients by stirring until creamy smooth.

4. Pour the dressing over the salad and top with the shredded daikon, carrots, and scallion.

Rice Salad with Walnuts and Grapes

This rice salad contains all the goodness of whole grains: fiber, B vitamins, many minerals, and protein. Here whole-grain rice is complemented by walnuts, which are lower in calories and fat than most nuts. (Although nuts tend to be high in fat—50 percent or more—they contain predominantly unsaturated fatty acids.) Walnuts contain calcium, iron, magnesium, phosphorus, potassium, and zinc, as well as vitamins A, B-complex, and E. They contain about 15 percent protein, which is a good match with the proteins of rice.

Serves 4

1 cup short- or medium-grain brown rice
3 cups water
1 cup red or green seedless grapes, sliced in half
½ cup slightly crushed walnuts
1½ teaspoons finely chopped parsley
3 tablespoons olive oil
3–4 tablespoons freshly squeezed lemon juice
2 teaspoons honey
1 garlic clove, minced
¼ teaspoon salt
Pinch of freshly ground black pepper

1. Place the rice in a medium pot. Add the water and a dash of salt and bring to a boil. Lower heat, cover, and simmer 35 minutes. Remove from heat and allow to cool.

2. In a large bowl, gently combine the cooled rice, grapes, walnuts, and parsley. Do not overcombine, as the starch from the rice will produce a sticky salad.

3. In a smaller bowl, combine the oil, lemon juice, honey, garlic, salt, and pepper. Add to the salad mixture. Lightly mix and serve or chill and serve.

Pasta Salad

This is a tasty warm-weather salad, loaded with vitamins, minerals, and plenty of complex carbohydrates from the pasta.

Serves 4

Pasta

> 8 ounces whole-grain, vegetable, or Jerusalem artichoke
> pasta (page 268)
> 2 tablespoons olive oil
> 1 red bell pepper, thinly sliced
> 1 zucchini, thinly sliced
> 1 yellow squash, thinly sliced
> 2 carrots, peeled and thinly sliced
> 2 tablespoons finely chopped fresh parsley
> 2 teaspoons finely chopped fresh basil

Dressing

> ½ cup sun-dried tomatoes
> 1 cup warm water
> 2 garlic cloves, minced
> ¼ cup olive oil
> 2 tablespoons apple cider vinegar
> 2 teaspoons soy sauce

1. Bring a large pot of water to boil, add the pasta, and cook until al dente. Drain well, toss with the olive oil, and set aside until cool, then combine with the vegetables, parsley, and basil.

2. Make the dressing: In a small bowl, combine the sun-dried tomatoes and the water. Set aside for 15 minutes, then drain the tomatoes, reserving 2 tablespoons of the liquid, chop them, and add them to the pasta and vegetables. Then whisk together the reserved liquid with the garlic, oil, vinegar, and soy sauce. Drizzle over the salad and serve.

Tofu Mock Egg Salad

Tofu is a very digestible form of protein and a good source of iron, phosphorus, and B-complex vitamins. Tofu by itself has a very bland taste; its magic is that it can easily mock the flavor of other foods. Here tofu acts as a substitute for eggs in this special salad.

Serves 4 to 6

> 16 ounces firm tofu
> 2 tablespoons poppy seeds
> 1 red onion, finely chopped
> ½ cup grated carrot
> ½ cup finely chopped celery
> 1 red or green bell pepper, cored, seeded, and finely chopped
> ¼ teaspoon turmeric
> ½ teaspoon celery seeds
> 1 teaspoon parsley
> 1 tablespoon sweet paprika
> ¾ cup mayonnaise or eggless mayonnaise
> ½ teaspoon salt
> ¼ teaspoon freshly ground black pepper

1. Empty the tofu into a colander or strainer and lightly press to remove excess water. With your fingers or a fork, break up the tofu into small pieces. It will resemble scrambled egg whites. Let drain while preparing step 2.

2. In a small skillet, lightly toast the poppy seeds over medium heat to release the aroma of the seeds. After about 3 minutes they will start to pop. Be careful not to put your face near the pan. Remove from heat.

3. In a large bowl, combine the tofu with the poppy seeds, then add the vegetables, turmeric, celery seeds, parsley, paprika, and mayonnaise. Add salt and pepper, mix, and refrigerate to chill. Serve atop lettuce, stuffed in pita breads, or on other breads for sandwiches.

Quinoa Asparagus Salad

Quinoa has a wonderful texture and nutty taste. Read more about it on page 111. It's very high in protein, particularly in several amino acids that are typically low in grains (such as lysine and methionine).

Fresh spring asparagus is a wonderful source of many nutrients, especially folic acid. Folic acid is part of the B complex of vitamins. Since it is water soluble it can be lost in cooking water, and this is why steaming asparagus is preferable to boiling it. Folic acid can contribute to good mental health, brain function, and a healthy appetite.

Serves 4 to 6

Salad

> 2 cups quinoa
> 4 cups water
> Pinch of salt
> 1 pound fresh asparagus, tough ends removed, chopped
> 2 carrots, peeled and finely chopped
> 1 tablespoon finely chopped fresh parsley
> 1 pound fresh spinach, preferably bought loose rather than bagged

Dressing

> 3 tablespoons extra virgin olive oil
> 1 tablespoon apple cider vinegar
> 1 garlic clove, minced
> 1 teaspoon dried thyme
> ½ teaspoon dried marjoram
> ½ teaspoon dried rosemary

1. Rinse the quinoa under the tap and drain it well. Place the quinoa in a medium pot, add the water and salt, and bring to a boil. Cover and reduce to a simmer. Cook 15 to 20 minutes, or until water is absorbed and quinoa is fluffy. Remove to a bowl and let cool.

2. Fill a medium pot with 3 inches of water and bring to a boil. Add the asparagus and carrots in a steamer or stainless steel colander that sits above the water level, cover, and cook 2 minutes. Drain and rinse in cold water.

3. In a large bowl, combine the quinoa, asparagus, carrots, and parsley.

4. Rinse the spinach and divide among 4 salad plates.

5. In a medium bowl, combine the oil, vinegar, garlic, thyme, marjoram, and rosemary. Add the dressing to the salad and toss. Serve at room temperature atop the greens on the salad plates.

White Bean and Tuna Salad

Here's a super protein meal. White beans are 25 percent protein and tuna is 80 percent protein. Protein is vitally important for those in recovery to rebuild every tissue of the body. It is also helpful in maintaining blood sugar balance and for regeneration of liver cells. This salad also provides B-complex vitamins and most major minerals.

Serves 4 to 6

> 3 tablespoons extra virgin olive oil
> 1 tablespoon Pommery mustard or 2 teaspoons regular
>   mustard plus 1 teaspoon mustard seed
> ½ teaspoon celery seed
> ½ teaspoon dried rosemary
> 2 garlic cloves, minced
> 2 6½-ounce cans tuna, packed in water
> 2 cups cooked white beans (see Bean Cooking Chart,
>   page 248)
> ¼ teaspoon salt
> ¼ teaspoon freshly ground black pepper

1. In a large bowl, combine the oil, mustard, celery seed, rosemary, and garlic.

2. Drain the tuna. In a small bowl, mash the tuna with a fork to break it into small pieces. Add the tuna to the larger bowl and stir to mix.

3. Add the beans to the large bowl and lightly mix together. Add salt and pepper to taste and serve.

Red Bean Salad

Red bean salad is high in protein and contains good amounts of phosphorus, potassium, calcium, and some B vitamins.

Serves 4 to 6

  2 tablespoons olive oil
  1 tablespoon lemon juice
  1 teaspoon honey
  2 garlic cloves, minced
  1 tablespoon chopped fresh dill
  3 cups cooked kidney beans (see Bean Cooking Chart, page 248)
  1 cup diced carrots
  ½ cup diced yellow squash
  ½ cup diced zucchini
  ½ cup fresh corn
  ½ teaspoon salt
  ¼ teaspoon freshly ground black pepper

1. In a large bowl, combine the olive oil, lemon juice, honey, garlic, and dill.

2. Add the beans and vegetables and lightly toss together. Season with salt and pepper and serve, or chill and serve.

Crab and Avocado Salad with Tomato Basil Vinaigrette

Crab, like most shellfish, is a great source of complete protein, and it is very low in calories and fat. Crab contains many essential minerals, particularly magnesium—which is involved in the regulation of body temperature, bone growth, and nerve and muscle functions.

Avocados are a good source of protein; fiber; minerals such as potassium, magnesium, iron, calcium, and phosphorus; and vitamins A, B-complex, and C. Avocados contain up to 22 percent fat, mainly monounsaturated, but no cholesterol. Those in recovery who wish to gain weight would do well to add more avocados to their diets rather than rich desserts or junk food.

Serves 4

Salad

> 1 large ripe avocado
> 1 teaspoon freshly squeezed lemon juice
> 1 large cucumber, peeled and chopped into ½-inch pieces
> 1 green bell pepper, cored, seeded, and chopped into
>   ½-inch pieces
> 1 large ripe tomato, seeded and chopped into ½-inch pieces
> ½ pound cooked lump crab meat
> 1 head Boston or butter lettuce, washed and separated into
>   leaves

Dressing

> 1 very ripe medium tomato, peeled, seeded, and chopped
>   (see page 269 for directions)
> 1 tablespoon balsamic vinegar or rice vinegar
> 1 tablespoon freshly squeezed lemon juice
> ¼ cup olive oil
> 2 teaspoons prepared mustard
> 2 garlic cloves, minced
> ¼ teaspoon salt
> Pinch of freshly ground black pepper
> 2 tablespoons finely chopped fresh basil

1. Peel the avocado and remove the pit. Chop into ½-inch pieces, then sprinkle with the lemon juice to keep it from turning brown. Combine the avocado, cucumber, green pepper, tomato, and crab in a large bowl.

2. To make the dressing, in a blender combine the tomato with the vinegar, lemon juice, olive oil, mustard, garlic, salt, and pepper. Blend at high speed 2 minutes, then add the fresh basil. Blend a second or two to mix the basil, then pour the dressing over the salad ingredients and toss. Divide the lettuce into 4 portions on salad plates or bowls and place a serving of salad atop each bed of lettuce.

Warm Shrimp Salad with Orange Vinaigrette

Mixing hot and cold ingredients in salads has become a new classic, and it's easy to see why once you've tried hot whole shrimp drenched in an orange vinaigrette.

Serves 4

18–20 large to medium shrimp
2 large leeks
1 bunch arugula or 1 head curly leaf lettuce
½ bulb fennel, top discarded, julienned and blanched

Vinaigrette

⅓ cup olive oil
2½ tablespoons apple cider vinegar
½ cup freshly squeezed orange juice, approximately
    2 oranges
1 tablespoon orange zest, blanched
½ teaspoon salt
Freshly ground black pepper to taste

1. Peel the shrimp. Place each shrimp on its side on a cutting board. Using a small knife, slice the skin along the outside curve. Stop at the tail, leaving it intact. Pull the black vein out. Rinse the shrimp and pat dry.

2. Remove root ends of the leeks. Cut away the tough dark green ends of the leeks, leaving the tender light green and white ends. Cut the leeks into long thin strips. Rinse well and pat dry.

3. Separate the arugula leaves, rinse, and shake or pat dry. Divide the arugula into 4 servings and place on 4 plates.

4. In a medium bowl, combine the oil, vinegar, orange juice, orange zest, salt, and pepper.

5. Heat a large skillet over medium heat and add 2 tablespoons of the vinaigrette. Add the leeks and fennel and cook, stirring frequently, until they are light golden in color. Add the shrimp. Cook 2 minutes, stir to toss, and cook 1 minute more. Add 3 more tablespoons of the vinaigrette. Heat 2 minutes, divide into 4 servings, and place atop the arugula.

Note: A medium onion can be substituted for the leeks.

Green Bean, Carrot, and Beet Salad

We could call this crisp salad the iron-rich anti-cancer salad with silicon. Silicon is a trace mineral that can be found in connective tissues of the body. It is thought to be important in the prevention of osteoporosis.

Serves 4

3 medium beets, washed and sliced into rounds
3 medium carrots, sliced into ¼-inch rounds
2 cups fresh green beans (see Note)
2 cups rinsed and torn spinach leaves

Dressing

⅓ cup apple cider vinegar or brown rice vinegar
⅓ cup toasted sesame oil
¼ cup canola or safflower oil
2 teaspoons prepared mustard
1 teaspoon salt or umeboshi vinegar
1 teaspoon honey
½ cup water

1. Fill a medium pot with 2 inches of water and bring to a boil. Add the beets in a steamer or stainless steel colander and bring to a boil. Cover and cook 4 to 5 minutes, then add the carrots and green beans. Cover and cook 3 minutes more; remove from heat.

2. Drop the vegetables into ice water to stop the cooking process.

3. In a large salad bowl, combine the vinegar, oils, mustard, and salt. Mix well and add the honey and water, mixing well again.

4. Add the beets, carrots, and green beans. Stir to coat with dressing. Add the spinach, toss, and serve.

Note: Haricots verts, the tiny French green beans, are good here.

Three Salad Dressings for Green and Raw Vegetable Salads

Light Dressing for Raw Vegetables

Makes ½ cup

> ¼ cup olive oil
> 2 teaspoons rice vinegar
> 1 tablespoon umeboshi vinegar
> Freshly ground black pepper
> ¼ cup water

1. In a medium bowl, whisk together the oil, vinegars, and pepper. Whisk in the water, then add the dressing to a bowl of vegetables or greens, toss, and serve.

2. Store the dressing separately for 1 to 2 weeks in a jar in the refrigerator. The dressing will become stronger in flavor over time.

Sesame Ginger Dressing

Makes 1 cup

> ⅓ cup canola oil
> ¼ cup rice vinegar
> 3 tablespoons dark sesame oil
> 1 tablespoon soy sauce
> 1 tablespoon apple juice
> 1 tablespoon toasted sesame seeds (see Note)
> 1 teaspoon minced fresh ginger root
> 1 garlic clove, minced

1. In a medium bowl, whisk together all the ingredients.

2. Add the dressing to raw vegetables such as carrots, celery, cucumbers, tomatoes, radishes, sprouts, and zucchini. The dressing can be stored for 1 week in a jar in the refrigerator.

Note: To toast sesame seeds, heat them in a dry skillet over low heat until light brown in color.

Herb Dressing for Greens
This is a great substitute for high-fat rich dressings.

Makes 3 cups

1 pound soft tofu
1½ cups water
2 tablespoons canola oil
2 tablespoons apple cider vinegar
2 tablespoons chopped fresh dill
1 tablespoon dried mustard
1 tablespoon chopped fresh basil
1 tablespoon chopped fresh mint
1 teaspoon dried thyme
1 teaspoon salt
½ teaspoon freshly ground black pepper

1. In a blender or food processor, combine all the ingredients. Blend until smooth and well mixed. Pour over salad.

2. The dressing can be stored in jars in the refrigerator up to 5 days.

Sandwiches

A recipe for a sandwich may seem like a contradiction. After all, sandwiches are probably the greatest of culinary improvisations—the first convenience food, the perfect carryall. Two pieces of bread with something tasty tucked in the center can be a complete meal in minutes (or less).

Sandwiches can be made from whole-grain breads, rolls, pitas, or flat breads. For spreads, try homemade salad dressing, soy mayonnaise, chutneys, salsas, creamy tahini, or nut butters. Stuff sandwiches with combinations of wholefoods. Imagination is your best guide when making a sandwich.

Sandwiches can be a great way to get lots of wholefoods in your diet. The following are a few of our favorites.

Stuffed Pita with Tahini Dressing

This nutrient-rich sandwich contains living enzymes from raw vegetables and sprouts. Sunflower seeds are extraordinarily nutritious. They provide vitamins A, D, E, and B-complex and traces of fluorine. They are only 20 percent fat, which is unsaturated.

Serves 2

> 1 small tomato, chopped
> 1 carrot, finely chopped
> 1 celery stalk, finely chopped
> 1 red or green bell pepper, seeded and finely chopped
> ½ cup shredded lettuce (green leaf, romaine, etc.)
> ¼ cup finely shredded red cabbage
> 2 whole-grain pitas, halved or split
> ½ cup sprouts
> ¼ cup sunflower seeds

Dressing

> ½ cup tahini
> ½ cup water
> 2 garlic cloves, minced
> 1 tablespoon soy sauce

1. Mix all the vegetables except the sprouts.

2. Blend the dressing ingredients in a blender.

3. Add the dressing to the vegetables and stuff the mixture into the pita. Stuff the top of each pita with some of the sprouts and sprinkle in the sunflower seeds.

Tuna Vegetable Salad on Toast

This is a high-protein sandwich that contains beta carotene, vitamin C, and B-complex vitamins.

Serves 2

> 1 6-ounce can white tuna packed in water
> 1 carrot, finely chopped
> 1 celery stalk, finely chopped
> 1 red bell pepper, seeded and finely chopped
> ½ scallion, finely chopped
> ¼ cup chopped peeled cucumber
> ¼ cup mayonnaise
> 1 teaspoon dried thyme
> ½ teaspoon mustard seeds
> ½ teaspoon rosemary
> ¼ teaspoon celery seeds
> Dash of freshly ground black pepper
> 4 slices whole wheat bread
> 2 large leaves romaine or green leaf lettuce

1. In a large bowl, combine the tuna, carrot, celery, red pepper, scallion, and cucumber.

2. In a small bowl, mix the mayonnaise, thyme, mustard seeds, rosemary, celery seeds, and black pepper. Add this to the tuna mixture and mix well.

3. Toast the bread.

4. Top 2 slices of bread with lettuce and tuna salad. Top them with the remaining 2 slices of toast, slice, and serve.

Tempeh Reubens with a Side of Carrot Raisin Salad

Grilled marinated tempeh makes a healthy low-fat, low-sodium reuben. It contains enzymes that make the soybeans very digestible. Tempeh provides valuable B vitamins. Both tempeh and sauerkraut are vegetarian sources of vitamin B_{12}.

Serves 2

> 6 ounces tempeh (page 107)
> ½ cup olive oil
> 2 tablespoons soy sauce
> 2 garlic cloves, crushed
> 4 slices rye bread
> 2 teaspoons prepared mustard
> ½ cup low-salt sauerkraut

1. Slice the tempeh into thin 2 x 2-inch pieces.

2. In a deep flat dish, combine the olive oil, soy sauce, and garlic. Place the tempeh in the soy mixture and gently turn the pieces to coat. Let them sit at least 10 minutes or refrigerate overnight.

3. Preheat the broiler. Place the tempeh on a baking sheet or broiling pan and broil 4 minutes on each side, or until crispy on the outside.

4. Take 2 slices of bread and brush one side of each slice with mustard; top with tempeh, sauerkraut, and the other slices of bread and serve.

Carrot Raisin Salad

Makes 2 cups

2 tablespoons oil
1 tablespoon freshly squeezed lemon juice or apple cider
   vinegar
4 large carrots, washed and shredded
½ cup golden raisins
½ teaspoon chopped fresh dill

1. Combine the oil and lemon juice in a bowl. Add the carrots, raisins, and dill and toss well.

2. Chill or serve at room temperature.

Tofu Salad Sandwich

A high-protein sandwich.

Serves 2

6 slices dark bread (rye or pumpernickel), toasted
4 crisp lettuce leaves, rinsed
1¼ cups of Tofu Mock Egg Salad (page 221)

1. Layer the sandwiches starting with 2 slices of toast, then lettuce and one-fourth of the salad on each slice. Top with another toast, repeat the lettuce and salad layer, and top with the third toast.

2. Cut the sandwiches into quarters and secure each piece with a toothpick.

Grilled Vegetable Sandwich

Grilling is a great way to serve vegetables, and these make for a special sandwich stuffing.

Serves 2

> 2 tablespoons olive oil
> 2 garlic cloves, crushed
> 1 red or green bell pepper, cut in half and seeded
> ½ small zucchini, sliced
> 1 medium onion, thinly sliced
> 2 6-inch pieces whole wheat baguette, sliced in half
>   lengthwise
> ½ cup Fresh Tomato Basil Sauce (page 269) or other
>   tomato sauce
> 2 slices soy cheese or mozzarella cheese (optional)

1. Preheat the broiler. Combine the oil and garlic in a medium bowl.

2. Place the pepper halves on a baking sheet or broiling pan skin-side up and broil until black. You may need to keep a close eye on them, since the time will vary from oven to oven. Remove and place in a paper bag.

3. Place the zucchini and onion slices in the bowl with the oil and garlic and toss to coat. Spread them on the baking sheet and cook until crispy, about 5 minutes. Turn them over and cook the other side. Remove.

4. Remove the pepper halves from the bag and peel. The black skin should slide off. Slice the pepper halves into 4 pieces each.

5. Place the opened baguettes on the baking sheet and brush generously with the tomato sauce. Place under the broiler for 4 minutes. Remove and top with the pepper, onion, zucchini, and cheese and return to the broiler for 2 minutes more. Remove and serve.

Italian Chicken Salad Sandwich

Serves 2

Vinaigrette

¼ cup olive oil
2 tablespoons canola oil
1 tablespoon vinegar (any kind)
1 tablespoon freshly squeezed lemon juice
2 garlic cloves, minced
1 teaspoon honey
1 tablespoon Pommery mustard
1 tablespoon finely chopped fresh basil or 1 teaspoon dried

2 cups chopped cooked chicken
½ medium cucumber, peeled, seeded, and chopped
10 black olives
2 8-inch pieces flat bread

1. In a large bowl, mix the oils, vinegar, and lemon juice together. Stir in the remaining vinaigrette ingredients.

2. Add the chicken, cucumber, and olives and toss.

3. Preheat the broiler. Spread one edge of the flat bread with half the chicken salad and roll closed. Place each roll on a baking sheet seam-side down so the sandwich doesn't roll open.

4. Place rolls under the broiler to toast the flat bread (this makes it cracker crispy and keeps it closed) and serve.

Pita Pizzas

The ever-popular pizza made home-style is a good use of the tomato sauce from last night's leftover spaghetti. It's also great sliced as a party canapé.

Serves 2

> ½ onion, thinly sliced
> ½ small zucchini, thinly sliced (substitute summer squash, ½ cup broccoli or eggplant, etc.)
> 2 whole-grain pitas
> 2–4 tablespoons olive oil
> ¾ cup Fresh Tomato Basil Sauce (page 269) or other tomato sauce
> ½ cup grated mozzarella cheese or mock mozzarella soy cheese

1. Preheat the broiler. Place the vegetables on a baking pan or sheet. Brush both sides with olive oil. Place under the broiler and lightly cook until golden, about 5 minutes, and remove.

2. Brush the pitas with 1 tablespoon olive oil. Toast the pitas under the broiler for 3 minutes. Remove and brush with tomato sauce, top with zucchini slices, then onions. Sprinkle the cheese on top and place back under the broiler until the cheese is melted and slightly golden. Slice into quarters and serve. These can be served chilled as well.

Cucumber Avocado Sandwich

The creamy, nutty avocados in this sandwich provide protein, beneficial fats, and fourteen minerals, including more potassium than in bananas. Avocados also have nutrients that aid blood and tissue regeneration. The sprouts add super nutrients and the sun-dried tomatoes heighten the flavor.

Serves 2

> 2 whole wheat croissants or whole-grain rolls
> 4–6 sun-dried tomatoes drenched in olive oil

½ cucumber, washed and sliced in ¼-inch pieces if
   organically grown, otherwise peeled and sliced
½ avocado, peeled and thinly sliced (see Note)
1 cup mixed sprouts

1. Slice the croissants open diagonally and top one side of each with the sun-dried tomatoes, cucumber, avocado, and sprouts.

2. Close and serve.

Note: Leave the pit inside the unused portion and use within 2 days.

Turkey Coleslaw Sandwich

Our favorite recovery sandwich. It contains protein, complex carbohydrates, fiber, vitamins A and B-complex, and the anti-cancer properties of cabbage.

Serves 2

Coleslaw

   2 tablespoons canola oil
   1 tablespoon apple cider vinegar
   1 teaspoon honey or rice yinnie (page 112)
   Dash of salt
   ½ teaspoon celery seeds
   1 cup shredded cabbage
   ⅓ cup shredded carrots

   2 large whole wheat rolls
   6 ounces sliced turkey breast
   2 slices Swiss cheese or soy cheese (optional)

1. In a large bowl, mix the oil, vinegar, and honey. Add the salt, celery seeds, cabbage, and carrot and let the flavors combine for 10 minutes or longer.

2. Slice open the rolls. Layer them with the coleslaw, turkey, and cheese. Close and serve.

Soyburgers

If you're trying to cut back on red meat, give this recipe a try. Soybeans are 38 percent protein, the highest in the vegetable kingdom; in fact, 1 cup of soybeans has more protein than a 4-ounce beef patty. Soybeans are also a good source of potassium, with 972 milligrams per cup. They contain calcium, phosphorus, iron, vitamin A, and 20 percent fat (mainly polyunsaturated). (Hamburger meat is anywhere from 30 to 50 percent saturated fat.) These burgers disappear pretty fast, so you can double the recipe and freeze half of them until use.

Serves 8

1 cup sunflower seeds
¼ cup alcohol-free soy sauce or tamari
2 cups cooked soybeans
½ cup cooked brown rice
½ cup cooked wild rice (see Note)
4 tablespoons finely chopped scallions
5 tablespoons finely chopped fresh parsley
1 carrot, peeled and finely chopped
1 celery stalk, finely chopped
2 garlic cloves, minced
2 eggs
¾ cup unbleached whole wheat pastry flour
¼ cup vegetable oil
1 teaspoon salt
⅛ teaspoon freshly ground white pepper
16 slices whole-grain bread
8 cups lettuce leaves
2 tomatoes, thickly sliced
2 cups sprouts
Mustard or mayonnaise
1 avocado, peeled, pitted, and sliced (optional)

1. Preheat the broiler.

2. In a medium skillet, toast the sunflower seeds for 5 minutes over medium-low heat, shaking the skillet back and forth to prevent the seeds from sticking and burning. Add the soy sauce and continue shaking the pan until the seeds have absorbed the sauce and are crispy, about 5 minutes.

3. In a food processor, meat grinder, or blender, process the sunflower seeds, soybeans, rice, scallions, parsley, carrot, celery, and garlic until they form a crumbly meal. Return the mixture to the skillet and cook over low heat 10 minutes, covered, then turn out into a large bowl.

4. In a small bowl, beat the eggs. Add the flour, oil, salt, and pepper and mix. Add this mixture to the soybean mixture and combine well. Shape into 8 small patties.

5. Broil for 10 minutes per side, flipping often to avoid burning the burgers. Serve on whole-grain bread with lettuce, tomato, sprouts, and either mustard or mayonnaise. A slice of avocado is a delicious addition.

Note: Instead of using the wild rice, you can increase the cooked brown rice to 1 cup.

Pinto Bean Burritos

Mexican pinto beans are often cooked in pork fat. This is a healthier version that's high in protein and fiber and low in fat. Serve with brown rice or millet.

Serves 4 to 6

2 tablespoons vegetable oil
1 large onion, chopped
3 garlic cloves, minced
2 teaspoons ground cumin
1 teaspoon ground coriander
1 red bell pepper, diced
1 jalapeño pepper, minced (only for those who like it hot)
1½ cups cooked black beans (see Note)
Salt and freshly ground black pepper
4–6 whole wheat burritos (available in frozen foods section of supermarkets or health food stores)
1 cup finely chopped or shredded lettuce
1 cup finely chopped tomato
1 cup finely chopped or shredded assorted vegetables, such as cucumbers, red onions, carrots, summer squash, or celery

1. In a large skillet, heat the oil. Add the onion and cook until golden. Add the garlic, cumin, coriander, and peppers, lower the heat, and cook 3 minutes. Add the beans and stir to combine. Add salt and pepper to taste. Cover and simmer until the beans are warmed, about 8 minutes.

2. Warm the burritos according to the package directions or in a warm oven for only a few minutes. Be careful not to warm them to a crisp, as burritos should be soft and pliable.

3. Spoon ¼ cup of the beans into the center of an opened burrito. Sprinkle on some lettuce, tomato, and mixed vegetables and serve. These are especially nice with a side dish of salsa and make a complete protein meal when served with a side dish of brown rice.

Note: Cook the beans until they are very soft, or puree half the cooked beans in a blender or food processor and then recombine.

Grains

Grains—including rye, oats, barley, brown rice, quinoa, and amaranth
—sustain much of the world's population. They can be tasty side
dishes, satisfying additions to soups and salads, and, when paired with
beans, complete-protein main dishes. Whole grains are complex carbohydrates that provide E and B vitamins, folic acid, and many minerals,
including chromium, magnesium, manganese, copper, molybdenum,
selenium, zinc, silicon, iron, calcium, and potassium. The nutrients in
whole grains contribute to the proper functioning of the entire body,
from the nervous system, to the digestive tract, to carbohydrate and
lipid metabolisms.

The following recipes will help you make whole grains an integral
and delicious part of your recovery diet.

17.1 GRAIN COOKING CHART

One Cup	Water (Cups)	Cooking Time	Yield (Cups)
Amaranth	2	25 min.	2
Barley			
Hulled	3	60 min.	3
Pearl	2	30 min.	2½–3
Buckwheat (kasha)	2	15 min.	2½
Bulgur	1½–2	15–20 min.	3
Millet	2	30–40 min.	3–3½
Rolled oats	2–2½	15–20 min.	2½
Quinoa	2	15–20 min.	4
Brown rice			
Short grain	2½	45–55 min.	3
Long grain	2	45–50	3
Rye	2	1½–2 hours	3½
Triticale	2	1½ hours	2
Wheat berries	3	1½–2	2½–3
Wild rice	3	1–1¼	3–3½

To cook grains, bring water to a boil, add grain and a pinch of salt, cover, and reduce heat to a simmer.

To pressure cook grains, reduce the water by one-third and cook 10 minutes for bulgur, 15 minutes for barley or brown rice, and 20 minutes for rye, triticale, wheat berries, or wild rice.

Bulgur can also be cooked by simply pouring boiling water over it in a bowl and covering the bowl for 15 minutes.

Millet and kasha can be toasted in a small amount of oil for 5 minutes until the aroma of the grain is strong before adding water. This adds a roasted taste and helps prevent the grains from becoming too mushy.

Wild Rice Pilaf

Wild rice is a rich source of vitamin B$_2$ (riboflavin). This pilaf goes well with chicken, duck, turkey, or fish and can also be used as a stuffing for poultry.

Serves 6 to 8

2 cups wild rice
5 cups stock (pages 198–200) or water
1 tablespoon vegetable oil
1 medium onion, finely chopped
2 garlic cloves, minced
1 cup finely chopped mushrooms
1 medium carrot, finely chopped
1 celery stalk, finely chopped
½ cup currants or raisins
¼ cup crushed pecans (optional)
1 teaspoon dried parsley
1 teaspoon dried sage
½ teaspoon dried rosemary
Salt
Freshly ground black pepper

1. Put the rice and stock in a medium pot, cover, and bring to a boil. Lower the heat and simmer for 45 minutes, or until the rice grains are tender and split open. Remove the pot from the heat and keep it covered for 10 minutes.

2. Heat the oil in a large skillet over medium heat. Add the onion and garlic and cook until golden. Add the mushrooms, carrot, celery, and currants and cook 5 minutes. Add the pecans and herbs and cook 4 minutes more. Then add the rice and stir well to combine. Add salt and pepper to taste. Serve.

Kasha

This recipe for kasha (roasted buckwheat) is a variation on a popular Eastern European dish. In addition to being great at dinner and lunch, kasha makes a good breakfast cereal. It is high in bioflavonoids (which are crucial for the absorption of vitamin C) and is also a good source of niacin.

Serves 4

1 tablespoon olive oil
1 medium red onion, finely chopped
1 cup mushrooms, finely chopped
2 carrots, peeled and finely chopped
1 tablespoon finely chopped fresh parsley
1 teaspoon dried thyme
1 cup kasha
2¼ cups water
Salt
Freshly ground black pepper

1. In a large skillet, heat the oil over medium heat. Add the onion and cook until golden. Add the mushrooms and cook 5 minutes until they are golden. Add the carrots, parsley, and thyme and cook 3 minutes.

2. Add the kasha and water. Cover and cook on low heat for 15 minutes. Salt and pepper to taste and serve.

Quinoa Pilaf

This pilaf is fast and easy. Quinoa cooks more quickly than other grains and yet has the highest protein value. It works well with fish main courses such as baked salmon steaks or red snapper. It can also be chilled and served on a bed of lettuce for a salad.

Serves 6

    4 cups stock (pages 198–200) or water
    2 cups quinoa, well rinsed
    1 tablespoon vegetable oil
    3 shallots, finely chopped
    2 carrots, peeled and finely chopped
    1 tomato, finely chopped
    1 tablespoon finely chopped fresh dill
    1 teaspoon dried basil
    1 teaspoon dried thyme
    Salt
    Freshly ground black pepper

1. In a medium pot, bring the stock or water and the quinoa to a boil over high heat. Reduce heat to low, cover, and cook 20 minutes.

2. In a large skillet, heat the oil over medium heat. Add the shallots and cook until dark golden. Add the carrots, tomato, dill, basil, and thyme and cook 5 minutes, or until most of the liquid from the tomato evaporates. Add the warm quinoa and stir to combine. Add salt and pepper to taste and serve.

New Orleans Red Rice

Red wehani rice is a rich and nutty-tasting natural in this New Orleans rice recipe. Often sold as Christmas rice, wehani is similar to cracked wheat when cooked and is a bit lighter in texture than brown rice. Serve with black or kidney beans or roasted chicken.

Serves 6 to 8

> 1 cup wehani (red) rice
> 2½ cups stock (pages 198–200) or water
> 2 bay leaves
> 1 tablespoon vegetable oil
> 1 medium yellow onion, finely chopped
> 2 garlic cloves, minced
> 2 celery stalks, finely chopped
> 1 green bell pepper, seeded and finely chopped
> 2 teaspoons finely chopped fresh parsley or 1 teaspoon
> dried
> 1 teaspoon dried thyme
> 1 teaspoon dried oregano
> ¼ teaspoon ground allspice
> ¼ teaspoon freshly ground black pepper
> Salt

1. Place the rice, stock, and bay leaves in a medium pot. Cover the pot. Bring to a boil, reduce heat, and simmer 45 minutes. Remove the pot from heat and let it sit 5 minutes. Remove the cover and fluff the rice with a fork. Remove the bay leaves.

2. In a large skillet, heat the oil over medium heat. Add the onion and garlic and cook until the onion is translucent, about 5 minutes. Add the celery, green pepper, parsley, thyme, oregano, allspice, and black pepper. Stir everything together and cook 5 minutes.

3. Add the rice to the skillet and lightly toss. Add salt to taste and serve.

Mexican Millet with Pinto Beans

After your gastrointestinal tract has begun to heal, it can be nice to wake up your taste buds with some mildly spicy Mexican food. Millet tastes a bit like corn and is rich in B_1, B_2, calcium, iron, niacin, phosophorus, and potassium. It also has up to three times the complex carbohydrates of most other grains. Pinto beans have one of the highest amounts of soluble fiber of the entire bean family. Like millet, pinto beans have generous amounts of B_1 (thiamine).

Serves 6

> 2 tablespoons vegetable oil, such as canola
> 1 large red onion, finely chopped
> 2 garlic cloves, minced
> 2 carrots, finely chopped
> 2 tomatoes, peeled, seeded, and coarsely chopped (see page 269 for directions)
> 1 red or green bell pepper, seeded and finely chopped
> 1 celery stalk, finely chopped
> 2 teaspoons ground cumin
> 1 teaspoon dried oregano
> 1 teaspoon ground coriander
> $1/2$ teaspoon turmeric
> 2 cups cooked millet
> 1 teaspoon salt
> $1/4$ teaspoon freshly ground black pepper
> 1 cup cooked pinto beans (page 248)
> 2 tablespoons finely chopped cilantro, for garnish (optional)

1. Preheat the oven to 350° F. In a large skillet, warm the oil over medium heat. Add the onion and garlic. Cook 4 minutes and add the carrots, tomatoes, pepper, celery, and spices and cook 5 minutes to blend the flavors.

2. Add the cooked millet and stir to combine. Add salt and pepper to taste. Add the pinto beans and gently stir to combine. Avoid overstirring, which will turn the beans to mush.

3. Bake for 30 minutes in a covered casserole dish or baking dish covered with aluminum foil. Remove from the oven and serve, garnished with cilantro if desired.

Saffron Rice with Raisins and Coconut

This Indian rice dish is delicately spiced and perfect with a curried chicken casserole, a roast turkey, or curried garbanzo beans.

Serves 4

¹⁄₂ teaspoon loosely packed saffron
1 cup hot water
1 cup stock (pages 198–200) or water
1 cup brown basmati rice or long-grain rice, rinsed
Salt
1 tablespoon vegetable oil
1 white medium onion, finely chopped
¹⁄₈ teaspoon ground cardamom seeds (see Note)
¹⁄₄ teaspoon ground cinnamon
1 red bell pepper, seeded and finely chopped
¹⁄₂ cup raisins
¹⁄₄ cup unsweetened dried shredded coconut
¹⁄₈ teaspoon freshly ground white pepper
¹⁄₄ cup chopped peanuts (optional)

1. Place the saffron in a small bowl. Cover with the hot water and let stand for 15 minutes.

2. Place the saffron water in a medium pot and add 1 cup of stock or water. Bring to a boil over high heat. And the rice and bring to a boil again. Add a dash of salt, cover, lower the heat, and simmer for 45 minutes. Remove the cover and fluff the rice with a fork.

3. In a large skillet, heat the oil and add the onion. Cook until translucent, about 5 minutes. Add the cardamom, cinnamon, red pepper, and raisins. Cook 5 minutes, or until the pepper is softened but still crunchy.

4. Add the rice, coconut, 1 teaspoon salt, and pepper. Stir gently to combine. Do not overstir or the rice will become sticky. Sprinkle with the peanuts.

Note: Press the whole cardamom open. Remove the seeds and discard the green hull. Grind the seeds with a mortar and pestle, coffee grinder, or food processor.

Beans

Beans are one of the least expensive and most nutritious wholefoods. They can be used in soups, salads, casseroles, or sandwich spreads or as side dishes with fish, poultry, or meat. They can even be added to homemade breads or muffins to increase their protein content. The nutritional content of specific beans varies, so eat many different types.

Beans come dried or in cans. The best choice is dried beans, but canned beans will do in a pinch (see the Prepared Foods list in chapter 15). Beans should not be cooked with salt or spice mixes that contain salt, since salt causes the beans' skins to harden and can even prevent cooking.

17.2 BEAN COOKING CHART

(after soaking)

One Cup	Cooking Time (Hours)	Water (Cups)	Yield (Cups)
Black beans	1½	4	2
Black-eyed peas	1	3	2
Chick peas (Garbanzos)	3	4	4
Kidney beans	1½	3	2
Lentils	½	3	2¼
Lima beans	1½	2	1¼
Pinto beans	2½	3	2
Split peas	1	3	2¼
White beans	1½	3	2

Beans can be cooked more quickly in a pressure cooker (see individual cooker for instructions). Beans often fall apart when cooked using this method, which is fine for soups and purees. Older beans will require a longer cooking time.

Dried beans must be soaked and drained before cooking. The ratio of water to beans should be three to one; you can either soak the beans overnight or bring them to a boil for 2 minutes and then let them soak for 1 hour. When cooking beans, we suggest adding a 3-inch piece of kombu to the pot to add a rich meaty flavor and increase the beans' digestibility.

Beans may be difficult to digest if you are unaccustomed to eating them. You can avoid this problem by adding them to your diet gradually and by using the special cooking methods described on page 105 in chapter 12.

White Beans and Fennel

The unusual taste combination of this dish of creamy white beans and crunchy anise-flavored fennel is one of our favorites. Serve with a simple pasta or grain dish or with salmon.

Serves 4

> 2 cups cooked white beans (either navy beans or large great northern beans; page 248)
> 2 tablespoons extra virgin olive oil
> 1 garlic clove, minced
> 1 fennel bulb, rinsed and julienned (save the green feathery tops for a garnish)
> Salt
> Freshly ground black pepper

1. Fill a pot with water and reheat the beans if they are not freshly cooked and hot. Rinse and keep warm.

2. In a skillet, warm the oil over medium heat. Add the garlic and fennel and cook over medium-low heat for 7 minutes, or until the fennel is softened but slightly crunchy. Do not let the oil smoke or the garlic brown during this process. Add the warm beans, salt, and pepper to the skillet and gently stir to combine. Serve and garnish with the green tops of the fennel bulb.

Lentil Pâté

This recipe was donated by Elis Tobin, a creative wholefoods chef from Brooklyn, New York. It's the best-tasting lentil pâté in Brooklyn, at the very least, and a favorite of recovery cooks everywhere.

Serves 8

⅓ cup safflower oil
3 medium leeks, washed and sliced
1 red medium onion, diced
Salt
1 teaspoon dried thyme
1 teaspoon garlic powder
1 tablespoon tamari
2 cups green lentils, rinsed and picked over
4½ cups water
1 bay leaf
1 tablespoon tahini
1 tablespoon white miso (page 107)
¼ bunch cilantro leaves, stems removed, finely chopped
¾ cup whole wheat bread crumbs (preferably Italian
    flavored)
Pinch of white pepper
Lettuce

1. In a 4-quart saucepan, heat the safflower oil on medium heat. Add the leeks and onion and a pinch of salt. Stir and then cover. Let the leeks and onion "sweat" for about 8 minutes, or until they are very soft. Add the thyme, garlic powder, and tamari. Stir for 2 minutes.

2. Add the lentils, water, and bay leaf to the pan. Bring to a boil, lower heat to medium, cover, and simmer 45 minutes. Stir the lentils once or twice while they are cooking.

3. Preheat the oven to 375° F. When the lentils are soft, remove the bay leaf and transfer the lentils to a food processor or blender. Puree for a few minutes. While the machine is running add the tahini, miso, and cilantro leaves through the feed tube of the food processor or blender. Slowly add the bread crumbs. Puree until smooth. Season with white pepper and salt.

4. Oil a 9 x 5-inch loaf pan and sprinkle with bread crumbs. Pour or spoon in the puree and bake for 1 hour, or until the top is browned. Allow the pâté to cool. It is best if it is refrigerated in the pan overnight before unmolding; the flavor and texture will be enhanced. Unmold onto a bed of lettuce, slice, and serve.

Chick Pea Tomato Curry with Spinach

Most curries contain ghee (clarified butter), but this version is much lower in fat. Chick peas served over basmati rice make complementary proteins that are nutritionally superior to either alone.

Serves 4

> 2 tablespoons vegetable oil
> 2 medium onions, chopped
> 4 garlic cloves, minced
> 1 1-inch piece ginger root, peeled and minced
> 1 tablespoon curry powder
> 2 cups cooked chick peas (page 248)
> 3 cups fresh spinach leaves, washed and patted dry
> 6 fresh tomatoes, peeled and chopped (see page 269 for directions), plus ½ cup tomato juice, or 1 12-ounce can whole tomatoes, with juice
> ½ cup green beans (optional)
> 3 cups cooked brown basmati rice

1. In a large sauté pan, heat the oil over medium heat. Add the onions and cook until golden, about 4 minutes. Add the garlic and ginger and cook 3 minutes. Add the curry powder and cook on medium-low heat for 3 minutes more.

2. Add the chick peas and spinach. Cover and cook until the spinach wilts. Add the tomatoes and simmer 20 minutes, stirring occasionally. Add the green beans for the last 5 minutes. Serve over the basmati rice.

Aduki Beans Oriental

Adukis (also called azukis or adzukis) contain carbohydrates, vitamins A and B-complex, iron, calcium, and phosphorus. In Oriental medicine aduki beans are said to strengthen the kidneys. This dish works well with sautéed greens for a meatless main meal or as a side dish with Sole Hazeldine (page 290).

Serves 4

2 cups uncooked aduki beans
1 2-inch piece kombu (optional)
1 teaspoon minced fresh ginger root
1 garlic clove, minced
6 cups unsalted vegetable stock (page 199) or water
1 tablespoon soy sauce

1. Soak the beans overnight. Discard the soaking liquid.

2. Put the beans, kombu, ginger, and garlic in a medium pot. Add the stock. Cover and simmer over medium heat for 45 minutes, or until the beans are soft. Add the soy sauce and serve.

Black-Eyed Peas with Tomatoes and Onion

Here's a new slant on an old Southern favorite. It supplies B-complex vitamins and vitamin C, calcium, magnesium, and phosphorus. Beans and onions have both been found to reduce cholesterol. Onions also have some of the antibacterial properties of garlic.

Serves 4

1 tablespoon olive oil
1 large onion, halved and sliced
4 ripe medium tomatoes, peeled, seeded, and chopped (see page 269 for directions), or 2 cups canned whole tomatoes, chopped
1 tablespoon coarsely chopped fresh parsley
3 cups cooked black-eyed peas (page 248)
2 teaspoons soy sauce
1 teaspoon oregano
Salt
Freshly ground black pepper

1. In a large skillet, warm the oil over medium heat. Add the onion and cook 2 minutes. Add the tomatoes and parsley.

2. Reduce the heat to a simmer, cook 5 minutes, then add the black-eyed peas, soy sauce, and oregano and simmer 5 minutes more. Add salt and pepper to taste and serve.

Pinto Beans with Apples and Vegetables

This is a healthy version of sweet Boston baked beans. Serve with roast chicken, turkey, or a whole-grain side dish.

Serves 4

> 2 tablespoons vegetable oil
> ½ cup finely chopped onion
> 1 apple, peeled, cored, and finely chopped
> 1 carrot, peeled and finely chopped
> 1 teaspoon salt
> 1 teaspoon dry mustard powder
> 2 very ripe fresh tomatoes, peeled, seeded, and chopped
>   (see page 269 for directions)
> ½ cup water
> 4 cups cooked pinto or kidney beans (page 248)

1. In a large skillet, warm the oil over medium heat and add the onion. Cook 2 minutes and add the apple and carrot. Cover and cook 5 minutes.

2. Add the salt and mustard powder and cook 2 minutes. Add the tomatoes, water, and beans. Cover and cook 40 minutes.

Red Bean Chili

A tasty mild chili that can warm you up in the winter and cool you down in the summer. Red beans are complemented here with fresh vegetables and grains for super protein. Red beans are a good source of thiamine.

Serves 4 to 6

2 tablespoons vegetable oil
1 large onion, finely chopped
3 garlic cloves, minced
1 tablespoon chili powder
½ teaspoon ground cumin
½ teaspoon ground coriander
½ teaspoon dried oregano
½ teaspoon dried thyme
3 carrots, finely chopped
2 celery stalks, finely chopped
1 green bell pepper, finely chopped
1 jalapeño pepper, seeded and finely chopped (see Note)
2 cups pureed tomatoes
1 large bay leaf
1½ cups cooked kidney beans (pinto beans work well also) (page 248)
⅓ cup cooked whole grains, such as barley, millet, brown rice, oats, or quinoa (page 241)
¾ cup stock (pages 198–200) or water
Salt
½ cup finely chopped fresh cilantro

1. In a large pot or deep skillet, heat the oil. Add the onion and cook until light golden. Add the garlic, chili powder, cumin, coriander, oregano, and thyme, and stir to mix ingredients. Cook over medium-low heat for 2 minutes, then add the carrots, celery, green pepper, and jalapeño pepper. Cover and cook for 15 minutes.

2. Add the tomatoes, bay leaf, beans, grains, and stock; stir to mix, cover, and cook for 20 minutes more. Add salt to taste and serve. Top with chopped fresh cilantro for an authentic Mexican flavor. Remove the bay leaf before serving.

Note: Use care removing the seeds. Wear gloves or wash hands immediately after cutting and don't put your hands near your eyes.

Vegetables

Vegetables are rich in vitamins, minerals, enzymes, and fiber. To maximize the nutritional value of vegetables, cook them as quickly as possible. Most vegetables contain water-soluble vitamins; when the vegetables are boiled, their nutrients are lost in the water. It's best to steam or roast them. All vegetables should be washed or rinsed well. If the vegetables are organically grown, use the peel.

Vegetables can be served raw in salads, pickled, pureed, stuffed, grilled, and more. Different preparation methods can really vary the flavor. For example, most people prepare beets by boiling them, but roasted beets are crispy and sweet. Cucumbers are typically served raw, but steamed cucumbers have a delightful nutty flavor. Some vegetable dishes are substantial enough to serve as entrées in their own right or make a meal when paired with grains and beans.

Steamed Greens

Greens are important in recovery diets as a rich source of fiber; vitamins A, B_2, B_6, C, and E; pantothenic acid; and the minerals magnesium, calcium, iron, manganese, choline, and silicon. Some greens require fairly long cooking times, while others cook quickly. Try this dish with Black-Eyed Peas with Tomatoes and Onion (page 252), or serve with a pasta or chicken dish.

Serves 4

   2 pounds greens, in any combination (spinach, mustard greens, beet greens, green beans, dandelion greens, Swiss chard, kale, dark leaf lettuce, etc.)

1. The greens should be properly cleaned by removing old or hardened stems and dropping the leaves into a large bowl of water. Remove the greens and empty the bowl of water to discard any sand in the bottom. Fill the bowl with water again and repeat the process, then shake the greens dry or pat dry and cut into 2- or 3-inch pieces. (Some cooks prefer to cut the greens before rinsing.)

2. Fill a large pot with a small amount of water and add a steamer basket. Place the longer-cooking greens (collard and kale) in the steamer, cover, and cook 4 minutes, then add quicker-cooking greens for 2 more minutes, or until the greens are wilted. Check the tougher greens for doneness. Serve hot.

Spinach Puree

Spinach is an iron-rich green that helps build blood. This preparation also uses lots of garlic. Recent evidence suggests that garlic may reduce LDL cholesterol, prevent some forms of stomach cancer, and boost the immune system. Garlic is a natural antibiotic that rids the body of certain harmful bacteria, fungi, and yeast. It also stimulates digestion.

Serves 8 to 10

   4 pounds fresh spinach leaves, tough stems removed
   3 tablespoons extra virgin olive oil
   16 garlic cloves, finely chopped
   1 teaspoon salt

1. Fill a large bowl with cold water and add the spinach. Soak to remove any sand. Shake excess water from the leaves and allow to drain.

2. Warm the oil in a large pot over medium heat. Add the garlic and cook, stirring frequently, 3 minutes. Do not let the garlic brown or it will taste bitter.

3. Add the spinach and salt, stir to mix with the garlic and oil, and cover. If the spinach does not easily fit into the pot, press down on the leaves; they will soon reduce as they cook. Cook 10 minutes, or until the leaves are tender. Puree in small batches in a blender or food processor, reheat the puree, and serve.

Spaghetti Squash

This squash gets its name from the stringy interior flesh of the squash. It's a great source of vitamin A, and it contains fair amounts of vitamin C, potassium, and calcium. Try spaghetti squash with Fresh Tomato Basil Sauce (page 269) or serve with Lemon Tarragon Chicken (page 283).

Serves 4 to 6

   1 3–4-pound spaghetti squash
   2–3 tablespoons olive oil
   1 teaspoon lemon juice
   1 tablespoon finely shredded fresh basil leaves, rinsed well
   1 garlic clove, minced

Salt
Freshly ground black pepper

1. Preheat the oven to 350° F. Bake the squash in a large baking pan with a little water in the bottom, about 25 minutes or until a fork easily pierces the skin.

2. In a small bowl, combine the oil, lemon juice, basil, and garlic.

3. Cut the squash lengthwise and gently scoop out the seeds, which are not to be eaten. Scoop out the strands of flesh from the center onto a platter. Separate the strands with 2 forks. It will resemble spaghetti. Toss lightly with the oil and lemon juice mixture. Add salt and pepper to taste and serve immediately (it cools very quickly).

Broiled Marinated Eggplant

Some individuals have difficulty digesting eggplant. The preparation method used in this recipe helps to mitigate this problem. Marinated eggplant works well with fish or simple grain dishes.

Serves 4

    1 medium eggplant
    1 tablespoon salt
    2 tablespoons olive oil
    1 tablespoon finely chopped fresh basil or 1 teaspoon dried
    1 teaspoon dried thyme
    1 tablespoon finely chopped fresh parsley or 1 teaspoon
       dried
    ½ teaspoon minced garlic

1. Cut the eggplant into thin slices and sprinkle with the salt. Put the eggplant in a colander and place a heavy plate on top to press the eggplant. Drain the covered colander over the sink for 15 minutes. Rinse thoroughly and pat dry.

2. In a medium bowl, combine the remaining ingredients. Add the eggplant and set aside for 10 minutes.

3. Preheat the broiler.

4. Broil the eggplant for 5 minutes, then turn and broil 3 to 4 minutes more, or until golden brown. Serve.

Roasted Root Vegetables

Roasting vegetables heightens their flavor. This recipe is a favorite of fried food lovers who have converted to healthier cooking methods.

Serves 4

> 2 medium red potatoes or 2 medium yellow Finn potatoes,
>   rinsed and cut into 2-inch pieces
> 2 small turnips, rinsed and quartered
> 2 carrots, peeled and sliced into 1-inch slices
> 1 parsnip, peeled and sliced into 1-inch slices
> 1 medium beet, washed, peeled, and cut into 1-inch pieces
> 1 medium yellow onion, sliced into wedges
> 8 garlic cloves, minced
> 2 tablespoons olive oil
> ½ teaspoon dried rosemary
> ½ teaspoon dried thyme
> ½ teaspoon dried tarragon
> ¼ teaspoon coarse or freshly ground black pepper
> 1 teaspoon salt

1. Preheat the oven to 350° F. In a large bowl, combine the vegetables.

2. In a small bowl, combine the oil, herbs, pepper, and salt. Add the herb mixture to the vegetables and toss.

3. Spread the vegetables in a baking dish and bake for 1 hour, or until a fork easily pierces the turnips and potatoes. Serve with chicken or fish.

Butternut Squash with Apple Kuzu Glaze

Butternut squash is a winter squash that contains carotenoids, a form of vitamin A. Kuzu (pronounced koo-zoo) is a white powder made from the concentrated starch of the kuzu root. It is very easily absorbed and converted into energy. Kuzu is a nutritious thickener used as an alternative to white flour or cornstarch. It provides relief from intestinal and digestive disorders and is quite beneficial for those in recovery.

Serves 4

1 medium butternut squash (about 1 pound), peeled,
    seeded, and cut into ½-inch squares
½ cup apple juice
1 teaspoon kuzu or arrowroot
¼ cup water
⅛ teaspoon cinnamon
Dash of salt

1. Put the squash in a medium pot and fill with just enough water to cover. Bring to a boil over high heat. Reduce the heat to medium low and cover. Cook 10 minutes, or until a fork pierces the squash but it is not mushy; drain.

2. While the squash is cooking, warm the apple juice in a medium saucepan over low heat. In a small glass, dissolve the kuzu in the water and add to the apple juice. Stir in the cinnamon and cook 5 minutes, or until the mixture is thick like syrup. Add the squash, season with salt, gently toss, and serve.

Mushrooms and Turnips

Turnips are transformed by this simple preparation. They contain vitamin C, potassium, calcium, and other trace minerals. Mushrooms contain vitamins B$_2$, B$_3$, and pantothenic acid, magnesium, potassium, and selenium.

Serves 4 as a side dish

2 tablespoons extra virgin olive oil
1½ teaspoons balsamic vinegar
2 teaspoons soy sauce
¼ pound mushrooms
2 small turnips (not baby turnips), rinsed and thinly sliced
    (include the highly nutritious greens if they are attached
    to the root)
Freshly ground black pepper

1. In a large bowl, combine the oil, vinegar, and soy sauce. Add the mushrooms and turnips.

2. Heat a medium skillet over medium heat and add the vegetable mixture. Cook until the mushrooms and turnips are crispy, about 10 minutes. Season with pepper and serve.

Garlic Mashed Potatoes

An exciting change of pace for potatoes. This recipe is smashing with chicken or fish. Potatoes are a good source of potassium. They also contain B vitamins and are virtually fat-free!

Serves 4

> 3 whole heads garlic
> 1 tablespoon olive oil
> 6 medium potatoes, peeled and diced
> Salt
> Freshly ground white pepper

1. Preheat the oven to 400° F. Coat the garlic with the olive oil, place on a baking sheet, and roast 40 minutes, or until the cloves are soft and pop out of their skins easily. Remove each clove by pressing the base of the head. They should slide right out.

2. In the meantime, place the potatoes in a large pot and cover with water. Cover the pot and bring to a boil over high heat. Reduce heat to a simmer, remove cover, and cook 20 to 30 minutes, or until the potatoes are very soft. Remove and drain the potatoes.

3. Combine the potatoes and garlic in a large bowl and mash by hand or blend both in a blender or food processor. Add a bit of the potato cooking water if the potatoes seem dry. Add salt and pepper to taste and serve.

Broccoli with Sesame Seeds and Ginger

This Chinese-style broccoli dish provides protection from many cancers. The sesame seeds provide more protein than any other seed as well as vitamins E and B_1 and niacin, and ginger is an expectorant that also stimulates blood circulation and the lungs.

Serves 4

> 1 medium head broccoli
> 1 tablespoon vegetable oil
> 2 teaspoons dark sesame oil, available in Oriental foods section of the supermarket or health food store
> 2 teaspoons minced fresh ginger root (peel the ginger before cutting)
> 1 tablespoon roasted sesame seeds
> Pinch of salt

1. Cut away the bottom 3 to 4 inches of the stem of the broccoli. Thinly slice the remainder of the stem, stopping at the base of each cluster of florets (tops). Pull the clusters apart. Place the stem slices and the florets in separate bowls of water. This allows any foreign matter to float to the top and removes some of the sprayed materials on nonorganic broccoli. Drain and set aside.

2. Fill a medium pot with 2 inches of water. Bring the water to a boil and add the stem slices in a steamer basket or place directly into the water and cover. When the stems begin to soften, add the florets and cook 2 minutes. Remove the broccoli, drain, and plunge into a bowl of cold water or ice water to prevent further cooking.

3. Heat the oils in a medium to large skillet. Add the ginger and stir to prevent burning. Quickly add the broccoli and continue stirring for 4 to 5 minutes. Add the sesame seeds and a pinch of salt or to taste. The broccoli should be bright green. Serve immediately for best results.

Steamed Cabbage and Onions with Caraway Seeds

*Cabbage, like broccoli and cauliflower, has anti-cancer proper-
ties that are currently under considerable research. Cabbage is a
good source of vitamins C and A and many minerals, but it may
cause digestive upset for those in the initial stages of recovery.
This mixture is great added to a little chicken broth.*

Serves 4

> ½ medium head white cabbage, rinsed and cut into
>   2-inch pieces
> ¼ cup chopped red cabbage, cut into 1-inch pieces
> 1 large yellow onion, chopped
> 1 tablespoon caraway seeds
> Olive oil (optional)

1. Fill a pot with 2 inches of water. Place a steamer basket in
the pot and add the vegetables.

2. Sprinkle the caraway seeds on top of the vegetables and
cover. Cook until the cabbage is soft and the onions are clear,
then serve. Sprinkle with a little olive oil if you miss fats.

Note: If a steamer is available, use a pot to fit the steamer, or use a
larger pot and substitute a stainless steel colander for the steamer.

Summer Stew

This stew is a meal in itself and is an excellent source of beta carotene; vitamins A, C, and B-complex; and calcium, magnesium, potassium, and other trace minerals.

Serves 4 to 6

2 tablespoons vegetable oil (canola is preferred)
8 pearl onions, peeled
8 cherry tomatoes, 4 whole and 4 coarsely chopped
2 garlic cloves, finely chopped
2 celery stalks, chopped into 1-inch pieces
½ teaspoon dried thyme
½ teaspoon dried marjoram
4 small new potatoes, chopped, or 1 cup chopped of any thin-skinned potato
1 ear tender fresh corn, cut into 1-inch pieces
1 large red bell pepper, seeded and cut into 1-inch pieces
4 baby carrots, peeled, or 2 thin carrots, peeled and chopped into 1-inch pieces
⅓ pound haricots verts (French beans), cut on the diagonal into 1-inch pieces
1½ tablespoons soy sauce or shoyu

1. Heat the oil in a large pot. Add the onions and brown lightly. Add ¼ cup of water. Cook for 3 minutes, or until the water is almost evaporated. Add the chopped tomatoes, garlic, celery, and herbs and cover. Cook over low heat for 4 minutes.

2. Add the remaining vegetables except the haricots verts. Cover the vegetables with just enough water to cover and simmer 20 minutes. Add the haricots verts and soy sauce. Simmer 3 minutes and serve.

Saffron Cauliflower with Sweet Peas

The subtle twist of flavor and a burst of color in this dish make the most of cauliflower. Fresh sweet peas are often paired with cauliflower in East Indian dishes.

Serves 4

½ teaspoon saffron (loosely packed)
1 head cauliflower, rinsed and cut into florets
1 cup shelled fresh peas
½ teaspoon salt
⅛ teaspoon freshly ground white pepper
2 tablespoons chopped fresh parsley

1. Place 1 cup water in a medium pot. Bring to a boil over high heat and add saffron. Stir, remove from heat, and set aside 15 minutes. Add 6 cups water, bring to a boil over high heat, and add cauliflower and peas. Reduce heat to medium and cook 7 minutes, or until the cauliflower begins to soften but is still crunchy.

2. Remove from heat and set aside about 5 minutes, or until the cauliflower has soaked up the bright yellow color of the saffron. Drain the cauliflower, season it with salt and pepper, place in serving dish, and garnish with the parsley.

3. This can also be served chilled in a salad or with a vegetable dip.

Stuffed Acorn Squash

Acorn squash contains large amounts of vitamins A and C and potassium. This vegetable dish can be served as an entrée, with soup or salad, or sliced into pieces and served with roast duck or turkey. Delicata squash can be substituted for the acorn squash.

Serves 4 as an entrée or 8 as a side dish

2 small green-skinned acorn squash, rinsed, halved, and seeded
2 tablespoons olive oil
1½ cups millet
3¼ cups water
Salt
1 small onion, finely chopped

1 small garlic clove, minced
1 carrot, peeled and finely chopped
1 celery stalk, finely chopped
1 bell pepper, seeded and finely chopped
2 teaspoons finely chopped fresh parsley
½ teaspoon dried thyme
¼ teaspoon dried rosemary
Freshly ground black pepper
1 cup tahini

1. Preheat the oven to 375° F.

2. Place the squash, cut-side down, on a deep baking sheet or pan. Pour water into the pan until the level is ½ inch deep. Bake until a fork easily pierces the outside skin of the squash, about 30 to 35 minutes.

3. In the meantime, warm 1 tablespoon of the oil in a large skillet over medium-low heat. Add the millet and toast 4 to 5 minutes, or until the grain smells aromatic. Do not brown the millet. Add the 3¼ cups water and a pinch of salt, then lower the heat, cover, and cook 25 to 30 minutes, or until the grain is light and fluffy.

4. In another skillet, warm the remaining tablespoon of oil over medium heat. Add the onion and sauté until golden brown. Add the garlic and stir 1 minute, then add the carrot, celery, pepper, and herbs. Cook 5 minutes. When the millet is cooked add it to the vegetable mixture. Season with pepper. Stir and turn off the heat.

5. When the squash is cooked remove it from the oven. Turn the squash over and stuff it with the millet mixture. If the squash halves seem too wobbly, slice a small piece off the bottom so each will sit flat. Press the stuffing mixture into the squash and let it spill off the sides. Drizzle the tahini over the tops and return the pan to the oven for 10 minutes.

Sea Vegetables

Sea vegetables contain many of the trace minerals that are rare in land vegetables and yet are essential for optimal health. They are also one of the only vegetable sources of complete protein and vitamin B_{12}. Sea vegetables also aid in detoxifying radioactive elements and toxic metals such as lead from the body.

Hijiki

Hijiki has more calcium per weight than any other sea vegetable —and more than milk. Hijiki also contains protein; vitamins A, B_1, and B_2; and iron and many other minerals. Use hijiki sprinkled on salads, in stir-fries, and with beans and rice or fish. When prepared with apple juice and soy sauce, hijiki has a slightly sweet, nonfishy flavor.

Serves 6 to 8

    1 package (2 ounces) hijiki (page 114)
    1 cup apple juice
    1 tablespoon soy sauce
    Spring water

1. Rinse the hijiki, cover with water in a bowl, and soak 15 minutes.

2. Rinse and place the hijiki in a medium pot. Add the juice, soy sauce, and spring water to cover. (Since hijiki expands, use a large enough pot.)

3. Simmer 30 minutes. Serve.

Note: Cooked hijiki can be served hot, at room temperature, or chilled, and it will keep for up to 9 days in the refrigerator.

Arame in Vegetable Sauté

Arame is a great source of protein, vitamins A and B-complex, and all the minerals.

Serves 4

    ½ cup arame
    1 cup apple juice

1 tablespoon soy sauce
½ cup sliced carrot
½ cup sliced daikon radish
2 cups broccoli florets
1 teaspoon toasted sesame oil
2 teaspoons olive oil
1 garlic clove, minced
1 teaspoon soy sauce (optional)

1. Rinse the arame, cover with water in a bowl, and soak 15 minutes. Rinse again and place in a large pot. Add juice to cover, soy sauce, and water to cover. Arame expands while soaking, so use a large enough pot.

2. Simmer 30 minutes. (At this point, arame can be served hot, at room temperature, or chilled. It can be kept in the refrigerator for up to 9 days.)

3. Fill a medium pot with 2 to 3 inches of water and bring to a boil. Add the carrot and daikon radish to a steamer basket and place it over boiling water. Cook covered for 3 minutes and remove. Add the broccoli to the steamer and cook, covered, for 2 minutes, then remove to the covered dish.

4. Heat the oils in a skillet over medium heat. Add the carrot, daikon, and garlic. Sauté 2 minutes and add the arame. Cook covered until the arame is hot. Add the broccoli, toss together, sprinkle in soy sauce, and serve.

Toasted Nori

Nori is typically used to wrap fish or vegetables in making sushi, but it is also a great high-mineral snack. Enjoy toasted nori alone or sprinkle it on salads, rice, or fish.

Serves 2

4 sheets of nori

1. Hold a sheet of nori 3 inches above a gas or electric element. Carefully hold for 2 seconds on each side. It will turn a lighter shade of green and become quite crispy.

2. Serve whole as a snack or tear into small pieces and sprinkle over food.

Pastas

Contrary to popular belief, pasta is low in calories and in fat, even though it is filling. Whole-grain pastas provide fiber, complex carbohydrates, protein, niacin, and phosphorus.

There are countless types of pastas and pasta dishes from virtually everywhere in the world. For example, pasta has been a staple of the Oriental diet for centuries, and the egg noodles we use in so many Eastern European dishes actually originated in the Orient. In Japan, soba noodles and udon noodles are immensely popular; while in China the universal favorites are mung bean noodles (often sold as bean thread or cellophane noodles). And in the Middle East, couscous—a tiny grain-like pasta made from wheat—is served with many traditional meat or vegetable dishes.

But pasta found its niche and reached its peak in Italy, where it can be found in dozens of shapes and forms. Although many of these popular pastas are made from highly processed flour (most notably durum semolina), there is an increasing variety of whole-grain pastas on the market. The healthiest choices are those made with whole-grain flours such as whole wheat, buckwheat, rice, soy, and quinoa, and also from vegetables such as spinach, beets, carrots, tomatoes, corn, Jerusalem artichokes, and potatoes. The recovery recipes rely on such whole-grain pastas to make healthy low-fat dishes that will satisfy the most hearty appetite.

Fresh Tomato Basil Sauce

Fresh tomatoes make this tomato sauce even better. Tomatoes are a good source of vitamin C and potassium. Serve over pasta or with fish, roasted chicken, zucchini, or eggplant.

Serves 8 to 10

> 12 medium or 10 large very ripe tomatoes, or 3 16-ounce cans of no-salt whole tomatoes (only in the winter when sweet fresh ones are not available)
> 1 tablespoon extra virgin olive oil
> 1 small onion, finely chopped
> 4 garlic cloves, minced
> 2 teaspoons honey (optional—for use with canned tomatoes)
> 1/4 cup finely chopped fresh basil
> 2 teaspoons finely chopped fresh parsley
> 1 teaspoon dried thyme
> 1 teaspoon dried oregano
> 1 teaspoon salt
> 1/4 teaspoon freshly ground black pepper

1. Fill a large pot with water and bring to a boil over high heat. With a small, preferably serrated, knife, make a large shallow X in the bottom of each tomato. Drop tomatoes, 1 or 2 at a time, into the water for 30 seconds, then remove with a slotted spoon and rinse under cold water. The skin should have curled a little around the incision and should slip off. Slice the top off each tomato and gently squeeze the seeds out. Then coarsely chop.

2. In a large heavy pot, warm the oil over medium heat. Add the onion and cook until light golden, about 7 minutes. Add the garlic and cook 3 minutes, then add the tomatoes and cook, uncovered, 15 minutes. Add the honey (if using), herbs, and salt and pepper, stir well, then cover and reduce to a simmer. Cook 20 minutes. Serve. This sauce can be refrigerated for 5 to 7 days or frozen for up to 3 months.

Angel-Hair Pasta with Scallops

Fine, light angel-hair pasta is well suited to bite-size scallops. Scallops provide protein and contain substantial amounts of the mineral selenium, which is a powerful antioxidant. It binds with toxic metals in the body and protects against the effects of radiation. Selenium also preserves the elasticity of our tissues. It works in conjunction with vitamin E to promote growth and fertility and in the treatment of angina.

Serves 4

> 3 tablespoons extra virgin olive oil
> 1 pound cleaned bay scallops (Slice any scallops that are larger than a quarter or more than a half-inch thick.)
> 3 garlic cloves, minced
> ½ cup vegetable stock (page 199) or water
> ⅓ cup thinly sliced fresh basil, plus whole basil leaves for garnish
> 12–16 ounces angel-hair pasta
> Salt
> Freshly ground black pepper

1. Fill a medium pot with water and bring to a boil over high heat.

2. In a large skillet, heat 2 tablespoons of the oil over medium heat. Add the scallops and cook over medium-high heat for 2 to 3 minutes on each side. They will turn a crispy golden color.

3. Add the garlic and cook 2 minutes. Add the stock and the basil and cook until most of the stock is evaporated, about 4 minutes.

4. In the meantime, cook the pasta in the boiling water until al dente, about 3 to 5 minutes. Strain the pasta and sprinkle with the remaining tablespoon of olive oil. Add the pasta to the scallops, toss together, season with salt and pepper, and garnish the serving platter or plates with a pair of fresh basil leaves.

Linguine with Mushrooms and Peas

Mushrooms are a good source of minerals such as potassium, magnesium, and chromium. Peas have almost no fat or sodium. One serving of fresh peas supplies the same amount of protein as an egg. They also provide vitamins C and B-complex, calcium, iron, phosphorus, and potassium.

Serves 4

12–16 ounces linguine or other noodles
2 tablespoons extra virgin olive oil
2 medium shallots, minced
½ pound mushrooms, sliced
2 cups fresh peas, cooked (see Note), or 2 cups fresh-frozen peas
1 tablespoon finely chopped fresh parsley
¼ teaspoon dried thyme
1 teaspoon finely minced fresh dill or ¼ teaspoon dried

1. Fill a large pot with water and bring to a boil over high heat. Add the pasta and cook until al dente. Drain well.

2. In the meantime, warm the oil over medium heat in a large skillet. Add the shallots and cook until golden brown, about 4 minutes, then add the mushrooms and cook until browned, about 6 minutes. If the pan gets too dry, add up to ¼ cup of stock or water. Add the peas and herbs, and cook, covered, for 5 minutes.

3. Top the pasta with the vegetable mixture.

Note: To cook fresh peas, bring a pot of water to a boil, drop in the peas, and cook 5 minutes, or until softened but still a bit crunchy, or prepare by cooking in a vegetable steamer.

Whole Wheat Couscous with Cashews

Couscous is a very tiny, grain-like pasta. This dish provides ample amounts of vitamins A, B, and C as well as protein, complex carbohydrates, iron, calcium, and many other minerals.

Serves 4

4 cups freshly squeezed orange juice
2 cups whole wheat couscous
1–2 tablespoons extra virgin olive oil
3 scallions, finely chopped
½ cup currants or chopped raisins
½ teaspoon ground allspice
½ teaspoon ground cumin
1 teaspoon finely chopped fresh parsley
½ cup cashews, finely crushed
½ teaspoon salt
Freshly ground white pepper

1. In a small pot, bring the orange juice to a boil. Place the couscous in a stainless steel or heat-resistant glass bowl. Add 2 cups of the hot juice and toss the couscous quickly, then cover and leave for 10 minutes. Repeat the procedure once more, using the remaining hot juice and covering for 5 to 10 minutes. Fluff with a fork.

2. In a medium skillet, heat the olive oil over low heat and add the scallions, currants, allspice, cumin, and parsley. Cook 3 minutes. Add the crushed cashews. Cook 2 minutes. Add the mixture to the couscous. Combine the ingredients, add salt and pepper to taste, and serve.

Udon Noodles with Mushrooms and Spinach

Serve this udon dish as a summer evening entrée with a fresh green salad, roasted herb chicken, or even sliced turkey breast. The preparation time is 15 minutes and the nutritional value is high in many vitamins and minerals.

Serves 4

    12–16 ounces udon noodles
    3 tablespoons plus 2 teaspoons extra virgin olive oil
    1½ cups very thinly sliced button mushrooms
    2 garlic cloves, minced
    1 pound broad-leaf spinach, tough stems removed, well
        rinsed, and coarsely chopped
    ½ teaspoon salt
    Freshly ground black pepper

1. Fill a large pot with water and bring to a boil over high heat. Add the noodles and 1 tablespoon of the oil. Cook 7 minutes, or until the noodles are cooked al dente (firm to the bite).

2. Meanwhile, heat 2 tablespoons of the oil in a large skillet over medium heat. Add the mushrooms and cook 10 minutes, or until the mushrooms are browned around the edges. Add the garlic and cook 3 minutes. Add the spinach, cover the pan, and simmer 4 minutes.

3. When the noodles are cooked, drain them and sprinkle lightly with 2 teaspoons of the olive oil. Add the noodles to the mushroom-spinach mixture. Stir to combine, season with salt and pepper, and serve.

Chicken Bolognese Sauce for Pasta

Bolognese sauce is traditionally made with beef, pork, and wine. This recovery version uses chicken and still tastes very rich although it's lower in fat and calories than traditional bolognese sauce.

This recipe requires a little work, so we suggest making it in large batches and freezing half.

Serves 10 to 12

> ¼ cup dried porcini mushrooms (available in the gourmet food section of supermarkets or specialty food shops)
> ⅓ cup plus 1 tablespoon extra virgin olive oil
> 2½ pounds uncooked ground chicken (if your butcher cannot grind it for you, use a meat grinder or food processor at home)
> 1 medium onion, finely chopped
> 1 large carrot, peeled and finely chopped
> 1 celery stalk, finely chopped
> ¼ cup white grape juice
> 1 teaspoon vinegar
> ¼ cup tomato paste
> ½ cup water
> 4 fresh tomatoes, peeled, seeded, and chopped (see page 269 for directions), or 2 16-ounce cans Italian whole tomatoes, drained and chopped
> ½ cup chopped fresh parsley
> 1 teaspoon dried thyme
> 1 teaspoon dried oregano
> ¼ teaspoon ground nutmeg
> ¼ teaspoon red pepper flakes
> ¼ teaspoon freshly ground black pepper
> 1 teaspoon salt

1. To remove any sand from the mushrooms, place them in a small bowl and cover with water. Remove the mushrooms after 15 minutes, finely chop, and set aside. Strain the liquid and set aside in a separate bowl.

2. In a large heavy pot, heat the oil over medium heat. Add ½ cup of the chicken and cook until browned, stirring frequently. Add the onion and cook until brown. Add the carrot, celery, and mushrooms and cook 4 minutes.

3. Add the mushroom liquid, grape juice, and vinegar and cook until the liquid is reduced by half.

4. Add the remaining chicken, chopping with a spoon or fork to break it up as it cooks over low heat 5 minutes.

5. In a small bowl, dissolve the tomato paste in the ½ cup of water. Add it with the tomatoes, parsley, thyme, oregano, nutmeg, red pepper flakes, black pepper, and salt to the pot. Cover and simmer 45 minutes (or longer, up to 2 hours; the flavors get stronger the longer it simmers). Toss the bolognese sauce gently with your choice of cooked pasta and stir to combine. Divide into portions or place on a large platter and serve.

Fettuccine with Broccoli Rabe

Broccoli rabe is a cousin of the broccoli we are all familiar with. It has small florets and slightly tart leaves.

Serves 3

> 8–10 ounces whole wheat, whole-grain, or spinach
>   fettuccine
> 3 tablespoons extra virgin olive oil, first cold press
> 4 garlic cloves, finely chopped
> 2 cups chopped broccoli rabe
> ⅓ cup finely sliced fresh basil (3 pairs of leaves reserved
>   for garnish)
> Salt
> Freshly ground black pepper

1. Fill a large pot with water and bring to a boil over high heat. Add the pasta and 1 tablespoon of the oil. Cook 7 minutes, or until the fettuccine is cooked al dente, or firm to the bite.

2. In the meantime, heat 1 tablespoon of the oil over low heat in a large skillet. Add the garlic and cook 3 minutes, or until the garlic becomes golden but not brown. Add the broccoli rabe and cook 5 minutes, or until the broccoli rabe is softened and bright in color but still crunchy.

3. Drain the fettuccine and add to the skillet of broccoli rabe. Add the basil and the remaining tablespoon of olive oil and toss. Add salt and pepper to taste and garnish each serving with a pair of basil leaves.

Tuna Tomato Sauce and Noodles

This is a favorite lunchtime meal in Italy and it's easy to see why. Tuna provides high amounts of protein; tomatoes provide vitamin C; and the whole-grain noodles add vitamin B-complex, fiber, and complex carbohydrates.

Serves 4

> 4 tablespoons extra virgin olive oil
> 1 large yellow onion, halved and sliced
> 2 garlic cloves, minced (optional)
> 1 cup canned whole peeled tomatoes, drained, or 4 fresh tomatoes, peeled, seeded, and chopped (see page 269 for directions)
> 2 6½-ounce cans white tuna in water, drained
> ½ teaspoon thyme
> ½ teaspoon marjoram
> 1 tablespoon finely chopped fresh parsley
> ½ teaspoon salt
> ⅛ teaspoon freshly ground black pepper
> 12–16 ounces noodles, shells, or any whole-grain or vegetable pasta

1. Heat 3 tablespoons of the oil in a medium saucepan over medium-low heat. Add the onion and raise the heat to medium. Cook the onion until it is golden brown. Add the garlic and tomatoes and cook 10 minutes, or until the tomatoes have lost most of their liquid. Add the tuna, crumbling it into little pieces as it's added. Add the thyme, marjoram, parsley, salt, and pepper and simmer over medium-low heat, covered, for 10 minutes.

2. Fill a large pot with water and bring to a boil over high heat. Add the noodles and cook 7 to 9 minutes, or until they are al dente (firm to the bite). Avoid overcooking the pasta always, but particularly in this dish. Drain the noodles and toss with the remaining 1 tablespoon of olive oil, then add to the tuna sauce and stir to combine. Serve at once.

Poultry

Poultry of almost any kind is an excellent source of low-fat complete protein (although some, most notably duck, can be fatty). Chicken is by far the most popular form of poultry; it is eaten in more countries than any other meat. As a result, there is a wealth of wonderful recipes for this versatile food—which can also be used in place of pork or veal in most recipes.

When buying chicken or other poultry, always try to buy a whole bird and have the butcher cut it up if the recipe calls for parts. Diseased birds are sometimes cut up and the diseased sections are discarded while the rest are sold as parts. When preparing raw poultry, remember to thoroughly clean the utensils and cutting boards in hot, soapy water before using them to prepare other foods. And always wash your hands well both before and after working with raw poultry.

All of the recovery recipes use aromatic herbs, vegetables, and spices to create healthy and interesting dishes that require very little cooking time. Most cooked dishes will keep for about two days in the refrigerator.

17.3 POULTRY COOKING CHART

Approximate Cooking Time at 350° F.*

Type	Weight	For Pieces	Whole Bird per Pound
Large roaster	up to 9 lbs.	50–70 min.	18–20 min.
Capon	4–7 lbs.	70–90 min.	18–20 min.
Stewing chicken (1 year and older)	3–7 lbs.	50–70 min.	(simmer, covered, 1½ hours)
Roasters (also Rock Cornish roaster)	3–5 lbs.	50–70 min.	18–20 min.
Turkey	18–25 lbs.		15–18 min.
	12–18 lbs.		15–18 min.
	5–18 lbs.		18–20 min.
	3–5 lbs.	70–90 min.	18–20 min.
Guinea fowl	1½–2½ lbs.		30–35 min.
Duckling	3–4 lbs.	35–40 min.	18–20 min.
Duck (10 weeks and older)	5 lbs. or more	as per chicken (legs may require 10–15 min. more)	18–20 min.
Goose	6–14 lbs.		18–20 min.
Rock Cornish game hen	1–2 lbs.		20–30 min.
Squab	12–16 oz.		20–30 min. (at 425° F.)

* To test for doneness, pierce the poultry flesh with a sharp knife; the juices should run clear.

Celebration Chicken

This pretty one-pot dish is great for company. It is quick and easy and is high in flavor and low in fat, calories, and cholesterol. Serve Celebration Chicken with a complex carbohydrate-rich food such as brown rice, quinoa, or whole-grain pasta for a nutritionally balanced meal.

Serves 4

2 tablespoons extra virgin olive oil
4 medium shallots, minced, or 2 small onions, finely chopped
2 garlic cloves, minced
1 cup sliced mushrooms
2 carrots, peeled and julienned
1 medium parsnip, peeled and julienned
6 sprigs fresh thyme or 1 tablespoon dried thyme leaves
2 boneless, skinless chicken breasts, split in half
1 red bell pepper, chopped
1¼ cups apple juice, preferably sparkling
¾ cup stock (page 200) or water
1 tablespoon freshly squeezed lemon juice
½ teaspoon salt
¼ teaspoon freshly ground black pepper

1. In a large skillet warm the oil over medium heat. Add the shallots and cook until lightly browned, about 3 minutes. Add the garlic and mushrooms and cook, stirring frequently, for 1 minute. Add the carrots, parsnip, and thyme. Stir for 2 minutes, push the vegetables to the side of the pan, and add the chicken. Brown on both sides (the chicken won't be cooked through) and add the red pepper, apple juice, stock, lemon juice, salt, and pepper. Cook about 4 minutes, or until the chicken is cooked through.

2. With a slotted spoon, remove the chicken and vegetables to a serving platter and keep warm. Stir the skillet juices, scraping up the brown bits at the bottom of the pan. Turn the heat to high and boil the juices until reduced by half, about 3 minutes. The sauce should look glossy and should thinly coat the back of a spoon. Pour the sauce over the chicken and vegetables and serve.

Broiled Chicken Breasts Brushed with Herbs

This crispy skinless chicken recipe is simple to prepare. Fresh herbs are usually well tolerated by those early in recovery, unlike spices, which tend to disturb digestion. Serve with Butternut Squash with Apple Kuzu Glaze (page 258) and a rice pilaf.

Serves 4

- 3 tablespoons extra virgin olive oil
- 2 teaspoons prepared mustard
- 2 teaspoons water
- 1 garlic clove, minced
- ¼ teaspoon ground cumin
- ½ teaspoon paprika (optional)
- 1½ teaspoons fresh thyme or ½ teaspoon dried
- ½ teaspoon finely chopped fresh rosemary or ¼ teaspoon dried
- ½ teaspoon finely chopped fresh parsley or ¼ teaspoon dried
- ½ teaspoon salt
- ¼ teaspoon freshly ground black pepper (optional)
- 4 skinless chicken breast halves

1. Preheat the broiler. Combine the oil, mustard, water, garlic, spices, herbs, salt, and pepper in a small bowl.

2. Place the chicken on a baking sheet and brush both sides with half of the oil-herb mixture. Broil the chicken bone-side up for 10 minutes. Turn and brush the remaining oil-herb mixture (reserving 2 tablespoons) on the top of the breasts and cook 7 minutes, or until the chicken is cooked (the juices will run clear when the breast is pierced with a fork). With a basting brush, brush the remaining marinade on the chicken for a moistened look. Remove and serve with Saffron Rice with Raisins and Coconut (page 247), Wild Rice Pilaf (page 242), or Quinoa Pilaf (page 244).

Braised Chicken with Cinnamon and Basil

A new take on chicken with gravy without the gravy calories, this is a real palate pleaser in any stage of recovery.

Serves 4

> 1–2 teaspoons vegetable oil
> ³/₄ teaspoon salt
> ¹/₂ teaspoon freshly ground black pepper
> 4–6 boneless chicken breasts or thighs, flattened and cut into 3-inch-long by 2-inch-wide strips
> 1 tablespoon finely minced shallot or white onion
> 3 tablespoons red grape juice
> 1 teaspoon freshly squeezed lemon juice
> 2 ripe medium tomatoes, peeled, seeded, and pureed (see Note)
> 1 cup chicken or vegetable stock (page 200, 199)
> 1 cinnamon stick (about 3 inches long) or 1 teaspoon ground cinnamon
> ¹/₄ cup chopped fresh basil or 1 tablespoon dried basil

1. Preheat the oven to 400° F. Heat the oil in a large skillet over medium heat. Lightly salt and pepper the chicken with ¹/₄ teaspoon of the salt and ¹/₄ teaspoon of the pepper. Add the chicken a few pieces at a time and quickly brown the outside without cooking the inside. Remove to a warm platter.

2. Add the shallot and cook until dark golden brown, about 10 minutes. Add the grape juice, lemon juice, pureed tomatoes, stock, the remaining salt and pepper, and the cinnamon. Bring the ingredients to a boil and allow the liquid to reduce by two-thirds.

3. Return the chicken pieces to the skillet, add the basil, and place in the oven for 7 minutes, or until the chicken is cooked. Remove from the oven and place the chicken on a platter or individual plates. Strain the sauce and drizzle it over the chicken. Serve with Wild Rice Pilaf (page 242) or pasta.

Note: To puree tomatoes, place them in a blender or food processor and mix until smooth.

Lemon Tarragon Chicken

The delicate flavor of tarragon and lemon are perfect for chicken. This recipe is fast, simple, tasty, and great for early recovery.

Serves 4

½ cup freshly squeezed lemon juice
¼ cup vegetable oil
4 teaspoons dried tarragon
4 split chicken breasts on the bone, skin removed, or 4
  medium skinless chicken legs
1 cup whole wheat flour (see Note)
½ teaspoon garlic powder
½ teaspoon thyme
½ teaspoon dried parsley
1 teaspoon paprika
1 teaspoon salt
¼ teaspoon freshly ground black pepper

1. Preheat the oven to 350° F. In a large glass dish, combine the lemon juice, oil, and 3 teaspoons of the tarragon. Add the chicken and marinate 15 minutes.

2. In a medium bowl, combine the flour, garlic powder, thyme, parsley, paprika, the remaining 1 teaspoon of tarragon, salt, and pepper. Put the combined ingredients in a large paper bag.

3. Drain the chicken and put one piece at a time into the paper bag. Shake well and place the chicken pieces on a baking sheet.

4. Bake for 25 minutes, or until the juices run clear when the chicken is pierced with a fork.

Note: Substitute rice flour if you are allergic to wheat.

Chicken Stir-Fry

The rich Chinese flavors in this stir-fry will keep you cooking in rather than ordering out. Try carrots, snow peas, corn, asparagus, cauliflower, or bean sprouts. Serve Chicken Stir-Fry by itself or on a bed of brown rice, plain soba noodles, or pasta.

Serves 4

> 1 pound boneless skinless chicken, light or dark meat, cut into thin 1-inch strips
> 1/3 cup soy sauce
> 2 tablespoons Oriental sesame oil
> 2 teaspoons minced fresh ginger root
> 2 teaspoons minced garlic
> 2 teaspoons rice vinegar or lemon juice
> 2 teaspoons honey, rice yinnie (page 112), or barley malt (page 110)
> 2 teaspoons vegetable oil
> 1 medium onion, sliced
> 1 red bell pepper, seeded and cut into thin 2-inch-long strips
> 1 cup chopped bok choy or broccoli florets
> 2 scallions, cut into thin 2-inch strips
> 1 cup thinly sliced Chinese cabbage or regular spinach
> 1 teaspoon arrowroot or kuzu

1. In a large bowl, combine the chicken, soy sauce, sesame oil, 1 teaspoon of the ginger, 1 teaspoon of the garlic, the vinegar, and the honey and marinate 15 minutes or longer. Refrigerate if marinating longer.

2. Heat a well-seasoned wok over medium-high heat and add the vegetable oil. Add the remaining ginger and garlic and, stirring constantly, cook 30 seconds. With a slotted spoon, add the chicken a small amount at a time and cook on high heat. Reserve the marinade. Quickly toss the chicken in the wok until the meat turns white on the outside.

3. Add the onion, pepper, bok choy, and scallions. Continue to toss the ingredients in the wok until the bok choy is soft but still crunchy, about 4 minutes. Then add the cabbage.

4. Dissolve the arrowroot or kuzu in ¼ cup of water.

5. Add the reserved marinade to the wok with the arrowroot or kuzu. Cook until the sauce thickens and creates a glaze over the chicken and vegetables.

Chicken and Bulgur

This makes a scrumptious meal in cold weather served hot or served chilled in the summertime. Bulgur is a cracked and par-boiled whole wheat that cooks up very quickly.

Serves 4

> 1 tablespoon vegetable oil
> 2 cups boneless, skinless chicken, cut into 1-inch strips
> 2 cups finely chopped onion
> 2 cups julienned carrot
> 1 teaspoon dried rosemary
> 1 teaspoon dried thyme
> 2 bay leaves
> 2 cups bulgur
> 1½ teaspoons maple syrup
> 2 tablespoons soy sauce (check alcoholic content if not "traditionally brewed")
> 4 cups chicken stock (page 200) or water

1. In a large skillet, warm the oil over medium heat. Add the chicken and quickly brown. Remove the chicken with a slotted spoon to a plate.

2. Cook the onion in the skillet until golden. Add the carrot, rosemary, thyme, bay leaves, bulgur, maple syrup, and soy sauce. Stir a few minutes to combine the ingredients, then add the stock. Cover and cook 10 minutes over medium-low heat.

3. Add the chicken and cook 5 minutes more. Remove the bay leaves. Remove from heat but leave uncovered. Fluff the mixture with a fork and serve.

Stuffed Baked Chicken or Turkey

Our favorite poultry dish. For the easiest of poultry recipes, omit the stuffing and start at step 3. This recipe is for any stage of recovery. Serve with Roasted Root Vegetables (page 258).

Serves 4 to 6

Stuffing

> 6 slices whole-grain bread
> 1 tablespoon vegetable oil
> 1 small onion or ½ medium onion, finely chopped
> 1 garlic clove, minced
> ½ cup finely chopped mushrooms (optional)
> 1 carrot, finely chopped
> 1 celery stalk, finely chopped
> ¼ cup currants (optional)
> ¼ cup walnuts, pecans, or chestnuts, chopped (optional)
> 1 tablespoon finely chopped fresh parsley or 1 teaspoon dried
> 1 teaspoon dried thyme
> 1 teaspoon dried sage
> ½ teaspoon dried rosemary
> ½ teaspoon salt
> ¼ teaspoon freshly ground black pepper
> ½ cup chicken or turkey stock (page 200) or water

Chicken or Turkey

> 1 3–5-pound chicken or turkey (increase the dressing recipe for larger birds)
> 2 tablespoons vegetable oil
> ¼ teaspoon cumin
> ½ teaspoon paprika
> ¼ teaspoon salt
> Freshly ground black pepper
> ½ teaspoon dried sage
> ½ teaspoon dried thyme
> ½ teaspoon dried marjoram

1. Preheat the oven to 350° F. Place the bread on a baking sheet and toast in the oven for 10 minutes (or toast bread in a toaster). Break up the bread into little pieces or pulse in a food processor or blender.

2. In a large skillet, heat the oil over medium-high heat. Add the onion and garlic and cook until onion is translucent. Add the mushrooms, carrot, celery, and currants and cook 5 minutes. Add the bread pieces, stir well to combine, then add the nuts, herbs, salt, and a dash of pepper. Add just enough of the stock to moisten the stuffing. Cover and cook 5 minutes more.

3. Rinse the bird inside and out with cool water and remove the inner parts and paper. Place in a roasting pan and stuff the bird three-quarters full of stuffing.

4. Combine the oil, cumin, paprika, salt, pepper, and herbs and brush the outside of the chicken with the mixture. Roast 1 to 1½ hours. The bird is done when the legs move freely, or when the juice flows clear when the thigh is pricked.

Chicken Teriyaki with Raspberries

Raspberries give Chicken Teriyaki a tart sweetness. This is a good recipe for chicken legs.

Serves 4

2 tablespoons vegetable oil
2 tablespoons minced onion
1 garlic clove, minced
2 tablespoons tomato paste
¾ cup white grape juice
3 tablespoons freshly squeezed lemon juice
¼ cup soy sauce
2 tablespoons rice vinegar
1 tablespoon grated fresh ginger root
¾ cup chicken stock (page 200) or water
1 tablespoon honey
½ cup raspberries (fresh or sugar-free frozen)
8 skinless chicken legs, or a combination of 8 chicken parts
   (breasts, thighs, legs, wings)

1. Preheat the oven to 375° F. In a large skillet, heat the oil, add the onion, and cook until light golden. Add the garlic and cook 2 minutes.

2. In a small bowl, dissolve the tomato paste in the grape juice and add to the skillet with the lemon juice, soy sauce, vinegar, ginger, stock, and honey. Simmer for 20 minutes, or until the sauce begins to thicken. Add half the raspberries and simmer 5 minutes more.

3. Place the chicken pieces in a baking dish and toss with half the sauce. Bake for about 30 minutes (leg pieces will take longer than other pieces). Spoon the sauce over the chicken two or three times during the cooking. Legs are done when the juices run clear.

4. Reheat the remaining sauce and drizzle over the chicken. Top with the remaining raspberries.

Fish

The key to delicious fish is timing. Frequently, home-cooked fish is overdone and dried out. Fish continues to cook once it's removed from the oven. So, the trick to a perfect fish meal is to have all the elements of the meal prepared (including setting the table) before the fish is cooked. The general rule of thumb is to allow 10 minutes per 1-inch thickness of fish. Always preheat the oven or stove top.

Our recovery recipes emphasize broiling, baking, poaching, or sautéing methods for cooking fish. Three forms of fish are used: whole fish (cleaned and scaled), fillets (the side slice of fish), or steaks (a crosswise cut of fish).

To check if fish is done, poke the thickest part of the fish with a sharp knife. It should be slightly translucent. The thinner parts should be opaque but not dry. The thickest parts will continue to cook.

Most fish requires little more than a brush of oil and herbs, but crushed nuts, mushrooms, onions, or other aromatic vegetables are excellent cooking companions. For additional information on choosing fish, see pages 145–148.

Sole Hazeldine

Here's a variation on sole almondine. Hazelnuts, substituted for almonds, are lower in saturated fat; higher in pantothenic acid, vitamins A, E, and B, and copper; and have twice the manganese. Sole is a delicate, white, mild-flavored fish that is low in fat and calories and contains many minerals. Serve with Fettuccine with Broccoli Rabe (page 276) or Quinoa Asparagus Salad (page 222).

Serves 4

1 cup shelled hazelnuts or sliced almonds
2 tablespoons extra virgin olive oil
4 garlic cloves, minced
2 tablespoons finely chopped fresh parsley
½ teaspoon onion powder
¼ teaspoon salt
Dash of freshly ground white pepper
4 4–6-ounce sole fillets
1 tablespoon freshly squeezed lemon juice
8 lemon slices, for garnish
4 parsley sprigs, for garnish

1. Place the hazelnuts in a heavy paper bag. Roll the bag closed, place it on a cutting board, and hit the bag with a rolling pin to crush the nuts to the size of rice. Turn out the nuts onto the cutting board and chop up any pieces that evaded your pounding. Set aside.

2. In a large frying pan, warm the oil over low heat. Add the garlic and cook 2 minutes, then add the hazelnuts, parsley, onion powder, salt, and pepper. Cook 5 minutes, or until the aroma of the nuts is strong. Push the nuts to the edges of the pan and add the sole to the pan. Cook 3 to 4 minutes per side, or until the fish flakes easily with a fork. Remove the sole to warm plates. Add the lemon juice to the pan, 1 teaspoon at a time, and stir it into the hazelnut mixture. Cook 1 minute, then top each fillet with some of the hazelnut mixture and garnish with 2 slices of lemon and a parsley sprig.

Poached Fish with Vegetables

Poached fish is the most soothing fish preparation. It is an easy-to-digest complete protein, appropriate for early stages of recovery. Boiled potatoes or cooked soba noodles are delicious with poached fish. Use any firm white fish for this recipe. Salmon also poaches well.

Serves 4

2 medium onions, sliced
2 leeks, rinsed well and sliced
2 carrots, thinly sliced
2 celery stalks, sliced
½ cup chopped fresh dill
1 tablespoon finely chopped fresh parsley
2 bay leaves
1 teaspoon dried thyme
½ teaspoon dried rosemary
½ teaspoon ground allspice
2 teaspoons salt
2 tablespoons freshly ground black pepper
1 cup brown rice vinegar or apple cider vinegar
5 cups water
4 4–6-ounce fish fillets (whitefish, cod, halibut, or salmon)

1. Place all the vegetables and herbs, the allspice, and the salt and pepper in a large pot, cover, and allow them to sweat for 5 minutes over low heat. After a minute or two, stir to prevent sticking and add a little water. This combines and releases the flavors of the vegetables and herbs.

2. Add the vinegar and water, cover, and simmer for 12 minutes.

3. Add the fish and cook over medium-low heat until the fish is flaky and solid white or pink, usually 10 minutes per 1-inch-thick piece. Using a spatula, remove each fillet to a large bowl. Remove the bay leaves and divide the vegetables and stock among the bowls.

Baked Italian Sole

All fish contain many vitamins, minerals, and trace minerals and elements, and sole is no exception. Zinc is an essential trace mineral found in sole and other fish. The vegetables here add vitamin C, calcium, and iron to this dish.

Serves 4

2 tablespoons olive oil, plus more for brushing the fish
3 garlic cloves, minced
4 medium tomatoes, diced
1 red or green bell pepper, diced
12 pitted black olives, minced
1 tablespoon finely chopped fresh parsley
Salt
Freshly ground black pepper
4 6-ounce sole or flounder fillets

1. Preheat the oven to 350° F. In a skillet, heat the oil over low heat. Add the garlic and tomatoes. Cook 5 minutes and add the bell pepper, olives, and parsley. Season with salt and pepper to taste. Cook 4 minutes more over medium-low heat.

2. Place the fillets in a baking dish and brush with olive oil. Top with the tomato mixture and bake 15 minutes. The fish is cooked when it is flaky and white all the way through. Serve with pasta or rice pilaf and steamed asparagus.

Baked Salmon Steaks

This is a great recipe for company. It looks elegant, tastes great, and is a snap to prepare. All fish contain some omega-3 fatty acids (EFA's), but the greatest concentration of these fatty acids is found in cold-water species such as salmon.

Serves 6

2 tablespoons olive oil
1 large onion, sliced
3 garlic cloves, minced
2 lemons, sliced
1 bunch fresh dill, minced
2 tablespoons finely chopped fresh parsley
2 teaspoons fresh cracked black peppercorns

¹/₂ teaspoon salt
6 3–4-ounce salmon steaks

1. Preheat the oven to 400° F.

2. In a bowl, combine the oil, onion, garlic, lemons, dill, parsley, pepper, and salt. Place half of this mixture in a long baking dish, place the salmon steaks on top, then sprinkle the remaining mixture on the fish. Bake 30–40 minutes, or until fish is opaque all the way through.

Moroccan Sea Bass Stew

Sea bass is high in omega-3 fatty acids, which are believed to lower LDL cholesterol and inhibit inflammatory agents. This recipe is flavorful without being too spicy.

Serves 4

2 tablespoons olive oil
1 large onion, cut into 1-inch-wide slices
3 bell peppers, cut into 2-inch pieces
2 carrots, cut into 1-inch slices
2 teaspoons chili powder
2 teaspoons paprika
1 medium zucchini, cut into 1-inch slices on the diagonal
1¹/₂ pounds sea bass fillets, cut into 1–2-inch squares
Salt
Freshly ground black pepper

1. Heat the oil in a large pot. Add the onion slices, bell peppers, and carrots. Cook over low heat for 4 minutes and stir once or twice to prevent sticking.

2. Add the chili powder, paprika, and zucchini. Cook 3 minutes and add the sea bass. Cover and simmer 10 minutes. Add salt and pepper to taste. Serve over couscous or millet if desired.

Halibut with Herb Bread Crumbs

This recipe is a variation on a Waldorf Astoria favorite. Halibut is a mild-flavored, firm-fleshed white fish. A three-ounce serving supplies an abundance of the B vitamin niacin. Niacin regulates delivery of oxygen to the brain, relieves insomnia, loosens stiff joints, and fuels digestion. Other firm white fish such as scrod, cod, or haddock work as well for this recipe. Serve with Roasted Root Vegetables (page 258) and Wild Rice Pilaf (page 242).

Serves 4 to 6

6 slices whole-grain bread, crusts removed
2 tablespoons extra virgin olive oil
1 small shallot, minced
1 garlic clove, minced
1½ tablespoons minced fresh parsley
1½ teaspoons minced fresh basil
1½ teaspoons minced fresh dill
1 teaspoon minced fresh tarragon or ¼ teaspoon dried
½ teaspoon dried rosemary
½ teaspoon dried thyme
¼ teaspoon salt
⅛ teaspoon freshly ground black pepper
4–6 6-ounce halibut fillets

1. Preheat the oven to 375° F.

2. Cut the bread into cubes and place on a baking sheet. Toast in the oven until crisp but not brown. Remove and cool.

3. In a medium skillet, warm 1 tablespoon of the olive oil over medium heat. Add the shallot and cook until translucent, then add the garlic and cook 2 minutes, stirring frequently. Remove from heat and cool.

4. In a blender or food processor, combine the bread cubes, shallot mixture, herbs, salt, and pepper. Process until the crumbs are very fine.

5. Place the fish in a baking dish. Drizzle the remaining tablespoon of olive oil over, then sprinkle the bread crumbs on top. Bake for 20 minutes, or until the fish is white all the way through.

Baked Trout with Thyme Stuffing

The mild but distinctive flavor of trout is enhanced by the sweet mild aroma of thyme. Trout is one of the fish highest in protein, with 21.5 grams per 3½-ounce serving. Trout is also a rich source of B vitamins including B_{12} as well as pantothenic acid.

Serves 4

> 2 tablespoons canola oil, plus more for greasing dish and
> brushing on fish
> 1 medium yellow onion, finely chopped
> 2 garlic cloves, minced
> 1½ tablespoons fresh thyme or 2 teaspoons dried
> 1 tablespoon minced fresh parsley or 1 teaspoon dried
> parsley
> 3 cups fine whole-grain bread crumbs
> ⅓–½ cup vegetable (page 199) stock or water
> ½ teaspoon salt
> Freshly ground black pepper
> 4 ¾–1-pound whole trout, cleaned, boned, and scaled
> (your fishmonger will do this for you)
> 4 sprigs fresh parsley or thyme, for garnish

1. Preheat the oven to 400° F.

2. In a medium skillet, warm the oil over medium heat. Add the onion and cook until translucent, about 5 minutes. Add the garlic and cook 3 minutes, being careful not to brown the garlic.

3. Add the thyme, parsley, and bread crumbs, stir well, then add just enough vegetable stock to moisten the mixture. If you are using dried herbs, add 2 more tablespoons of liquid to the skillet. Add salt and pepper to taste and remove from heat.

4. Spoon ¼ of the mixture into the pocket along the bottom of each fish. Place the fish in a lightly greased baking dish and brush the tops with oil. Bake 35–40 minutes, or until the fish is white all the way through. Serve garnished with sprigs of parsley or thyme.

Baked Red Snapper with Amaranth Stuffing

Amaranth makes a delicious stuffing for a mild-flavored fish like snapper. Like fish, it is high in protein, including two amino acids—lysine and methionine—that are rare in grains. It is also a fine source of fiber, calcium, iron, and, remarkably, vitamin C, which is not present in most grains.

Serves 4

Stuffing

> 1 tablespoon olive oil
> ½ cup finely chopped shallots
> 1 cup amaranth
> ½ cup finely chopped carrots
> 2 celery stalks, finely chopped
> 2 teaspoons finely chopped fresh parsley
> 1 tablespoon finely chopped fresh thyme or 1 teaspoon dried
> ½ teaspoon tarragon
> ½ teaspoon savory
> 2 cups vegetable stock or water

Fish

> 2 tablespoons olive oil
> 1 tablespoon lemon juice
> 2 shallots, peeled and sliced
> ½ teaspoon dried thyme
> ½ teaspoon dried tarragon
> 1 teaspoon salt
> ⅛ teaspoon freshly ground black pepper
> 4 6-ounce red snapper fillets or 1 2-pound whole red snapper, cleaned, scaled, and sliced lengthwise

1. Make the stuffing. In a large skillet, warm the oil over medium heat. Add the shallots and cook until lightly golden. Add the amaranth and stir until toasted, about 3 minutes. Add the carrots, celery, and herbs and stir to combine. Add the stock or water, cover the skillet, and cook over medium heat 15 minutes. Remove from heat and set aside.

2. Preheat the oven to 350° F. In a small bowl, combine the oil, lemon juice, shallots, thyme, tarragon, salt, and pepper.

3. Place the snapper on a baking sheet and brush both sides

with the oil mixture. Place 2 fillets skin-side down and top them with the stuffing, then place the other 2 fillets on top, skin-side up. For a whole snapper, stuff the inside with the stuffing and place the remaining stuffing around the outside of the fish. Bake the fillets 20 minutes; bake the whole fish 40 minutes, or until the flesh is white and flaky. Remove and place on a platter.

Garlic Shrimp with Fettuccine

This classic pasta dish is a rich and flavorful meal that doesn't rely on heavy sauces to please the palate. With a side salad or vegetable, it makes a satisfying lunch or dinner.

Serves 4

¾ pound medium shrimp
12–16 ounces fettuccine, preferably spinach fettuccine
3 tablespoons extra virgin olive oil
6–8 garlic cloves, minced
1 tablespoon minced fresh parsley or 1 teaspoon dried
Dash of freshly squeezed lemon juice
½ teaspoon salt
⅛ teaspoon freshly ground black pepper

1. Rinse the shrimp and peel off the shells and tails. Devein the shrimp by making a small, shallow incision along the back of the shrimp, then pulling out the vein.

2. Fill a large pot with water and bring to a boil over high heat. Add the fettuccine and 1 tablespoon of the olive oil. Cook 7 to 8 minutes, or until cooked al dente (firm to the bite). Drain and place in a large serving bowl. Toss with 2 teaspoons of the olive oil and cover.

3. In a large skillet, warm the remaining olive oil over medium heat. Add the garlic and cook 1 minute, stirring constantly. Add the shrimp and sauté by stirring and/or shaking the pan while cooking, so that the shrimp cook evenly and do not stick to the bottom of the pan. After 3 minutes add the parsley, lemon juice, salt, and pepper and cook 1 minute more. Place the shrimp on top of the pasta and serve.

Island Tuna

This tropical dish provides large amounts of protein. In fact, tuna provides more complete protein than any other fish. Serve this dish with Rice Salad with Walnuts and Grapes (page 219), couscous, or soba noodles and a choice of vegetables.

Serves 4

2½ cups apple cider vinegar
2 tablespoons fresh rosemary or 1 tablespoon dried
½ cup soy sauce or shoyu
1 tablespoon paprika (Hungarian sweet paprika if available)
1½ cups pineapple juice (fresh is best)
4 4–6-ounce tuna steaks, 1–2 inches thick
2 tablespoons oil

1. In a small saucepan, bring the vinegar and rosemary to a boil. Reduce the heat to a gentle boil and cook 7 minutes. Strain the liquid into a bowl and add the soy sauce, paprika, and pineapple juice. Add the tuna steaks and marinate 15 minutes in the refrigerator.

2. Preheat the oven to 200° F. In a large skillet, heat half the oil. Add 2 tuna steaks and cook over medium-high heat for 4 minutes. Turn and cook 2 minutes, then add 2–4 tablespoons of the marinade and cook 4 minutes more, or until the fish is cooked. Place in the oven to keep warm and repeat the process for the remaining steaks without washing the pan. Finish by removing the last steaks and adding the remaining marinade to the skillet. Turn the heat to high and cook until it reduces to a thick sauce. Pour over the fish and serve immediately.

Sweet Endings: Desserts

Serving a dessert can be a tasty and nutritious way to make a meal last a little longer. Unlike most traditional desserts, which are high in sugar and refined carbohydrates, the recovery recipes are made from hearty whole-grain flours, fresh fruits, nuts, and other wholefoods ingredients. There are also wheat-free, egg-free, and even no-bake recipes.

The recovery desserts provide an abundance of vitamins, minerals, and enzymes. Unlike many desserts, these recipes do not rob the body of nutrients but rather enhance a recovery diet.

Poached Apples and Pears with Berry Sauce

An easy dessert recipe for those who have trouble eating fresh fruit every day. This dish can be served hot or cold; chilling the fruit and serving it with hot berry sauce is delicious. This dish also works without the berries, during times when berries are not in season.

Serves 4

4 cups apple juice or apple raspberry juice
1 cup finely chopped strawberries or raspberries
2 slices lemon
1 1-inch cinnamon stick
½ teaspoon alcohol-free vanilla extract
2 whole golden or red Delicious apples, peeled
2 whole Bosc pears, peeled

1. In a medium saucepan, combine the apple juice, berries, lemon slices, cinnamon stick, and vanilla extract. Bring to a boil over high heat, then reduce to a simmer, add the apples and pears, cover, and cook 12 minutes. The fruit is done when a fork slides easily into the flesh. Remove the fruit with a slotted spoon and set aside in a covered dish to keep warm, or bring to room temperature and chill.

2. Continue cooking the juice and berries until the liquid is reduced to a thick sauce, about 25 minutes. Divide the fruit among 4 plates and drizzle the sauce over each serving.

Fresh Fruit Pie with a Nut Crust

This is a mouth-watering, no-cook pie full of sweet fruit in a crunchy crust. It supplies lots of vitamins C and B-complex, bioflavonoids, folic acid, copper, manganese, phosphorus, and pantothenic acid. Nuts are a vegetarian source of protein.

Serves 8

Nut Crust

> 1 cup almonds
> 1 cup hazelnuts or walnuts
> ⅓ cup raisins
> ¼ cup apple juice

Filling

> 2 bananas
> 1 tablespoon freshly squeezed lemon juice
> 2–3 kiwifruits
> 1 quart fresh strawberries

1. Place the nuts and raisins in a blender or food processor and pulse until they are chopped well but not too fine. They should resemble small pebbles, not flour. Add the apple juice and pulse on and off for a few seconds. Pour the nut mixture into a glass pie plate and press out to shape a crust.

2. Slice the bananas and spread them inside the bottom of the nut crust, pressing slightly. Sprinkle with the lemon juice to prevent the bananas from turning brown. Slice the kiwifruits and add atop the bananas, pressing slightly. Slice the strawberries and add atop the kiwis, pressing slightly.

3. Chill the pie for at least 1 hour. Carefully slice and serve.

Apple Pie

Real old-fashioned apple pies had hearty whole-grain crusts just like this one. The walnuts add crunch and many vitamins and minerals. Use the pie crust for other fruit pies such as peach, berry, or rhubarb.

Serves 8

Crust

    2 cups whole wheat pastry flour
    Dash of salt
    4 tablespoons vegetable oil
    ¼ cup iced apple juice

Filling

    8 McIntosh apples, peeled, cored, and sliced
    2 tablespoons arrowroot
    ½ teaspoon ground cinnamon
    ⅛ teaspoon nutmeg
    ½ teaspoon salt
    2 tablespoons freshly squeezed lemon juice
    2 tablespoons honey
    1 cup chopped walnuts

1. Make the crust. In a large bowl, combine the flour and the salt. Add the oil and mix with a fork until the mixture resembles small peas. Add the iced apple juice a little at a time, adding only enough so that the dough pulls away from the sides of the bowl and forms a rough ball. Turn out onto a lightly floured board and gently knead a few strokes, then wrap in a plastic bag and set aside 10 to 15 minutes at room temperature.

2. Preheat the oven to 350° F.

3. Make the filling. In a large bowl, toss the apples with the arrowroot, cinnamon, nutmeg, and salt. In a smaller bowl, mix together the lemon juice, honey, and walnuts. Add the mixture to the apples and stir to combine.

4. Remove the dough from the plastic bag and cut into 2 even pieces. Roll each out on a floured board into 2 10-inch, ⅛-inch-thick circles. Carefully place one circle in an 8-inch pie plate, add the apple mixture, and top with the other circle. Crimp the edges together and prick the top several times with the tines of a fork. Bake about 20 minutes, or until golden brown.

Banana Cream

This recipe is for homemade ice cream the real easy way. The taste is incredible and is loved even by those who don't consider themselves to be banana lovers. Bananas are high in potassium and low in calories and fat. For variation, add a frozen fresh peach or ¼ cup of frozen fresh berries. Substitute pecans or almonds for the walnuts, or substitute orange juice for the water.

Serves 4

> 6 very ripe bananas
> 3 tablespoons cold water
> ½ cup chopped walnuts

1. Peel the bananas and place on a dish in the freezer. Leave until frozen. (Freeze overnight or put them in in the morning to serve in the evening.)

2. Place in a food processor or blender and quickly puree. Add water 1 tablespoon at a time until the bananas are the consistency of ice cream. Divide into 4 portions, sprinkle with walnuts, and serve immediately.

Apple-Blueberry Crisp

This is a nutritious low-fat recipe. This crisp is high in fiber, biotin, and manganese. Any favorite fruit combinations will do.

Serves 10

> 1½ cups whole wheat flour or ¾ cup barley flour
>   and ¾ cup soy flour
> ½ cup oats
> ½ teaspoon salt
> 2 tablespoons vegetable oil
> ½ cup iced apple juice
> 2 tablespoons apple juice
> 10 apples, preferably McIntosh, peeled, cored, and sliced
> 2 cups blueberries
> ½ cup crushed walnuts or pecans

1. Preheat the oven to 350° F.

2. In a medium bowl, combine the flour, oats, and salt. Add the oil and with a fork stir the mixture until it resembles small peas. Add the iced apple juice a little at a time, adding just enough so that the dough pulls away from the sides of the bowl into a rough ball. Press together with your hands, then return the dough to the bowl and set aside 10 minutes.

3. Break the dough into tiny pieces and place on a greased baking sheet. Bake 10 minutes, or until the dough is crunchy.

4. In a large pot, bring the apple juice to a boil over high heat. Add the apples and blueberries, reduce heat to a simmer, and cook 5 minutes. Remove from heat and pour into an 8 x 8 x 2-inch baking dish.

5. Sprinkle the cooked dough and nuts over the fruit. Bake 35 to 40 minutes. You may want to put a piece of foil or a baking sheet under the pan, since the juices may bubble up and out of the pan onto the oven floor.

Variation: Peach-Strawberry Crisp

Substitute 12 peaches, peeled, pitted, and sliced, and 2 cups sliced strawberries for the apples and blueberries. Substitute ½ cup crushed pecans for the walnuts.

Variation: Pear Crisp

Substitute 10 pears, peeled, cored, and sliced, for the apples.

Strawberry Plum Tart

This low-fat, naturally sweet tart gives all the satisfaction of a rich dessert with none of the guilt, and the contrast of the crisp crust and rich red filling is as pleasing to the eye as it is to the palate.

Serves 8 to 10

Crust

¼ cup vegetable oil
2½ cups whole wheat pastry flour
½ teaspoon salt
Dash of ground cinnamon
⅓ cup ice water

Filling

1 cup apple juice
1 cup sliced strawberries
1 teaspoon honey, rice yinnie (page 112), maple syrup, or
  other sweetener
½ teaspoon alcohol-free vanilla extract
1½ pounds plums, pitted and sliced

1. Make the crust. Chill the oil in the refrigerator until cold. In a large bowl, combine the flour, salt, and cinnamon. Stir in the oil and combine with a fork until the mixture resembles small peas. Stir in the ice water a little at a time, adding just enough so that the crust pulls away from the sides of the bowl into a rough ball. Turn out onto a lightly floured board and briefly knead into a ball. Cover with a plastic bag and chill 15 to 20 minutes.

2. In a small saucepan, combine the juice, half of the strawberries, honey, and vanilla extract. Bring to a boil over medium heat, then reduce to a simmer and cook until the juices have reduced and the sauce is syrupy, about 20 minutes.

3. In the meantime, preheat the oven to 400° F.

4. Remove the dough from the wrap and roll out on a lightly floured board into a 10-inch circle, ⅛ inch thick. If the crust is too crumbly and falls apart, press it back into a ball and knead it briefly, then start rolling it out again. Place the tart pan over the dough circle and cut around it, 2 inches wider

than the pan all around. Gently press the crust into the tart pan and roll the rolling pin over the top to trim the edges. Set aside.

5. Add the plums to the strawberry sauce and cook 2 minutes. Remove from heat, allow to cool, then pour into the tart crust. Place the remaining strawberries around the outer circle of the tart and bake 20 minutes.

Fresh Fruit Compote

The fruit in this compote contains several types of fiber. Some fiber is soluble, such as pectin in apples and pears. Pectin forms a gel in the gastrointestinal tract that slows food absorption and provides a feeling of fullness. Some fiber is insoluble—cellulose, for example. It also absorbs many times its weight in water, so it provides a feeling of fullness to dieters. This compote is also a source of vitamin C, carbohydrates, and natural sweeteners. It can be served hot or cold over hot cereal or pancakes, or alone as a dessert.

Makes 4 cups

> 4 cups apple juice or any apple juice combination, such as apple-strawberry, apple-pear, etc.
> 2 apples, preferably golden Delicious or red Delicious, cored and coarsely chopped
> 1 pear, cored and coarsely chopped
> 1 peach or fresh apricot, pitted and coarsely chopped (if unavailable, use another pear)
> 1 fresh fig, or 4 dried unsulfured figs, coarsely chopped
> ½ cup seasonal berries
> ¼ cup raisins
> 1 1-inch cinnamon stick or ½ teaspoon ground cinnamon
> Sprigs of fresh mint (optional, for garnish)

1. Place all the ingredients (except the mint) in a medium pot and bring to a boil over high heat.

2. Reduce heat to a simmer and cook until the fruit is very thick and syrupy, about 30 minutes. Garnish with mint before serving.

Mock Mocha Pudding

A great substitute for chocolate pudding, this rich but light dessert is a favorite of students at the Natural Gourmet Cookery School in New York City and comes from Annemarie Colbin, the school's founder.

Serves 4

2 cups apple juice
1 bar or 4 tablespoons agar flakes (available at health food stores)
1 teaspoon alcohol-free vanilla
2 tablespoons instant cereal coffee (that is, coffee-free cereal drinks such as Cafix, Pero, or Postum)
1 tablespoon tahini
4 teaspoons chopped almonds

1. Place the juice in a small saucepan. Rinse the agar bar and shred it into the juice or sprinkle the flakes over the juice. Simmer until dissolved, about 2 to 3 minutes. Stir in the vanilla and the cereal coffee.

2. Pour into a shallow pan and chill to set, about 2 hours.

3. Remove from the refrigerator, cut up, and place in a food processor or blender. Add the tahini and process until creamy. Pour into individual serving bowls, garnish with almonds, and serve.

Brown Rice Pecan Cookies

These cookies are wheat- and dairy-free and make for a nutritious quick snack.

Makes 1 dozen

1 cup brown rice flour
1/4 teaspoon ground ginger
3 tablespoons vegetable oil, plus more for brushing the pan
1/4 cup honey or rice yinnie (page 112)
1/4 teaspoon alcohol-free vanilla extract
3 tablespoons ice water
1 cup crushed pecans

1. Preheat the oven to 350° F. In a medium bowl, combine the flour and ginger. Add the oil, honey, vanilla, water, and pecans. Stir until the mixture forms into small pea-shaped balls.

2. Lightly coat a baking sheet with vegetable oil. Press table-spoonfuls of the dough into 2-inch rounds and place on the baking sheet 2 inches apart. Bake 10 minutes. Remove from the oven and let cool on the rack. These cookies should be crunchy.

Peanut Oat Clusters

The clusters are chewy, gooey, and good. Peanuts are very high in protein. They do contain fat, but most of it is unsaturated. They are very high in biotin, which is necessary for the utilization of protein, B_{12}, folic acid, and pantothenic acid.

Makes 1 dozen

> ½ cup organic peanut butter
> ¼ cup honey
> 2 tablespoons vegetable oil, plus more for greasing the pan
> 2 egg whites
> 1 cup oats
> ¼ cup chopped walnuts
> ¼ cup unsweetened coconut

1. Preheat the oven to 375° F.

2. In a large bowl, cream together the peanut butter, honey, oil, and egg whites. Stir in the oats, nuts, and coconut. Drop from a tablespoon onto a lightly greased cookie sheet. Bake about 15 minutes, or until lightly browned and cooked through.

Hot Weather Coolers for Dessert

Strawberry Sun Cooler

A perfect drink for after dinner that's high in vitamin C and digestive enzymes.

Serves 2

>   1 cup crushed ice
>   ½ cup pineapple juice
>   ½ cup apple juice
>   ½ cup strawberries, hulled
>   ⅔ cup freshly squeezed orange juice

Blend the ingredients in a blender and serve in chilled glasses.

Mellow Mint Cooler

A real summer refresher that contains good amounts of iron and potassium. Remember that potassium regulates intercellular fluids and works with sodium to maintain the body's water balance.

Serves 2

>   1 cup crushed ice
>   1 cup sparkling mineral water
>   2–3 tablespoons chopped mint
>   1 finely chopped fig
>   1 banana, peeled
>   ½ cup freshly squeezed lemon juice

Blend the ingredients in a blender and serve in chilled glasses.

Tropical Passion Cooler

Fresh juices are superior in nutritional value to anything in a can or bottle. Papaya has received the highest nutritional rating of any fruit by the Washington-based Center for Science in the Public Interest. It contains vitamin A, vitamin C, folic acid, potassium, and lots of fiber.

Serves 2

1 cup pineapple juice
Juice from 2 oranges
Juice from 1 lemon
½ cup crushed ice
½ cup chopped papaya

Blend the ingredients in a blender and serve in chilled glasses.

Perky Apple Cooler

Here's a cleansing, stimulating drink that's even great hot.

Serves 2

2 cups apple juice
1 cup sparkling apple juice
½ teaspoon finely shredded fresh ginger root

Blend the ingredients in a blender and serve over ice, or heat and serve.

18 *People and Food: Finding the Spiritual Connection*

This book has addressed an area largely ignored in most recovery programs: the unique and critical connection between the body and the mind, and the ways in which food can influence this connection. We have examined some of the processes that break down as a result of drug and alcohol addiction and eating disorders. We have explored how good nutritional practices—including a diet of wholefoods, exercise, and nutritional supplementation—can correct this damage and bring about a truly complete recovery. And we have provided specific information on how you can change your eating habits and lifestyle to enhance your own recovery process.

But there is another, less tangible way in which food can work for recovery. Few human activities are more creative, communal, and life-affirming than preparing and eating meals. Food is at the center of many religious ceremonies and cultural traditions, from the Passover seder, to the Thanksgiving feast, to the communion rites of various Christian groups. Food is more than just a source of physical sustenance. It has an emotional and spiritual resonance as well.

The concept of a spiritual connection between humans and their food is nothing new. It has been acknowledged, respected, and maintained through a variety of large and small mealtime rituals. Some, such as the traditions mentioned above, are major events that are part of our shared culture. Others are carried out on a personal or family basis—such as saying grace or "always" having pot roast on Sundays—that give us a sense of comfort and security within the smaller cultural parameters of our families or individual households. Whatever the specific tradition, the rituals we practice at mealtimes indicate the significance we give to food in our lives and, by extension, the significance we give to caring for ourselves and others through food.

In the days when people worked in the fields and literally took their foods from the soil, the complex relationships between nature, food, and our physical and emotional well-being were clear and incontrovertible. Our ancient (and not-so-ancient) ancestors were aware of the precious balance between a good life and a good crop. They worshipped the sun, the wind, and the rain and even endowed the crops themselves with divinity.

Today, most of us are completely removed from these natural sources of our foods. We buy foods that are encased in plastic, wax, cardboard, and metal. Food doesn't come from the earth—it comes from supermarket shelves or hurried waiters. Is it surprising that our relationship with food has become distant and distorted? Strange though it may seem, reestablishing our spiritual connection with food is an integral part of the recovery process.

The prevalence of eating disorders in our society indicates that many people do indeed have intense relationships with food—albeit unhealthy ones. Distorted emotional and spiritual links to food are the root of many eating disorders: In the absence of an understanding of food and its effects, people eat the wrong foods, at the wrong times, in the wrong amounts, and suffer the biochemical and physical consequences. Avoiding these pitfalls, and establishing a healthy alliance with food, requires an understanding of the physical and psychological aspects of our relationship with food and eating.

Analyzing Your Relationship with Food

If you were to ask most people how they relate to food, you'd probably get one of two responses: "I don't know" or "Love/hate." Food occupies such a unique and confusing place in our society that our relationships with food have become equally complex. Do we love foods because of the satisfaction they provide or hate them for "making us fat?" Do we love dining out because it is an enjoyable social occasion or hate it because it is expensive and we're not sure what fork to use? Do we love holiday meals for the camaraderie with family and friends, or hate them for the stress of preparation and the tension of some interpersonal relationships?

We use a sort of psychological litmus test when working with clients and patients, to assess their feelings about food. Sit down in a comfortable chair at a table, with a paper and pen in front of you. Close your eyes and relax for a few moments. Then say the word "food" aloud. Open your eyes and write down the very first word, thought, or image that came to mind. Don't edit yourself or stop to think about what your response might mean. Repeat these steps twelve times.

One of our eating disorder clients conducted this test when she was several months into recovery. Her responses were "love," "sex," "nurturing," "chicken," "orange," "Jell-O," "fast," "angry," "cook," "alone." After some consideration, she realized that her responses were a capsule history of her eating disorder. She had often substituted food for "sex" and "love." When she was a child, her grandmother showed her love by feeding her roasted "chicken" and "orange" "Jell-O." She often ate "fast" or at "fast" food restaurants, which left her feeling "angry." She wanted to learn to "cook" good foods for herself when she was "alone."

Try this experiment for yourself. It may reveal some interesting things in your relationship with food. If nothing is immediately apparent, try doing the experiment several times, and tack your responses to the refrigerator so that you can refer to them over time. Perhaps you, like many of our clients, will find that there are old associations/memories associated with food that are affecting your eating habits now. Perhaps you became engaged while eating chocolate cake, or received a promotion while sipping hot coffee with your boss. Memory and emotion are deeply connected with taste and smell, so it is likely that whenever you eat or even smell these foods they evoke pleasant sensations. Conversely, foods that are associated with unpleasant events and experiences are likely to evoke unpleasant sensations and cause you to avoid these foods.

The goal of this exercise is to sort through your emotional reactions to food in general (and specific foods in particular), and analyze and discard those that are obstacles to eating well. If you hate spinach because your mom forced you to eat it when you were a child, maybe it's time to learn how to deal with spinach as an adult.

Putting Food in Perspective

In analyzing your relationship with food, it is important to examine when, where, and how you eat your meals. Try keeping a meal journal for a couple of weeks. Note when you eat, where you eat, what you eat, and how long you actually spend enjoying your meals. Do you bolt down your food on the run, or while watching television, or while standing at a corner hot dog stand? Do you ever think about what you are eating and where it came from? If not, it's time to make some changes.

Take steps to change some of your bad habits. Wake up a little earlier and eat breakfast: Boil an egg or cook some oatmeal while showering. At lunchtime, find a park or green area to eat in. If you can't leave work and find it too busy in the lunchroom, try to eat a bit later after the crowd has dispersed. Dinnertime finds many in recovery too tired to cook. To overcome this, try to cook grains or beans in advance so that all you have to do is reheat them and quickly steam a vegetable or make a salad.

Remember to eat. Skipping meals puts the body into a starvation mode in which it will turn any food into fat for storage. More frequent, smaller meals seem to work best for those in recovery because this pattern gives the body a chance to absorb all the nutrients. Make sure to vary your diet as well so that you receive a variety of nutrients. Before eating, close your eyes for a moment and rid your body of its everyday stresses.

It is also important to examine any rituals you may associate with food and the taking of meals. Try asking yourself the following questions to discover what your rituals are and how you can change them to make a more healthy connection with food.

Do you shop daily, weekly, monthly?

Do you shop in a supermarket or outdoor farmer's market?

Do you shop differently for holidays and weekends than you do for weekdays?

What is the method of your preparation?

Do you envision pleased guests when stirring a sauce?

Do you watch television when you eat or do you concentrate solely on your dinner?

Do you put your answering machine on during meals?

Do you eat alone or with others?

Do you ever reflect on the source of your food?

Mealtime rituals are important not only because they heighten or mark events for us, but because they separate the activity of mealtime from other activities in our lives. It is at this moment that a spiritual connection can be made, when we stop and take time to meditate or pray in acknowledgment of the source of our food. This time serves another function as well. It gives us an opportunity to release daily tensions, thereby readying our bodies to receive the maximum amount of nutrients from our food.

The manner in which we take our meals reflects more about us than we might care to admit. However, keep in mind that nothing is more life-affirming than eating. Keep looking at ways to create loving rituals around your meal and its preparation. Creating new rituals or reviving lost rituals can help our progress toward healthful eating habits and maintaining them.

For truly complete recovery it isn't enough to know the why and what of the dietary and lifestyle changes needed to become well. Each recovering person also needs to figure out how he or she can best make those changes, by looking carefully at existing relationships with food and identifying the areas that need change.

A key step is learning to shop and prepare fresh wholefoods. This is the foundation for developing a healthy biochemical balance. Maintaining the recovery process requires a recognition of the connection each of us has to our food source—the spiritual connection.

If you have been in recovery and are unsatisfied or unhappy, if you suspect there's more to life in recovery than what you're feeling, you're right. There *is* a higher level of recovery. But it does not come without its cost. The price of this higher level of recovery is change—a change to a healthier lifestyle. For some it's a fairly easy transition or extension of their current path, and for others it's a strange and more difficult road. But if you take the changes one day at a time and allow yourself to be open to the newness of life, you'll be greatly rewarded with a healthier, happier, and more energetic life. Good luck.

Appendixes

Appendix A

Potential Drugs of Dependency

Classification	Drug	Trade/Street Name(s)
STIMULANTS	amphetamines	Benzedrine
	methamphetamines	Methadrine
	dextroamphetamine	Dexedrine
	methylenedioxy-amphetamine	MDA
	diet aids	Preludin, Tenuate, Fastin, Lonamine, Dexatrim
	cocaine	coke, crack
	caffeine	found in: coffee, tea, cola, over-the-counter wake-up pills, some analgesics
	nicotine	found in: tobacco
SEDATIVE-HYPNOTICS	Barbiturates: secobarbital pentobarbital amobarbital	Seconal Nembutal
	Piperidinediones: glutethimide methyprylon	Doriden Noludar
	Quinazolones: methaqualone	Quaalude, Mequin

Classification	Drug	Trade/Street Name(s)
	Tertiary Alcohol: ethchlorvynol	Placidyl

	Benzodiazepenes:
	  alprazaolam
	  chlordiazepoxide
	  clonazepam
	  clorazepate
	  diazepam
	  flurazepam
	  halazepam
	  lorazepam
	  oxazepam
	  prazepam
	  temazepam
		
		Xanax
		Librium
		Klonopin
		Tranxene
		Valium
		Dalmane
		Paxipam
		Ativan
		Serax
		Centrax
		Restoril

	Carbamates:
	  meprobamate
	  tybamate
		
		Miltown

	Halogenated hydrocarbons: chloral hydrate	chloral hydrate
OPIATES AND OPIOIDS	opium	
	codeine	
	morphine	
	heroin	
	hydro-morphine	Dilaudid
	oxycodone	Percodan
	methadone	Dolophine
	propoxyphene	Darvon
	meperidine	Demerol

Classification	Drug	Trade/Street Name(s)
HALLUCI-NOGENS	Lysergic acid diethylamide	LSD
	Laphophora williamsii	mescaline
	Psilocybe cubensis	psilocybin
	Tetrahydrocanna-binol	THC (found in marijuana)
	2, 5-dimethoxy-4-methyl-amphetamine	STP, DOM
	Methylenedioxy-amphetamine	MDA
	Dimethyltryptamine	DMT
	Phencyclidine	PCP

Appendix B

Alcohol Content of Common Medications

Item	Use	Manufacturer	Alcohol %
Ambenyl	cough suppressant	Forest	5.0
Ambenyl-D	cough suppressant, decongestant, expectorant	Forest	9.5
Amytal Elixir	sedative	Lilly	30.0
Asbron G Elixir	antiasthmatic	Sandoz	15.0
Astring-D-Sol	mouthwash	Breon	70.0
Benadryl-Elixir	antihistamine	Parke-Davis	14.0
Benylin Cough Syrup	cough suppressant	Parke-Davis	5.0
Breacol	cough	Glenbrook	10.0
Betalin Complex Elixir	vitamin	Lilly	17.0
Bronchol-Tussin	cough	First Texas	40.0
Bronkolixir	antiasthmatic	Winthrop	19.0
Cepacol	mouthwash	Lakeside	14.5
Ce-Vi-Sol Drops	vitamins	Mead-Johnson	5.0
Cheracol D Cough Syrup	cough suppressant	Upjohn	4.75
Chlor-Trimeton Syrup	antihistamine	Schering	7.0
Choledyl Elixir	antiasthmatic	Parke-Davis	20.0
Colace Liquid	laxative	Mead-Johnson	1.0
Colgate 100	mouthwash	Colgate-Palmolive	15.3
CONTAC Nighttime	cold medicine	SmithKline & French	25.0
Co-Tylenol Liquid	cold-allergy	McNeil	7.0
Day Care Liquid	cough	Vicks	7.5
Dilaudid Cough Syrup	cough suppressant, analgesic	Knoll	5.0
Dimetane Elixir	cold/allergy	Robins	3.0
Dimetane Expectorant	cough	Robins	3.5
Dimetapp Elixir	cold/allergy	Robins	2.3
Diural Oral Suspension	diuretic	Merck Sharp & Dohme	0.5
Donnatal Elixir	antispasmodic	Robins	23.0
Dristan Liquid	cough	Whitehall	12.0
Elixophyllin-KL-Elixir	antiasthmatic	A.H. Robins	23.0

Item	Use	Manufacturer	Alcohol %
Feosol Elixir	iron supplement	SmithKline & French	5.0
Fergon Elixir	iron supplement	Winthrop	6.0
Geriplex-FS	vitamins	Parke-Davis	18.0
Geritol Liquid	vitamins	Beecham Labs.	12.0
Halls Cough Syrup	cough	Warner-Lambert	22.0
Hycotuss	expectorant	DuPont	10.0
Iberet Liquid	vitamins	Abbott	1.0
Imodium A-D	antidiarrheal	McNeil	5.25
Lanoxin Elixir Pediatric	cardiac medicine	Burroughs Wellcome	10.0
Larylgan Aerosol Spray	mouthwash	Ayerst	94.0
Lasix Oral Solution	diuretic	Hoechst-Roussel	11.5
Lavoris	mouthwash	Vicks	5.0
Listerine	mouthwash	Warner-Lambert	26.9
Lomotil Liquid	antidiarrheal	Searle	15.0
Lufyllin Elixir	bronchodilator	Wallace	20.0
Marax-DF Syrup	bronchodilator	Roerig	5.0
Mediatric Liquid	estrogen	Wyeth-Ayerst	15.0
Mellaril Oral Solution	antipsychotic	Sandoz	3.0
Modane Liquid	laxative	Warren-Teed	5.0
Mol-Iron Liquid	vitamin	Schering	4.0
Naldecon DX Drops	decongestant	Bristol Labs.	0.6–5.0
Nembutal Elixir	sedative	Abbott	18.0
Neo-Synephrine Elixir	cold/allergy	Winthrop	8.0
Novahistine Elixir	antihistamine, decongestant	Lakeside	5.0
Nucofed Expectorant	cough suppressant, decongestant, expectorant	Beecham Labs.	12.5
Nyquil Cough Syrup	cough suppressant	Vicks	25.0
Organidin Elixir	expectorant	Wallace	21.75
Pamelor Oral Solution	antidepressant	Sandoz	3.0–5.0
Peri-Colace Syrup	laxative	Mead-Johnson	10.0
Permitil Oral Concentrate	antipsychotic	Schering	1.0
Phenergan Expectorant	cough suppressant	Wyeth-Ayerst	7.0
Phenergan Syrup	antihistamine	Wyeth-Ayerst	1.5
Phenobarbitol Elixir	sedative	Roxane	13.5
Prolixin Elixir	antipsychotic	Princeton	14.0
Proval Elixir	analgesic	Reid-Provident	10.5

Item	Use	Manufacturer	Alcohol %
Quiet Nite Syrup	cough	Rexall	15.0
Rexall Cold Sore Lotion	cold sore	Rexall	90.0
Robitussin Syrup	cough	Robins	3.5
Romilar CF Syrup	cough	Black	10.0
Rondee D.M.	cough	Ross	0.6
Scope	mouthwash	Procter & Gamble	18.5
St. Joseph Fever Reducer for Children	analgesic	Plough	9.5
St. Joseph Cough Syrup for Children	cough	Plough	0.6
Sominex Liquid	sleep aid	Beecham Labs.	10.0
Theo-Organidin Elixir	cough	Wampole	15.0
Tylenol	cough	McNeuk	7.0
Valadol Liquid	cough	Squibb	9.0
Vicks Formula 44	cough	Vicks	10.0
X-Prep Liquid	laxative	Gray	7.0

Appendix C

Alcohol-Free Medications

Item	Use	Manufacturer
Actifed Syrup	decongestant	Burroughs Wellcome
Bentyl Syrup	antispasmodic	Lakeside Pharmaceuticals
Chloraseptic Liquid	anesthetic and antiseptic mouthwash/gargle	Richardson-Vicks
Colace Liquid	laxative	Mead-Johnson
Gly-Oxide	oral anesthetic, anti-inflammatory	Marion
Haldol Concentrate	antipsychotic	McNeil
Kaopectate	antidiarrheal	Upjohn
Kwelcof Liquid	cough suppressant	B.F. Ascher & Co.
Liquiprin Drops & Elixir	analgesic	Norcliff Thayer
Maalox Suspension	antacid	Rorer
Mylanta Liquid	antacid, antigas	Stuart
Mysoline Suspension	anticonvulsant	Wyeth-Ayerst
Naldecon CX Adult Liquid	cough suppressant, expectorant	Bristol Labs.
Naldecon DX Adult Liquid	decongestant, expectorant, cough suppressant	Bristol Labs.
Naldecon Senior EX	expectorant	Bristol Labs.
Nucofed Syrup	cough suppressant, decongestant	Beecham Labs.
Pepto-Bismol	antacid, antigas, antidiarrheal	Procter & Gamble
Periactin Syrup	antihistamine	Merck Sharp & Dohme
Proventil Syrup	antiasthmatic	Schering
Scot-Tussin DM Cough & Cold Medicine	cough suppressant, decongestant	Scot-Tussin
Sinequan Oral Concentrate	antidepressant	Roerig
Slo-Phyllin Syrup	antiasthmatic	Rorer
Stelazine Concentrate	anxiolytic, antipsychotic	SmithKline & French
Sudafed Plus Liquid	decongestant, antihistamine	Burroughs Wellcome
Sumycin Syrup	antibiotic	Squibb
Theolair Liquid	antiasthmatic	3M Riker
Theolair-Plus Liquid	antiasthmatic	3M Riker

Item	Use	Manufacturer
Thorazine Syrup	antipsychotic	SmithKline & French
Triaminic Cold Syrup	decongestant, antihistamine	Sandoz
Triaminic-DM Cough Formula	cough suppressant, decongestant	Sandoz
Tussirex Sugar-Free, Alcohol-Free & Dye-Free	cough suppressant	Scot-Tussin
Vicks Children's Cough Syrup	cough suppressant, expectorant	Richardson-Vicks
Vicks Children's Nyquil	cough suppressant, decongestant, antihistamine	Richardson-Vicks
Vistaril Oral Suspension	anxiolytic	Pfizer

Appendix D
Diagnostic Criteria for Addictions

According to the American Psychiatric Association's *Diagnostic and Statistical Manual of Mental Disorders* (the DSM III-R), a person is chemically dependent if he or she shows at least three of the following behavior patterns or symptoms for at least one month (or has displayed them intermittently for a long while).

*The substance is taken in larger doses or for longer periods than originally intended.

*There have been repeated and unsuccessful attempts to cut down or eliminate use of the substance.

*The bulk of the person's time is spent getting, using, or recovering from the substance.

*Major role obligations at work, school, home, and so forth are neglected because of intoxication with or withdrawal from the substance.

*Normal social, recreational, and occupational activities are neglected or abandoned due to substance use.

*Substance use is continued despite obvious negative physical, psychological, and social effects.

*Substance is used even when it is physically dangerous (for example, drinking and driving).

*More of the substance is required in order to become intoxicated or achieve the desired "high." (This phenomenon is also known as tolerance.)

*Physical and psychological withdrawal symptoms (anxiety, tremors, nausea, etc.) are experienced when the substance is not taken.

*The substance is used in order to stave off withdrawal symptoms (rather than for recreational purposes).

There are several questions you can ask yourself (or another) to determine if you have become addicted to a particular substance, be it alcohol or coffee. These include:

*Have you stopped eating regular meals? (Food is one of the first things to fall by the wayside in addicted individuals.)

*Have you been eating more sugar and sweets? (Sugary foods become substitutes for the real nutrition the body requires, particularly in alcoholics.)

*Have you recently gained (or lost) weight for no apparent reason?

*Are you able to use the substance without seeming intoxicated? (Tolerance is one of the surest signs of addiction.)

*Have you increased the amount you take?

*Do you take the substance every day, in a regular pattern? (As addiction progresses, the addict needs to maintain a constant level of the substance in order to feel even vaguely normal or functional.)

*Have you begun to experience strange fluctuations in mood, or inappropriate reactions to relatively common events? (Hypoglycemic episodes and disrupted neurochemical balance can cause dramatic emotional and psychological "peaks and valleys.")

*Have you been feeling depressed, or considered suicide?

*Have you lost interest in sex? (Addictions, particularly alcoholism, disrupt the hormones and brain regions that regulate sexual activity, causing impotence and loss of sexual drive.)

*Have you been experiencing motor problems, such as dropping things or bumping into things?

*Have you been having trouble sleeping? (Addictions can disturb the brain regions that regulate sleep, leading to a pattern of restless and limited sleep time.)

If the answer to six or more of these questions is yes, you are probably addicted. If you're in doubt, try answering the following questions (culled from the Michigan Alcoholism Screening Test, or MAST). The number of points to be credited for each yes answer is in parentheses at the end of each question.

#1. Do you feel you are a normal user of this substance? (no: 2)

#2. Have you ever forgotten events that occurred when you were under the influence of this substance? (yes: 2)

#3. Have your spouse or parents complained about your substance use? (yes: 1)

#4. Can you easily stop using the substance after taking a small amount (such as two drinks)? (no: 2)

#5. Have you ever apologized for (or felt bad about) your substance use? (yes: 1)

#6. Do your friends and relatives consider you to be a normal substance user? (no: 2)

#7. Have you ever tried to limit your use of this substance to certain times of day or certain places? (0)

#8. Can you stop using the substance whenever you like? (no: 2)

#9. Have you ever attended an Alcoholics Anonymous (or similar group) meeting? (yes: 5)

#10. Have you gotten into fights when under the influence of this substance? (yes: 1)

#11. Has your substance use created problems in your marriage or relationships? (yes: 2)

#12. Have any of your family members gone to Al-Anon or similar groups? (yes: 2)

#13. Has your substance use caused problems at work? (yes: 2)

#14. Have you lost a lover because of your substance use? (yes: 2)

#15. Have you lost a job because of your substance use? (yes: 2)

#16. Have you been absent from work or school for more than two days in a row because of your substance use? (yes: 2)

#17. Do you use the substance before noon? (yes: 1)

#18. Have you ever had liver trouble? (yes: 2)

#19. Have you ever had physical symptoms after not using the substance for awhile? (yes: 2)

#20. Have you ever gone for counseling about your substance use? (yes: 5)

#21. Have you ever been hospitalized for substance abuse? (yes: 5)

#22. Have you ever been hospitalized in a psychiatric facility because of your substance use? (yes: 2)

#23. Have you ever been arrested for behaviors caused by (or related to) your substance (such as drunk driving, possession of a controlled substance, or drug dealing)? (yes: 2)

A score of five points or more is considered a positive indicator of addiction.

Appendix E
Diagnostic Criteria for Eating Disorders

Eating disorders are unique in that the substance being abused is absolutely essential for human life. In eating disorders, abstinence is not an option. Instead, the *relationship* with food must be evaluated and changed.

Although there are many overweight men, and a small percentage of men suffer from anorexia and bulimia, women are far more likely to suffer from eating disorders. It has been estimated that more than 90 percent of anorexics and bulimics are female. For this reason, we will be using the female pronoun when discussing these disorders.

Compulsive Overeating

Most people overindulge in food at one time or another. But a truly compulsive eater does so all the time, eating the wrong foods, at the wrong times, in the wrong amounts. Food (usually candy, cakes, or some other sweet) is the first thing the compulsive eater reaches for in a crisis situation. Eating has little or nothing to do with real physical hunger.

When an individual eats compulsively, food serves not as sustenance, but as a substance—much like alcohol, heroin, or any of the other drugs of abuse. The individual uses food as a panacea for a variety of psychological, social, emotional, and physical problems. When the compulsive overeater consumes lots of sugary processed foods (as most do), the chemistry of the brain is also affected, so that a true physical addiction develops.

Bulimia (or Binge-Purge Syndrome)

Bulimics are the psychological cousins of compulsive overeaters, with one crucial difference. Although the bulimic may *ingest* large quantities of food, she will not *digest* them. Instead, she will force the food (and dreaded calories) out of her system, using a number of methods, including vomiting, enemas, laxatives, diuretics, and compulsive exercise.

Because the bulimic does not actually absorb most of the calories she consumes, most bulimic individuals are at or slightly below normal weight. Superficially, bulimics can appear fairly healthy, although they may show some signs of the damages of purging, such as:

> *skin disorders on the hand used to induce vomiting (due to contact with gastric acids)
>
> *bad breath
>
> *discolored and/or decaying teeth (due to corrosion of dental enamel by gastric acids)
>
> *shin splints, stress fractures, or other injuries as a result of compulsive exercise.

According to the *Diagnostic and Statistical Manual of Mental Disorders,* a person is diagnosed as bulimic if she displays the following patterns or symptoms:

> *constant preoccupation and concern with weight and body shape
>
> *frequent episodes of binge eating, in which large amounts of food (such as a gallon of ice cream) are eaten in a short amount of time (such as fifteen minutes)
>
> *a loss of control over the eating behavior during these binges ("Once I started, I just couldn't stop.")
>
> *regular use of self-induced vomiting, laxatives, diuretics, fasts, or abnormally vigorous exercise to offset binges and prevent weight gain
>
> *at least two binges a week for at least three months.

Anorexia

In anorexia, food of any kind is the enemy, and eating is seen to be a failure. Although some anorexics are also bulimic, in general the anorexic's goal is not to eat at all. Anorexics typically have no idea what they really look like and believe that they are "fat" even when they are emaciated and drawn. Anywhere from 5 percent to 18 percent of anorexics die of this disorder, as a result of the extensive metabolic and physical effects of prolonged starvation.

The DSM-III (R) sets the following diagnostic criteria for anorexia:

* excessive anxiety over gaining weight and becoming fat, regardless of actual weight

* refusal to maintain the body weight appropriate for age and height; weight is 15 percent or more below normal

* disturbed and inaccurate perception of the body; claims to be fat even when gaunt

* loss of menstrual cycle (in females) for at least three consecutive months.

Appendix F
Treatment Guidelines

Not all treatment programs are created equal. Some pay a great deal of attention to the biological needs of patients, and others completely ignore them. Whether you are looking for a long-term inpatient facility or a coordinated program of outpatient care, there are certain "must haves" in the treatment of addictions and eating disorders. Without them, your chances of achieving a serene and long-term recovery are definitely reduced.

Diagnosis

Treatment is only as good as the information on which it is based. This information is gathered through careful testing and analysis, including:

* chest X ray

* full blood workup, including:
  – complete blood count
  – protein metabolism
  – lipid metabolism
  – carbohydrate metabolism

> –vitamin and mineral assays (if available)
> –toxic metal screen

*complete urinalysis, including:
> –drug and alcohol screen
> –evaluations for blood, bile, sugar, albumin, and acetone
> –evaluations of pH and specific gravity

*EKG (within 24 hours of admission)

*PAP smear (for women, if not done within the past year)

*allergen testing of blood sample (preferably using the RAST screening method) in persons with preexisting allergic symptoms, such as:
> –asthma
> –chronic gastroenteritis
> –adverse food reactions
> –rashes
> –wheezing
> –chronic fatigue

More detailed immunological evaluation, using a skin test and other techniques, should be performed. Food, chemical, and environmental sensitivities should be thoroughly investigated.

Psychological testing and diagnoses should be avoided until the patient is stable and has been detoxified for at least five days. While it is important to know if a patient is a threat to himself or herself or others, strict psychiatric labeling should be avoided until some of the biological damage of addiction has been addressed.

Treatment

The information gathered through such physical and psychological testing should be used to develop an individualized treatment plan for the recovering person. Whether inpatient or outpatient, every recovery program should incorporate the kind of Body-Mind-Spirit approach delineated in this book (and in the early work of Alcoholics Anonymous). Such a program would include:

*nutrition education

*immunological and neurological restoration

*exercise programs

*individual and group counseling

*behavioral retraining (such as role playing) to help the recovering patient learn new ways to handle situations in which he or she used to abuse drugs, alcohol, or food

*family therapy.

Persons in recovery must literally learn a whole new way of life. From the way we eat to the way we handle stress, we must learn to replace the unhealthy patterns of our addiction with the healthy patterns of recovery. This relearning is a long-term process, so a recovery program should provide long-term support and care—both medical and psychological. No patient should simply be released from a hospital or outpatient program and left to sink or swim on his or her own. In the first year or so of sobriety, the recovering person needs more than 12-Step meetings.

Specifically, there should be regularly scheduled *medical* follow-ups, complete with lab tests and urinalyses, to track the progress of physiological recovery. Medications, exercises, and nutritional supplements should be adjusted to meet the patient's changing needs. Regular visits to a physician trained in treating addictive diseases will ensure quick identification and treatment of any physical, nutritional, or immune system complications during recovery.

Such follow-up medical care should dovetail with continuing education, counseling, and group involvement and should last for at least one year. Some programs use "contracts" with patients to ensure that they understand the importance of continuing care. Others use "contingency contracts" in which the patient agrees to some sort of mild penalty for not complying with the follow-up (for instance, having to donate money to an organization he or she finds particularly offensive).

Appendix G

Finding a Doctor

Despite the prevalence of addictions and eating disorders, many physicians are not well versed in how to recognize or treat these problems. Coincidentally, many physicians are not well versed in the rather unique needs of persons in recovery. For those in recovery, then, choosing a physician can be a somewhat tricky proposition.

Although medicine still has a way to go in the area of addiction and recovery, there are an increasing number of medical programs and individual doctors who are becoming adept at handling such patients. A national medical organization—the American Society of Addiction Medicine (ASAM)—specifically trains physicians in the identification and treatment of addictive disorders of all kinds. Physicians are certified by examination as specialists in addiction medicine and are kept up to date on advances in the field of addiction.

The national office of ASAM maintains a state-by-state listing of its members. You can contact this office to get the names and numbers of physicians near you who are specifically trained in addiction medicine. For additional information, write or call:

> *The American Society of Addiction Medicine*
> *12 West 21st Street*
> *New York, New York 10010*

Your local medical association can also provide information on physicians in your area, and groups such as Alcoholics Anonymous, Overeaters Anonymous, and Narcotics Anonymous are always good sources of information and referrals.

Appendix H

Smoking

Smoking is a deadly habit and giving it up is an integral part of a complete recovery program. However, since nicotine is one of the most addictive of all drugs, and withdrawal from it can be very stressful, some addiction professionals advise recovering individuals to wait a year before trying to quit smoking. Ultimately, the choice is yours and should be made after careful consideration of your degree of addiction, your fears of withdrawal, and the advice of your doctor or treatment team.

Nicotine, like most stimulants, increases the level of epinephrine (one of the body's natural stimulants) and generally speeds up many of the body's processes. Heart rate and pulse go up after smoking a cigarette. Even the digestive tract is affected, since nicotine increases the muscular action of the colon.

When you stop smoking, these processes are reversed, causing the symptoms of withdrawal:

   *headaches

   *muscle aches

   *constipation

   *decreased energy

   *impaired concentration

   *lowered blood pressure and heart rate

   *sore gums and tongue

   **severe* craving.

The physical symptoms of nicotine withdrawal are compounded by the sheer force of the smoking habit. You will find yourself reaching for a cigarette at the times you usually smoked—while on the phone, after a meal, with a cup of coffee, etc. You'll discover that reaching for a cigarette can be as automatic as tying your shoes, and just as difficult to unlearn.

The first step in tackling your tobacco habit is defining the severity of your addiction. Most people don't realize when, or how often, they smoke. If you are going to successfully conquer this addiction, you'll need to know just what you are dealing with.

First, develop a chart of how, when, and why you smoke. For several days (two or three at least), keep a log of every cigarette. Don't try to change the pattern or avoid smoking, just observe and document your own smoking behavior. Note the following:

   *when you lit the cigarette

   *where you lit the cigarette

   *what you were doing just prior to lighting the cigarette

   *why you wanted the cigarette.

At the end of the observation period, figure out how many cigarettes (or packs) you smoke each day. Remember, the more frequently you dose yourself with nicotine, the more severe your dependence. Then look over your log and check to see if there are any consistent patterns in your smoking habit. Do you always smoke when you are on the phone? Do you smoke after meals? Do you smoke when you are nervous? What are the social, emotional, and just plain habitual cues that prompt you to go for a cigarette?

Go over your smoking pattern chart with your doctor and evaluate which cigarettes you can eliminate. Set a schedule for gradually reducing the number of cigarettes you smoke each day. At the same time, set a target date for giving up cigarettes entirely. Make sure the target date is reasonable. Ideally, you should have cut your smoking down by at least half before the target date. If you are a very heavy smoker, you will want to cut your consumption by even more. Give yourself the time to get your cigarette consumption down to a reasonably low level before you cut cigarettes out of your life entirely.

Cutting back requires a great deal of self-awareness. You may find you need some sort of substitute to occupy your hands and mouth. *Don't* get in the habit of popping candies or sugared gums into your mouth. Try noncaloric alternatives such as sugarless chewing gum, cinnamon sticks, or anise root.

While you are cutting back, follow the general program of biological restoration outlined in this book. The better your overall health, the less difficult the withdrawal process.

If you start having physical problems during the reduction period, make sure to tell your doctor. If necessary, there are some nonaddictive medications that he or she can prescribe to ease your discomfort. Make certain that your doctor knows you are in recovery, and that you are not given medications that have addictive potential, such as tranquilizers.

When you reach the day you will give up cigarettes entirely, you may still need medical support to deal with the physical aspects of nicotine withdrawal. The most common method of helping a patient with nicotine withdrawal is *nicotine replacement therapy*. This technique gives the patient gradually decreasing doses of nicotine in a form other than tobacco to help ease him or her through the withdrawal process. The two most popular methods are nicotine patches and nicotine gum.

The nicotine patch is preferred to nicotine gum, since it is less addictive, and it comes in a variety of dosages so that your physician can control the amount of nicotine you are getting. The patch is placed on the body (usually the arm), where the nicotine is absorbed into your system through the skin. This means a fairly constant supply of nicotine is being fed to your addicted cells, and the amount of nicotine is reduced with each new patch.

Nicotine gum is a strong, rather unpleasant-tasting gum that delivers a dose of nicotine through the mucus tissues of the mouth, in much the same way chewing tobacco does. It is a medication, *not* a candy, and you should be trained in how and when to use it. Smoking at the same time that you are taking nicotine gum can lead to a toxic reaction, so be certain that you are completely cigarette-free if you go onto this therapy. The average dosage schedule for nicotine gum is seven to fifteen pieces per day.

You should chew the first piece in front of your doctor. Avoid swallowing the saliva generated when you chew the gum, since it may still contain nicotine. In general, you should follow these basic rules:

*Keep the gum with you at all times.

*For the first week, chew one piece an hour regardless of withdrawal symptoms.

*Coffee and other beverages should not be consumed immediately before or after chewing the gum. (Caffeine can negate the gum's effects.)

*Gum use immediately after eating may result in hiccuping, nausea, or gastric distress.

*Each piece should last approximately 30 minutes. Chew slowly.

*When a tingling sensation is felt, stop chewing the gum until the sensation subsides, then resume chewing.

Over time, your doctor will have you reduce the number of pieces of gum you chew each day, much as you reduced your intake of cigarettes. A word of warning, however: Nicotine gum can be addictive and habit-forming in its own right, so follow your doctor's instructions to the letter, lest you get caught in another form of nicotine addiction.

Some physicians will prescribe both the patch and the gum for the first week or so after the target date, and additional medications are occasionally prescribed as well. Whether you use gum or a nicotine patch to aid in your withdrawal, it is important that you maintain a program of total physical restoration while you are giving up smoking. A well-nourished, nontoxic, and physically fit body will bounce back from nicotine withdrawal far more quickly than will a toxic and mal-nourished one.

Appendix I

Nutritional Supplementation in Recovery

Your specific nutritional needs in recovery will be affected by a variety of factors, most notably your

*unique genetic programming

*previous medical history

*allergy status

*extent of physical damage.

In general, nutritional supplements in recovery should contain a balance of the known essential nutrients, including:

*vitamins

*minerals

*the essential amino acids

*fatty acids

*antioxidant enzymes.

In choosing a supplement, refer to the list of essential nutrients in chapter 2, and pick a formulation that includes all or most of those listed. A private company is now marketing a comprehensive nutritional supplement called Physicians' Recovery Formula for recovering individuals, based on the science discussed in this book. For more information on these formulations, contact:

Swanson Health Products
1318 19th Street NW
Fargo, North Dakota 58102
1-800-787-0230

In addition to a multi-nutrient supplement, there are a few specific supplements that can be particularly useful for people in recovery, most notably the amino acid l-glutamine (which can help reduce cravings for sweets and alcohol) and the essential fatty acids. Specific fatty acid supplements include:

*EPA (eicosapentaenoic acid) and DHA (docosahexaenoic acid) are two fish oils that have been associated with decreased risk of cardiovascular disease. You can buy EPA-DHA supplements in some pharmacies and most health food stores.

*Evening primrose oil has also received a great deal of attention. It is derived from a traditional medicinal plant and contains GLA (gamma linolenic acid)—a fatty acid the only other nutritional source of which is mother's milk. It is also the crucial "second step" in the production of prostaglandins from linoleic acid. Taking an evening primrose oil supplement may help the body bypass the enzyme block that some individuals have inherited.

For those who wish to learn their specific nutritional needs, the lymphocyte assay technology discussed in chapters 9 and 10 is now available. Interested patients and their physicians can get information on the test from:

SpectraCell Laboratories, Inc.
515 Post Oak Blvd. (Suite 830)
Houston, TX 77027
1-800-227-5227

Remember, as you become more physically stable in your recovery, your nutritional needs will change. If you do have this test, it is a good idea to be evaluated several times over the first few years of recovery, and to adjust your vitamin supplements accordingly.

Taking supplements alone will not "cure" the physiological damages of addictions and eating disorders, and supplements should *never* be a substitute for maintaining a healthy diet and lifestyle. Following the general principles outlined in this book, and getting to know your own specific needs through techniques such as lymphocyte testing and allergy testing (including at-home methods such as the oral food challenge), are the backbone of your recovery program.

Appendix J

Assessing Food Sensitivities

As we noted earlier in chapter 8, continual exposure to foods and chemical additives that prompt an immunological reaction can cause the immune system to go on something of a sit-down strike. The "Stone Age" diet relieves by eliminating the most common problem foods and replacing them with other natural, chemical-free wholefoods. Once the body has been relieved of such immunological stress, it can respond appropriately when presented with a suspect food during the oral food challenge.

The diet should be followed closely for *no less than four and no more than seven days,* during which you should eat *only* the following foods:

* fresh fruit (well rinsed to remove any pesticides, colorings, or other chemical residues)

* fresh poultry or fish

* fresh vegetables (except corn)

* fresh nuts (*not* dry roasted or salted), excluding peanuts

* fresh and/or bottled *unsweetened* juices (fructose is an added sweetener and should be avoided)

* bottled water or unflavored seltzer

* cold-pressed oils: canola, olive, or safflower.

Steam or braise foods whenever possible, and use only the allowed oils when cooking. Do not use prepared condiments such as mayonnaise or ketchup, and avoid salt and other spices. Be certain to drink at least six to eight glasses of filtered or bottled water (or unflavored seltzer) every day, since this will keep you from becoming dehydrated.

For the duration of the diet you should *strictly avoid* the following:

* all dairy products

* all processed meats (bologna, sausage, etc.)

* all grains (wheat, corn, rye, oats, rice, barley, etc.) and foods containing them (breads, cereals, crackers, etc.)

* coffee and tea, caffeinated or decaffeinated

*sugar of any kind, including artificial sweeteners

*all alcoholic beverages

*tobacco in any form

*prepared foods of any kind.

Before you start to complain (as almost all of us do) about how this leaves you nothing to eat, turn to chapters 13 and 14 and examine the fruits, vegetables, fish, and other foods you *can* eat with abandon on this diet. And keep in mind that it will only last four to seven days!

Once you have been on the diet for a day or two, don't be surprised if you find yourself feeling simply awful and craving precisely the foods you are not supposed to have. As we noted in chapter 8, food allergies are unique in that they often metamorphose into food addiction. The cravings, aches, and generally lousy feeling that afflicts many people around day two of the detoxification diet is a manifestation of that addiction. It is, quite literally, withdrawal. If you stick it out, however, you will find that by day three or four you will feel better than you have in quite some time.

Oral Food Challenge

Around the fifth day of the diet it is time to perform the oral food challenge. You will "challenge" your body with the suspect food in its purest form and monitor the reaction. Since the process is time-consuming and reactions can sometimes be dramatic, pick a day when you have nothing pressing to do and can easily remain at home.

Step 1. Fix a large portion of the suspect food. Do not add salt, sugar, or flavorings of any kind. To test milk, for example, drink a large glass of whole milk. To test wheat, use *plain* Wheatena.

Step 2. Eat or drink the entire portion (do not take more than 20 minutes).

Step 3. Monitor how you feel at 10, 20, 30, and 60 minutes after finishing the food, and write it down. Make sure to note symptoms that are not "classic" allergy symptoms, such as

*headache
*drowsiness
*depression
*itchy ears
*itchy chest.

Step 4. If at the end of the first hour you have not experienced any symptoms, eat another portion that is *half* the original serving.

Step 5. Repeat Step 3.

Step 6. If there still is no change, go about your normal daily activities, but *eat and drink nothing but water.*

Step 7. At dinnertime, eat a meal of "safe foods" *plus* a normal portion of the test food.

Step 8. Monitor symptoms before bedtime and the next morning.

Since adverse reactions to foods can be delayed, it is important to carry out the whole day of the food challenge to get an accurate response. If you have reactions at any point during the day (or the following morning), consider the food positive.

Rotating Your Diet

A rotation diet is one in which no food is eaten more than once every four to seven days. That may sound simple, but when the food in question is milk, or wheat, or sugar—all of which are found in almost every prepared food on the market—setting up a rotation diet becomes a little more challenging. In these cases, switching to wholefoods is critical. The recipes in this book use a variety of grains, few dairy products, and little to no sugar to accommodate those who have such food allergies or sensitivities. The following chart is an example of the foods that can be eaten during a typical four-day rotation cycle.

	BREAKFAST	SNACK	LUNCH	SNACK	DINNER	SNACK
DAY 1	oatmeal w/maple syrup	kiwifruit chestnuts	scallops broccoli	walnuts	lamb kale millet	figs pecans
DAY 2	eggs wheat toast prunes apple butter	pear almonds	chicken Swiss chard	apple sesame seeds	beef spinach mushrooms wheat pasta tomatoes	apricot cherries
DAY 3	corn grits	peanuts raisins	rice beans avocado	melon	flounder asparagus rice	popcorn
DAY 4	barley cereal orange or grapefruit	pistachio nuts	turkey	cheese celery	scrod carrots butternut squash	yogurt blueberries

<u>Appendix K</u>	
Food Families	
<u>Examples of "Related" Foods</u>	
Food Family	**Notable Family Members**
Produce	
Carrot	angelica, anise, caraway, carrot (carrot syrup), celeriac (celery root), celery (celery seeds and leaves), chervil, coriander, cumin, dill (dill seed), fennel (finocchio, Florence fennel), parsley, parsnips, sweet cicely
Composite	artichoke, burdock root, chamomile, chicory, coltsfoot, dandelion, endive, escarole, goldenrod, Jerusalem artichoke (artichoke flour), lettuce, romaine, safflower, sunflower (seeds, meal, oil), tansy, tarragon, French endive, wormwood (absinthe), yarrow
Fungi	baker's yeast, brewer's yeast, mold (in certain cheeses), morel, mushroom, puffball, truffle
Gourds	chayote, Chinese preserving melon, cucumber, gherkin, muskmelons (cantaloupe, casaba, Cranshaw, honeydew, Persian melon), pumpkin (pumpkin seeds, pumpkin meal), squashes (acorn, buttercup, butternut, Boston marrow, caserta, cocozelle, crookneck, cushaw, golden nugget, pattypan, turban, spaghetti squash, zucchini), watermelon
Grasses	barley (malt, maltose), bamboo shoots, corn (cornmeal, corn oil, cornstarch, corn sugar, corn syrup, hominy grits, popcorn), lemongrass (citronella), millet, oats (oatmeal), rice (rice flour), rye, sorghum grain (sorghum syrup), sugarcane (cane sugar, raw sugar, molasses), sweet corn, triticale, wheat (bran, bulgur, gluten flour, graham flour, patent flour, whole wheat flour, wheat germ), wild rice

Food Family	Notable Family Members
Produce	
Laurel	avocado, bay leaf, cassia bark, cinnamon, sassafras
Legumes	Alfalfa (sprouts), beans (fava, lima, mung, navy, string, kidney), black-eyed peas, carob (carob syrup), chick peas, fenugreek, gum acacia, gum tragacanth, jicama, kudzu, lentil, licorice, pea, peanut (peanut butter, peanut oil), red clover, soybeans (soy milk, soy flour, soy grits, soy oil, lecithin), tamarind, tonka bean (coumarin)
Lily	asparagus, chives, garlic, leeks, ramp, sarsaparilla, shallot, yucca
Mint	apple mint, basil, bergamot, catnip, chia seed, clary, horehound, hyssop, lavender, lemon balm, marjoram, oregano, pennyroyal, peppermint, rosemary, sage, spearmint, summer savory, thyme, winter savory
Mustard	broccoli, Brussels sprouts, cabbage, cardoon, cauliflower, Chinese cabbage, collards, colza shoots, curly cress, horseradish, kale, kohlrabi, mustard greens, mustard seed, radish, rapeseed (canola oil), rutabaga (swede), turnip, upland cress, watercress
Nightshade	egglant, ground cherry, pepino (melon pear), peppers (bell, sweet, cayenne, chili, paprika, pimiento), potato, tomato, tomatillo, tree tomato
Palm	coconut (coconut meal, coconut oil), dates (date sugar), palm cabbage, sago starch
Parsley	anise, caraway seed, carrot, celery, parsley, parsnips
Plum	almond, apricot, cherry, peach, plum
Rue (Citrus)	citron, grapefruit, kumquat, lemon, lime, orange, pomelo, tangelo, tangerine

Food Family	Notable Family Members
Seafoods	
Codfish	scrod, cusk, haddock, hake, pollack
Sea Bass	grouper, sea bass
Croaker	croaker, drum, sea trout, silver perch, spot, weakfish (spotted sea trout)
Mackerel	albacore, bonito, mackerel, skipjack, tuna
Marlin	marlin, sailfish
Flounder	dab, flounder, halibut, plaice, sole, turbot
Herring	herring, shad (roe)
Sunfish	black bass (all types), sunfish (all types, pumpkinseed), crappie
Perch	sauger, walleye, yellow perch
Poultry	
Dove	dove, pigeon (squab)
Duck	duck (eggs), goose (eggs)
Pheasant	chicken (eggs), peafowl, pheasant, quail
Turkey	turkey (eggs)
Meats	
Bovine	Beef: including by-products found in gelatin, oleomargarine, rennet (used in cheese), sausage casings, suet Milk products: including butter, ice cream, lactose, spray-dried milk, yogurt Veal Buffalo (bison)

Food Family	Notable Family Members
Meats	
Bovine (cont.)	Goat (cheese, ice cream, milk) Sheep (lamb, mutton, milk, cheese)
Deer	caribou, deer (venison), elk, moose, reindeer
Hare	rabbit
Horse	horse
Swine	hog (pork, bacon, ham, lard, pork-based gelatin, sausage, scrapple)

Derived from Ensminger, et al., eds., *The Food and Nutrition Encyclopedia, Volume I.* (Clovis, Calif.: Pergus Press, 1983), 49; and from N. Golos, F. G. Golbitz, and F. S. Leighton, *Coping With Your Allergies* (New York: Simon & Schuster, 1979), 108–116.

<u>Appendix L</u>
Establishing an Oasis

The quality of our recovery is affected not only by the quality of our food and water supplies, but by the quality of our overall environment. While some environmental conditions are beyond our individual control, it is possible to set up at least one area in which we can enjoy several hours of relative environmental purity. Such an oasis can be a tremendous boon to recovery.

The guidelines listed here are for a fairly strict oasis setup. The degree to which you can fulfill them will vary. In general, your oasis room should be:

> *free of furniture and decorations that will collect dust: no rugs, little to no upholstery, a minimum of knickknacks, etc.

> *free of all house plants

> *off limits to pets and smokers

> *away from the garage.

To establish an ideal oasis, we recommend the following measures:

1. Remove carpeting and replace it with wood or ceramic tiles. If this is not possible, vacuum the carpeting frequently and thoroughly.
2. Do not use rug cleaners, waxes, or polishes. Mop frequently using a biodegradable, chemical-free cleaning formula (see box below for specific names).
3. Air the room frequently, at all times of the year. Do not seal the windows.

ENVIRONMENTALLY KIND CLEANERS
Bon Ami
Power Plus (laundry detergent)
E-Z Maid
Soil Away
Karpet Kleen
Auto Dish Detergent
Super Clean

4. Install an air purifier that is capable of filtering air particulates, dust, mold, pollens, and chemicals (such as formaldehyde). Portable models are available that will work for most bedrooms. Additional purifiers can also be placed in other rooms to reduce environmental contaminants (see box below for some specific manufacturers).

AIR PURIFIERS
Enviracaire
Companion Aire
Airstar
Maetinaire
Puridyne

5. Use 100 percent cotton bedding (wash new bedding three or four times before use).
6. Use cotton or dacron pillows, *not* foam rubber or down.
7. Pillow covers should be cotton or dacron barrier cloth.
8. Air pillows frequently and/or fluff them in the dryer at high temperature.
9. Wash bedding frequently in one of the environmentally kind soaps listed above.

10. Use 100 percent cotton draperies—*without* rubber backing.
11. Furnish with real wood furniture as much as possible, not with fiberboard or particle board that has been veneered.
12. Clean furniture with a damp cotton rag, not with polish or wax.
13. Keep house plants in other rooms.
14. Keep the closet closed when not in use. If possible, keep clothes in another room entirely.
15. Remove all toiletries (cosmetics, perfumes, soaps, powders).
16. If the bathroom is adjacent to the oasis room, keep the door closed when not in use and use only nonscented, nonaerosol toiletries.
17. Have only one book in the room at a time.
18. Keep all animals out of the oasis room.
19. Do not smoke in the oasis room.
20. Air and dust the room frequently.

Appendix M

Mail-Order Wholefoods Sources

Alabama

Pearly Gates Natural Foods
2308 Memorial Parkway SW
Huntsville, AL 35801
(205) 534-6233
Natural and organic foods, over 600 bulk herbs.

Alaska

Whole Earth Grocery
Box 80228
Fairbanks, AK 99708
(907) 479-2052
Fresh produce, soy products, oils.

Arizona

Oak Creek Orchards Country Market
Box 132–236
Copper Cliffs Drive
Sedona, AZ 86336
(602) 282-2726
Fresh produce.

Tucson Co-op Warehouse
1716 E. Factory Avenue
Tucson, AZ 85709
(602) 884-9951
Whole grains, cereals, flours, rice, breads, fresh fruit, vegetables and legumes, nuts and nut butters, dried fruit, soy products, fruit juices.

Arkansas

Mountain Ark Trading Co.
120 South East Avenue
Fayetteville, AR 72701
(501) 442-7191
Organic coffee, condiments, dried beans, dried fruit, whole grains, flour and meal, herbs, nuts, nut butters, oils, soy products, sweeteners, soups, teas, sea vegetables.

Eagle Agricultural Products, Inc.
407 Church Avenue
Huntsville, AR 72740
(501) 738-2203

Dried beans, fresh fruit, whole grains, fresh vegetables, flours and meals, rice, pastas, condiments, fruit juices.

California

Healthfood Express
Lin Martin
181 Sylmar
Clovis, CA 93612
Mail to:
PO Box 8357
Fresno, CA 93747
(209) 252-8321
Meat substitutes, granola products, and dried fruits.

Lee Anderson's Covalda Date Company
PO Box 908
51–392 Highway 86
Coachella, CA 92236
(619) 398-3551
Dates, citrus fruits, and pecans.

Great Date in the Morning
Jim Dunn
PO Box 31
85–710 Grapefruit Boulevard
Coachella, CA 92236
(619) 298-6171
Dates, melons, strawberries, fresh vegetables, and spices.

Gravelly Ridge Farms
Star Route 16
Elk Creek, CA 95939
(916) 963-3216
Fresh fruit, dried fruit, vegetables, and grains.

Capay Canyon Ranch
Leslie Ranch
PO Box 508
Esparto, CA 95627
(916) 662-2372
FAX (916) 662-2306
Fresh apricots, cherries, and grapes, dried fruit, nuts, nut butters.

Black Ranch
Dave and Dawn Black
5800 Eastside Road
Etna, CA 96027
(916) 467-3387
Whole grains, rose hips, whole-grain flour, six-grain cereal.

Kozlowski Farms-Sonoma County Classics
Cindy Kozlowski-Hayworthy
5566 Gravenstein Highway
Forestville, CA 95436
(707) 887-1587
FAX (707) 887-9650
Jams, jellies, fruit butters, chutneys, vinegars, mustards, syrups, fresh and frozen berries, apple cider.

California Health Foods
115 E. Commonwealth
Fullerton, CA 92632
Fresh fruits, dried fruits, vegetables, nuts, grains, cereals, breads, flour, rice, pasta, oils, beans, soy products, cheeses, spices.

Van Dyke Ranch
7665 Crews Road
Gilroy, CA 95020
(408) 842-5423
Dried fruit and fresh fruit.

Mountain Peoples Warehouse
110 Springhill Boulevard
Grass Valley, CA 95959
(916) 273-9531
Baked goods, coffee, condiments, dairy products, dried beans, fresh fruit, whole grains, flour and meals, herbs and spices, nuts and nut butters, soy products, oils, sweeteners, vegetables.

Timber Crest Farms
4791 Dry Creek
Healdsburg, CA 95448
(707) 433-8251
Organic dried fruits and vegetables.

Licata's California Nutrition Centers
5242 Bolsa Avenue, Suite 3
Huntington Beach, CA 92647
(714) 893-0017
Cereals, flours, oils, beans, dried
fruit, soy products, beverages.

Albert's Organics Inc.
4605 S. Alameda Avenue
Los Angeles, CA 90058
(213) 234-4595
Wide variety of organically grown
fruits and vegetables.

Melissa's Brand
PO Box 21407
Los Angeles, CA 90021
(213) 588-0151
Beans, fresh fruit, spices, vegetables,
noodles, wild rice, tofu.

Mendocino Sea Vegetable Company
PO Box 372
Navarro, CA 95463
(707) 895-3741
Sea vegetables.

Spectra
484 Lake Park #163
Oakland, CA 94610
(415) 834-8731
Organic juice, yogurt, and herbs.

Lundberg Family Farms
5370 Church Street
PO Box 369
Richvale, CA 95974
(916) 882-4551
Rice products.

Be Wise Ranch
9018 Artesian Road
San Diego, CA 92127
(619) 756-4851
Fresh fruit and vegetables.

Appleseed Ranch
1834 High School Road
Sebastopol, CA 95472
(707) 823-4408
Baked goods, dried fruit, fresh fruit,
herbs and spices, juices, seeds,
sweeteners, teas, fresh vegetables.

**Santa Barbara Olive Oil Co. Inc. and
The Olive House**
1661 Mission Drive
Solvang, CA 93463
(805) 688-9917
Olives, olive oils, sesame oil,
vinegars, condiments.

Jaffe Bros. Inc.
PO Box 636
Valley Center, CA 92082
(619) 749-1133
Beans, grains, dried fruit, nuts and
nut butters.

Colorado

Allergy Resources Inc.
195 Huntington Beach Drive
Colorado Springs, CO 80921
(719) 488-3630
Condiments, baking goods, baking
substitutes, flours, milk substitutes,
wheat- and gluten-free products,
grains and meals, dried rice and
beans, oils, pasta, cereals.

Malachite School and Small Farm
ASR Box 21
Pass Creek Road
Gardner, CO 81040
Honey, dried herbs, sourdough
starter.

Suzanne's Specialties
116 9th Street
Steamboat Springs, CO 80487
(303) 879-5731
Coffee, tea, seasonal fruit juices,
organic vegetables.

Connecticut

Aux Fines Herbes
PO Box 9500
Dimock Lane
Bolton, CT 06043
(203) 224-3724
Herbs and vegetables.

Cricket Hill Farm
670 Walnut Hill Road
Thomaston, CT 06787
(203) 283-4707
Garlic and onions.

Florida

Orange Blossom Cooperative Warehouse
1601 NW 55th Place
Gainesville, FL 32606
(904) 372-7061
Wholefoods and organic produce, coffee, condiments, beans, fruit, grains, flour, meals, herbs, spices, juices, nuts, nut butters, oils, seeds, soy products, sweeteners, teas.

Sprout Delights Inc.
13090–2702 NW 7th Avenue
Miami, FL 33168
(305) 687-5880
Over 90 percent organic—cakes, snacks, crackers, cookies, breads.

Tree of Life Corp.
27 Styertown Road
St. Augustine, FL 32085
(904) 824-8181
Baked goods, condiments, beans, dried fruit, fresh fruit, herbs, spices, juices, nuts, nut butters, oils, seeds, soy products, sweeteners.

Monroe Health Foods
5025 E. Fowler Avenue, Suite 13
Tampa, FL 33617
(831) 988-7788
Grains, cereals, breads, flours, rice, pasta, dried beans, miso, tempeh, tofu, soy milk, soy sauce, cheeses, nuts and nut butters, oils, spices, dried fruit, fruit juices, coffee, tea.

Georgia

Harry's Farmers Market
1180 Upper Hembree Road
Roswell, GA 30076
(404) 664-6300
Baked goods, bread.

Hawaii

Hawaiian Exotic Fruit Co., Inc.
Box 1729
Pahoa, HI 96778
(808) 965-7154
Fresh fruit, fresh vegetables, dried fruits.

Illinois

Strathmore Farm
2400 Spring Creek Road
Algonquin, IL 60102
(312) 550-5077
Dried beans, whole grains, meat.

New City Market
1810 N. Halsted Street
Chicago, IL 60614
(312) 280-7600
Complete assortment of whole-food grocery items and fresh organic produce.

Green Earth
2545 Prairie Street
Evanston, IL 60201
(800) 322-3662
Organic produce, grains, meats.

Indiana

Good Earth Natural Food Store
6350 N. Guilford Avenue
Indianapolis, IN 46220
(317) 253-3609
Grains, cereals, flour, bread, meat, poultry, nuts and nut butters, rice, oils, soy products, dried fruit, fresh fruit and vegetables, fruit juices, herbs and spices.

Iowa

Paul's Grains
2475–B 340 Street
Laurel, IA 50141
(515) 476-3373
Whole grains and grain products, apples, beans and nuts, beef, lamb, chicken, turkey.

Kansas

Cross Seed Co.
H.C. 69, Box 2
Bunker Hill, KS 67626
(913) 483-6163
Grains, flour, beans.

Cheyenne Gap Amaranth
H.C. 1, Box 2
Luray, KS 67649-9743
(913) 698-2457
Amaranth grain, flour, planting seed.

Maine

Fiddler's Green Farm
RR 1, Box 656
Belfast, ME 04915
(207) 338-3568
Organic baking mixes and cereals.

Wood Prairie Farm
RFD 1, Box 164
Bridgewater, ME 04735
(207) 429-9765
Fresh organic vegetables and fruits.

Maine Coast Sea Vegetables
Shore Road
Franklin, ME 04634
(207) 565-2907
Sea vegetables, sea chips, sea
seasonings, and condiments.

Maryland

Organic Foods Express
11003 Emack Road
Beltsville, MD 20705
(301) 937-8608
Cereals, juices, beans, nuts, nut
butters, fruits, vegetables, dried fruit,
dairy and soy products, herbs.

Massachusetts

Northeast Cooperatives
5 Cameron Avenue
Cambridge, MA 02140
(617) 389-9032
Coffee, dairy products, dried beans,
dried fruit, fresh fruit, whole grains,
flour and meals, herbs and spices,
juices, nuts and nut butters, oils,
seeds, sweeteners, soy products, teas,
fresh vegetables, organic cheese.

Berkshire Mountain Bakery Inc.
PO Box 785
Housatonic, MA 01236
(800) 274-3412

Michigan

**Michigan Federation of Food
Cooperatives**
727 W. Ellsworth Street
Ann Arbor, MI 48108
(313) 761-4642
Coffee, condiments, dried beans,
dried fruit, whole grains, spices,
juices, nuts and nut butters, pasta,
seeds, soy products, sweeteners, teas.

Harvest Health Inc.
1944 Eastern Avenue SE
Grand Rapids, MI 40507
(616) 245-6268
Baked goods, beans, breads, cereals,
flours, soy products, rice, pasta, oil,
dairy products, fruit juices, dried
fruits, nuts, spices.

Minnesota

Life-Renewal Inc.
Highway 18, Box 92
Garrison, MN 56450
(612) 692-4498
Processed and fresh beans, teas,
breads, popcorn, cereals, flour, dried
fruit, oils, pasta, grains, nuts, spices
and medicinal herbs.

Linden Hills Co-op
4306 Upton Avenue S.
Minneapolis, MN 55410
(612) 922-1159
Cookies, corn chips, muffins,
beans, beverages, breads, cereals,
dairy products, flour, fruit juices,
fresh and processed vegetables
and spices, rice, soy products.

Diamond K Enterprises
R.R. 1, Box 30
St. Charles, MN 55972
(507) 932-4308
Dried and fresh beans, flours, meals, grains, nuts, seeds, oils, dried fruits.

Brandt's Market
6525 Delmar Street
St. Louis, MO 63130
(314) 727-3663
Beans, coffee, sodas, teas, breads, cereals, dairy products, flour, juices, nuts, oils, pasta, rice, soy products, vegetables, dried and fresh fruit, spices.

Plumbottom Farm
Route 3, Box 129
Willow Springs, MO 65793
Organic produce.

Montana

Real Food Store
1090 Helena Avenue
Helena, MT 59601
Wide variety of organic and wholefoods, bulk herbs.

Great Grains Milling Co.
PO Box 427
Scobey, MT 59262
(406) 783-5588
Stone-ground wheat products.

Nebraska

Do-R-Dye Organic Mill
Box 50
Rosalie, NE 68055
(402) 863-2248
Grains, oatmeal, flour.

Nevada

Ira's Organic Foods Market
5643 W. Charleston Boulevard #3
Las Vegas, NV 89102
(702) 258-4250
Wide variety of organic produce and wholefoods, yeast-free bread.

New Jersey

Simply Delicious
243-A N. Hook Road, Box 124
Pennsville, NJ 08070
(609) 678-4488
Wide variety of wholefoods items, fresh produce.

Victory Market
31 W. Front Street
Red Bank, NJ 07701
(201) 747-0508
Wholefoods and natural produce.

New Mexico

Semilla Natural Foods
510 University Avenue
Las Vegas, NM 87701
(505) 425-8139
Fresh produce, beans, beverages, dairy products, dried fruit, grains, turkey, chicken, nuts, soy products, spices, baked goods, oils.

New York

Bread Alone
Route 28
Boiceville, NY 12412
(914) 657-3328
Whole wheat breads.

Earth's Harvest
1244 Hicksville Road
Seaford, NY 11783
(516) 797-0700
Full line of organic foods.

Hawthorne Valley Farm
R.D. No. 2, Box 225A
Ghent, NY 12075
(518) 672-7500
Fresh fruits and vegetables, dried fruit, fruit juices, beans, grains, baked goods, breads, cereals, oils, rices, pasta, dairy products, nuts and nut butters, spices, soy products.

Deer Valley Farm
RD #1
Guilford, NY 13780
(607) 764-8556
Dried beans, dried fruit, whole grains, flours and meals, sweeteners, fresh vegetables, baked goods.

Good Life Natural Foods
339 S. Broadway
Hicksville, NY 11801
(516) 935-5073
Natural groceries and produce.

Integral Yoga Natural Foods
229 W. 13th Street
New York, NY 10011
(212) 243-2642
Fresh organic produce, wholefoods, and macrobiotic foods.

Whole Foods SoHo
117 Prince Street
New York, NY 10012
(212) 673-5388
Wholefoods and produce.

North Carolina

Macrobiotic Wholesale Company
799 Old Leicester Highway
Asheville, NC 28806
(704) 252-1221
Macrobiotic products.

New American Food Company
PO Box 3206
Durham, NC 27705
(919) 682-9210
Baked goods, beans, beverages, cereals, whole wheat flour, apple juice, nuts, oils, pasta, soy products, salsa.

Nature's Storehouse
Highway 108, PO Box 69
Lynn, NC 28750
(704) 859-6356
Breads, beans, beverages, cereals, dairy products, dried fruit, nuts, oils, peanut butter, rice, soy products, grains, spices, sprouts.

Zoolie's Natural Food Market Inc.
208 Haywood Square
PO Box 869
Waynesville, NC 28786
Baked goods, fresh beans, beverages, cereals, dairy products, flour, dried fruit, nuts, nut butters, oils, pasta, rice, soy products, grains, spices.

Ohio

Millstream Natural Health Supplies
1310–A E. Tallmadge Avenue
Akron, OH 44310
(216) 630-2700
Baked goods, condiments, dairy products, dried beans, dried fruit, fresh fruit, grains, flours, meals, herbs, spices, juices, nuts, nut butters, oils, seeds, soy products, sweeteners, teas, fresh vegetables.

Federation of Ohio River Cooperatives
320 Outerbelt Street
Columbus, OH 43210
(614) 861-2446
Coffee, condiments, dairy products, dried beans, dried fruit, fresh fruit, grains, flours, meals, herbs, juices, oils, seeds, soy products, sweeteners, fresh vegetables.

Silver Creek Farm
7097 Allyn Road
Hiram, OH
(216) 569-3487
Fresh blueberries, popcorn, poultry, basil, dill, mushrooms, peppers, squash, shallots, and honey.

Oregon

Oregon Spice Co. Inc.
3525 SE 17th Avenue
Portland, OR 97202
(503) 238-0664
Coffee, teas, all culinary herbs and spices, and salt-free seasoning.

Pennsylvania

Millennial Health & Books
1718 12th Avenue
Altoona, PA 16601
(814) 949-9108
Yogurt, bulk herbs, snack foods, coffee, teas, juices.

Neshaminy Valley Natural Foods Distributor Ltd.
5 Louise Drive
Ivyland, PA 18974
(215) 443-5545
Organic beans, cereals, flour, grains, breads, baked goods, dried fruit, fruit juices, oils, pasta, rice, fresh fruit and vegetables, dairy products, soy products, nuts and nut butters, beverages, candy and sweeteners.

Kimberton Hills Farmstore
Box 155
Kimberton, PA 19442
(215) 935-0214
Seasonal fresh fruit and vegetables.

Krystal Wharf Farms
RD 2, Box 191 A
Mansfield, PA 16933
(717) 549-8194
Organic fruits and vegetables.

Rising Sun Organic Produce
Box 627 1–80 and Pa–150
Milesburg, PA 16853
(814) 355-9850
Fresh fruit, vegetables, dried fruit, grains, flour, cereals, pasta, nuts, beans, soy products, cheese, yogurt, fruit juices, jellies, oils, bread, herbs and spices, beverages.

Walnut Acres
Walnut Acres Road
Penns Creek, PA 17862
(717) 837-0601
Baked goods, dried beans, whole grains, flours, pasta, rice, cheese, oils, nuts and nut butters, dried fruit, soy products, spices, fruit juices.

Freshlife
2300 East 3rd Street
Williamsport, PA 17701
(717) 322-8280
Natural groceries and produce.

Rhode Island

Harvest Natural Foods
1 Casino Terrace
Newport, RI 02840
(401) 846-8137
Wholefoods and organic produce.

South Dakota

Willow Hill Italian Veal
PO Box 16
Olivet, SD 57052
(605) 387-2307
Natural, free-range veal.

Tennessee

Nature's Pantry
4928 Homberg Drive
Knoxville, TN 37919
Wholefoods grocery items.

Honeysuckle Health Foods
4741 Poplar
Memphis, TN 38117
(901) 682-6255
Wholefoods grocery items and organic produce in season.

Texas

Arrowhead Mills Inc.
PO Box 2059, 110 South Lawton
Hereford, TX 79045
(806) 364-0730
Beans, grains, cereals, flours, seeds, brown rice, oils.

Virginia

Integral Yoga Natural Foods
923 Preston Avenue
Charlottesville, VA 22901
Organic produce, wholefoods items, and macrobiotic foods.

Hatch Natural Foods Corporation
PO Box 888
Warrenton, VA 22186
(703) 987-8551
Baked goods, dairy products, dried
beans, dried fruit, fresh fruit and
vegetables, whole grains, cereals,
flour, meals, breads, pasta, rice,
herbs, spices, nuts, nut butters, oils,
seeds, soy products, fruit juices.

Vermont

Northeast Cooperatives
PO Box 1120, Quinn Road
Brattleboro, VT 05301
(802) 257-5856
Coffee, dairy products, dried beans,
dried fruit, fresh fruit, whole grains,
flour and meals, herbs and spices,
juices, nuts and nut butters, oils,
seeds, soy products, sweeteners, teas,
fresh vegetables, organic cheese.

Organum Natural Foods
227 Main Street
Burlington, VT 05401
(802) 863-6103
Wholefoods grocery items, bulk
items, organic produce.

Vermont Northern Growers' Co-op
Box 125
East Hardwick, VT
(802) 472-6285
Organic fruit and vegetables.

Longwind Farm
Box 203
East Thetford, VT 05043
(802) 785-2793
Organic vegetables, berries, and
basil.

Washington

Cascadian Farm
PO Box 568
Concrete, WA 98237
(206) 853-8175
Fruit, vegetables, condiments, whole
grains, sweeteners.

Heritage Flour Mills
2925 Chestnut
Everett, WA 98020
(206) 258-1582
Mixes, beans, teas, cereals, flour,
fruit drinks, oils, pastas, rice.

Ener-G Foods Inc.
PO Box 84487
Seattle, WA 98124
(206) 767-6660
Dietetic foods, baked goods, breads,
cereals, flour, grains, nuts and nut
butters, oils, pasta, brown rice,
tapioca, soybean milk.

West Virginia

Mother Earth Foods
1638 19th Street
Parkersburg, WV 26101
(304) 428-1024
Wholefoods grocery items and some
organic produce.

Wisconsin

**Common Health Warehouse
Cooperative Association**
1505 N. 8th Street
Superior, WI 54880
(715) 392-9862
Cereal, flour, breads, oils, pasta, rice,
beans, soy products, dried fruit, fresh
fruit and vegetables, nuts, nut
butters, meat, poultry, seafood, dairy
products, baked goods, herbs, spices,
juices.

Wyoming

Mosher Products
PO Box 5367
Cheyenne, WY 82003
(307) 632-1492
Whole wheat grain and flour.

Appendix N

Some Common Additives and Their Side Effects

These are a sample of the many chemicals added to our food. Although many are necessary, or at least benign, others serve no nutritional or safety purpose and have potentially serious health effects. To learn more about additives, refer to Ruth Winter's *A Consumer's Dictionary of Food Additives* (Crown, 1989), or subscribe to the *Nutrition Action HealthLetter* (published by the Center for Science in the Public Interest, in Washington, D.C.).

Additive	Uses	Possible Adverse Effects
Acesulfame K (Sunette, Sweet One)	artificial sweetener	Tumor formation (in lab animals)
Acacia gum (or gum arabic)	thickening agent, keeps sugar from crystallizing	Allergic reactions (including asthma attacks)
Amyl acetate	flavoring agent	Skin irritation, headaches, tiredness, CNS depression, sore and runny nose
Aspartame (Nutrasweet, Equal)	artificial sweetener	Headaches, dizziness, seizures, menstrual problems, prenatal damage
Benzoic acid (Benzoate, Sodium Benzoate	preservative (teas, jams and jellies, soft drinks, margarine, etc.)	Allergic reactions (gastrointestinal irritation and red eyes). Very taxing on the liver. Those sensitive to aspirin are often sensitive to this.
Benzoyl peroxide	bleaching agent (flours, cheese, and milk)	Allergic reactions. Toxic if inhaled. May also destroy vitamins A, C, and E.
Butylated hydroxyanisole (BHA)	preservative (baked goods, soups, lard, shortening, cereals, ice cream, candy)	Allergic reactions, kidney & liver problems. Animal studies have found neurological and reproductive damage and increased cancer incidences.

Additive	Uses	Possible Adverse Affects
Butylated hydroxytoluene (BHT)	preservative (same foods as BHA, as well as refined and enriched rice and rice products, freeze-dried meats)	Kidney toxicity. Animal studies have shown impairments in fat metabolism and blood clotting. May combine with steroid hormones or oral contraceptives to form carcinogens.
Bromates (calcium bromate and potassium bromate)	used in the process of making flour and bread	Kidney failure, nervous system disorders, skin eruptions
Brominate vegetable oil	demulsifier and clouding agent	May build up in the body's fat cells.
Calcium disodium EDTA	preservative (soft drinks, canned vegetables, mayonnaise)	Associated with muscle cramps, GI problems, and kidney damage.
Caramel	Coloring (soft drinks, candies, baked goods, etc.)	Caramel made with sulfite and ammonia have caused GI problems.
Monosodium glutamate (MSG)	flavor enhancer, widely used	Causes brain damage in young lab animals (no longer used in baby food). Associated with mood changes in some humans. Reduced fertility in lab animals.
Nitrites	color fixatives, inhibit botulinum spores (bacon and cured meats)	Combines with chemicals in stomach (and in other foods) to form carcinogenic nitrosamines.
Propyl gallate	antioxidant (mayonnaise, various oils, potato flakes and mashed potatoes, citrus flavorings)	May cause stomach or skin irritation in asthmatics.
Propylene glycol	emulsifier (confectionery goods, ice creams, meat products	In animals, high doses have been associated with kidney changes and depression.
Saccharin	artificial sweetener (diet soft drinks)	Known animal carcinogen, suspected human carcinogen.

Bibliography

Chapter 1: Body-Mind-Spirit

Beasley, J. D., et al.: Follow-up of a cohort of alcoholic patients through 12 months of comprehensive biobehavioral treament. *Journal of Substance Abuse Treatment* 1991; 8 (2): 133–142.

Becker, J. T., and Jaffe J. H.: Impaired memory for treatment-relevant information in inpatient men alcoholics. *Journal of Studies on Alcohol* 1984; 45 (4): 339–343.

Emrick, C. D.: A review of psychologically oriented treatment of alcoholism: II. The relative effectiveness of different treatment approaches and the effectiveness of treatment versus no treatment. *Quarterly Journal of Studies on Alcohol* 1975; 36, (1): 88–108.

Fatis, M., et al.: Following up on a commercial weight loss program: Do the pounds stay off even after your picture has been in the newspaper? *Journal of the American Dietetic Association* 1989; 89: 547–548.

Field, H. L.: Conspectus: Eating disorders. *Comprehensive Therapy* 1989; 15: 3–11.

Gordis, E., et al.: Outcome of alcoholism treatment among 5,578 patients in an urban comprehensive hospital based program: Application of a computerized data system. *Alcoholism: Clinical and Experimental Research* 1981; 5 (4): 509–522.

Guenther, R. M.: The role of nutritional therapy in alcoholism treatment. *International Journal of Biosocial Research* 1983; 4 (1): 5–18.

Helzer, J. E., et al.: The extent of long-term moderate drinking among alcoholics discharged from medical and psychiatric treatment facilities. *The New England Journal of Medicine* 1985; 312 (26): 1678–1682.

Jonas, J. M.: Eating disorders and alcohol and other drug abuse: Is there an association? *Alcohol Health & Research World* 1989; 13 (3): 267–271.

Mendelson, J. H., et al.: Hospital treatment of alcoholism: A profile of middle-income Americans. *Alcoholism: Clinical and Experimental Research* 1980; 6 (3): 277–383.

Pettinati, H. A., et al.: The natural history of alcoholism over four years after treatment. *Journal of Studies on Alcohol* 1982; 43 (3): 201–215.

Russell, G. F. M., and Treasure, J.: The modern history of anorexia nervosa: An interpretation of why the illness has changed. In: Schneider, L. H., Cooper, S. J., and Halmi, K. A. (eds.): *The Psychobiology of Human Eating Disorders: Preclinical and Clinical Perspectives.* New York: The New York Academy of Sciences, 1989.

Trulson, M. F., Fleming, R., et al.: Vitamin medication in alcoholism. *Journal of the American Medical Association* 1954; 155: 114–119.

Williams, B.: *The Vitamin B-3 Therapy: A Second Communication to AA Physicians.* Published privately, Feb. 1968.

Williams, R. H.: Treatment of alcoholism. *Consumers Research* 1985; December: 16–19.

Williams, R. J.: The etiology of alcoholism: A working hypothesis involving the interplay of hereditary and environmental factors. *Quarterly Journal of Studies on Alcohol* 1947; 7: 567–589.

Winokur, G., et al.: Alcoholism, III: Diagnosis and familiar psychiatric illness in 259 alcoholic probands. *Archives of General Psychiatry* 1972; 128: 122–126.

Chapter 2: What Is Nutrition?

Bricklin, M., and Stocher, S. (eds.): *The Natural Healing and Nutrition Annual.* Emmaus, PA: Rodale Press, 1992.

Brody, J.: *Jane Brody's Nutrition Book.* New York: W. W. Norton & Co., Inc., 1981.

Colbin, A.: *Food and Healing.* New York: Ballantine Books, 1986.

Drummond, K. E.: *Nutrition for the Food Service Professional.* New York: Van Nostrand Reinhold, 1989.

Dunne, L. J.: *Nutrition Almanac* (3d ed.). New York: McGraw-Hill, 1990.

Gaull, G. E. (ed.): *The Future of Food and Nutrition.* New York: John Wiley & Sons, 1991.

Haas, E. M.: *Staying Healthy with Nutrition.* Berkeley, CA: Celestial Arts, 1992.

Werbach, M. R.: *Nutritional Influences on Illness.* New Canaan, CT: Keats Publishing, 1990.

Chapter 3: The Macro-Nutrients

Bellerson, K. J.: *The Complete and Up-to-Date Fat Book.* Garden City Park, NY: Avery Publishing Group, 1991.

Erasmus, U.: *Fats and Oils.* Vancouver: Alive Books, 1986.

Harrison, L.: *Making Fats & Oils Work for You: A Consumer's Guide for a Healthier Life.* Garden City Park, NY: Avery Publishing Group, 1990.

Wurtman, J.: *The Carbohydrate Craver's Diet.* New York: Ballantine Books, 1983.

Chapter 4: The Micro-Nutrients

Editors: Iron. *The Edell Health Letter* 1991; 10 (7): 6.

Kleiner, S. M.: Tap the protective power of vitamin C. *Executive Health Report* 1991; 27 (4): 7.

Lieberman, S., and Bruning, N.: *The Real Vitamin & Mineral Book.* Garden City Park, NY: Avery Publishing Group, 1990.

Prevention (eds.): *The Complete Book of Vitamins.* Emmaus, PA: Rodale, 1984.

Schroeder, H.: *The Trace Elements and Man.* Old Greenwich, CT: Devin Adair, 1973.

Chapter 5: Making It Work

Blundell, J. E.: Impact of nutrition on the pharmacology of appetite. In: Schneider, L. H., Cooper, S. J., and Halmi, K. A. (eds.): *The Psychobiology of Human Eating Disorders; Preclinical and Clinical Perspectives.* New York: The New York Academy of Sciences, 1989.

Chapter 6: The Impact of Addictions

Dornhorts, A., and Ouyang, A.: Effect of alcohol on glucose tolerance. *Lancet,* October 30, 1971: 957–959.

Geokas, M. C., Lieber, C. S., et al.: Ethanol, the liver, and the gastrointestinal. *Annals of Internal Medicine* 1981; 95: 198–211.

Gold, P. W., Kaye, W., et al.: Abnormalities in plasma and cerebrospinal fluid arginine vasopressin in patients with anorexia nervosa. *The New England Journal of Medicine* 1983; 308 (19): 117–123.

Goldstein, D. B: Ethanol-induced adaptation in biological membranes. *Annals of the New York Academy of Sciences* 1987; 492: 103–111.

Lieber, C. S.: Metabolic effects of ethanol in the liver and other digestive organs. *Clinics in Gastroenterology* 1981; 10 (2): 315–342.

Lieber, C. S.: The metabolism of alcohol. *Scientific American* 1976; 234 (3): 25–33.

Marks, V.: Alcohol & changes in body constituents: Glucose & hormones. *Proceedings of the Royal Society of Medicine* 1975; 68 (6): 377–380.

Mezey, E.: Alcohol abuse and digestive diseases. *Alcohol Health and Research World* 1985; 10 (2): 6–9.

Serenyi, G., and Endrenyi, L.: Mechanism and significance of carbohydrate intolerance in chronic alcoholism. *Metabolism* 1978; 27 (9): 1,041–1,046.

Sherlock, S.: Nutrition and the alcoholic. *Lancet* 1984; 1 (8374): 436–439.

Chapter 7: Diet and the Mind

Abrahamson, E. M., and Pezet, A. W.: *Body, Mind, and Sugar.* New York: Holt, Rinehart & Winston, 1971.

Asberg, M., Thoren, P., et al.: "Serotonin depression"—a biological subgroup within the affective disorders? *Science* 1976; 191: 478–480.

Ballenger, J., Goodwin, F., et al.: Alcohol and central serotonin metabolism in man. *Archives of General Psychiatry* 1979; 36: 224–227.

Blum, K., and Trachtenberg, M. C.: Neurochemistry and alcohol craving. *California Society for the Treatment of Alcoholism & Other Drug Dependencies News* 1986; 13 (2): 1–7.

Brown, G. L., Ebert, M. H., et al.: Aggression, suicide, & serotonin: Relationships to CSF amine metabolites. *American Journal of Psychiatry* 1982; 139 (6): 741–746.

Collins, M. A., Nijm, W. P., et al.: Dopamine-related tetrahydro-isoquinolones: Significant urinary excretion by alcoholics after alcohol consumption. *Science* 1979; 206: 114–116.

Genazzani, A. R., Nappi, G., Facchinetti, F., et al.: Central deficiency of beta-endorphin in alcohol addicts. *Journal of Clinical Endocrine Metabolism* 1982; 55 (3): 583–586.

Govoni, S., Pasinetti, G., et al.: Heavy drinking decreases plasma met-enkephalin concentrations. *Alcohol and Drug Research* 1987; 7 (2): 93–98.

Hamilton, M. G., Blum, K., et al.: Identification of an isoquinoline alkaloid after chronic exposure to alcohol. *Alcoholism, Clinical and Experimental Research* 1978; 2 (2): 133–137.

Hoebel, B. G., Hernandez, L., et al.: Microdialysis studies of brain norepinephrine, serotonin, and dopamine release during ingestive behavior: Theoretical and clinical implications. In: Schneider, L. H., Cooper, S. J., and Halmi, K. A. (eds.): *The Psychobiology of Human Eating Disorders: Preclinical and Clinical Perspectives.* New York: The New York Academy of Sciences, 1989.

Kent, T. A., Campbell, J. L., et al.: Blood platelet uptake of serotonin in men alcoholics. *Journal of Studies on Alcohol* 1985; 46 (4): 357–359.

Liebowitz, S. F.: Hypothalamic neuropeptide Y, galanin, and amines: Concepts of coexistence in relation to feeding behavior. In: Schneider, L. H., Cooper, S. J., and Halmi, K. A. (eds.): *The Psychobiology of Human Eating Disorders: Preclinical and Clinical Perspectives.* New York: The New York Academy of Sciences, 1989.

Maher, T. J.: Natural food constituents and food additives: The pharmacologic connection. *The Journal of Allergy and Clinical Immunology* 1987; 79 (3): 413–422.

Padus, E.: *The Complete Guide to Your Emotions and Your Health.* Emmaus, PA: Rodale Press, 1986.

Woods, S. C., and Gibbs, J.: Regulation of food intake by peptides. In: Schneider, L. H., Cooper, S. J., and Halmi, K. A. (eds.): *The Psychobiology of Human Eating Disorders: Preclinical and Clinical Perspectives.* New York: The New York Academy of Sciences, 1989.

Wurtman, J.: *Managing Your Mind and Mood Through Food.* New York: Harper & Row, 1988.

Chapter 8: Adverse Food Reactions and Food Addictions

Bjarnason, L., Ward, K., et al.: The "leaky gut" of alcoholism: Possible route of entry for toxic compounds. *Lancet* 1984; 1 (8370): 179–182.

Closson, W.: Levels of IgE antibodies in hospitalized alcoholics vs. nonalcoholic elective-surgery controls. Unpublished paper, 1985, Brunswick Hospital Center.

Kushi, M.: *Allergies: A Natural Approach.* Tokyo: Japan Publications, 1985.

Marsh, M. N.: *Immunopathology of the Small Intestine.* New York: John Wiley & Sons, 1987.

Metcalfe, D. D.: Diseases of food hypersensitivity (editorial). *The New England Journal of Medicine* 1989; 321 (4): 255–257.

Rajkovic, I. A., and Williams, R.: Mechanisms of abnormalities in host defenses against bacterial infection in liver disease. *Clinical Science* 1985; 68: 247–253.

Sugerman, A. A., Southern, L., and Curran, J. F.: A study of antibody levels in alcoholic, depressive, and schizophrenic patients. *Annals of Allergy* 1982; 48: 166–171.

Chapter 9: Biological Individuality

Anson, B. J.: *Atlas of Human Anatomy.* Philadelphia: W. B. Saunders Co., 1951.

Begleiter, H., Porjesz, B., et al.: Event-related brain potentials in boys at risk for alcoholism. *Science* 1984; 225 (4669): 1,493–1,496.

Blum, K., Noble, E. P., et al.: Allelic association of human dopamine D2 receptor gene in alcoholism. *Journal of the American Medical Association* 1990; 263 (15): 2,055–2,060.

Cadoret, R. J., Cain, C. J., et al.: Development of alcoholism in adoptees raised apart from biologic relatives. *Archives of General Psychiatry* 1980; 37: 561–563.

Diamond, I., Hrubel, B., et al.: Basal and adenosine receptor-stimulated levels of cAMP are reduced in lymphocytes from alcoholic patients. *Proceedings of the National Academy of Science* 1987; 84: 1,413–1,416.

Gabrielli, Jr., W. F., Mednick, S. A., et al.: Electro-encephalograms in children of alcoholic fathers. *Psychophysiology* 1982; 19 (4): 404–407.

Goodwin, D. W., Schulsinger, F., et al.: Alcohol problems in adoptees raised apart from alcoholic biological parents. *Archives of General Psychiatry* 1973; 28: 238–243.

Holland, A. J., et al.: Anorexia nervosa: A study of 34 twin pairs and one set of triplets. *British Journal of Psychiatry* 1984; 145: 414–419.

Hrubec, S., and Omenn, G. S.: Evidence of genetic predisposition to alcoholic cirrhosis & psychosis: Twin concordances for alcoholism & its biological end points by zygosity among male veterans. *Alcoholism, Clinical & Experimental Research* 1981; 52: 207–215.

Nagy, L. E., Diamond, I., et al.: Cultured lymphocytes from alcoholic subjects have altered cAMP signal transduction. *Proceedings of the National Academy of Science* 1988; 85: 6,973–6,976.

Pollock, V. E., Volavka, J., et al.: The EEG after alcohol administration in men at risk for alcoholism. *Archives of General Psychiatry* 1983; 40: 857–861.

Schuckit, M. A.: Biological markers: Metabolism & acute reactions to alcohol in sons of alcoholics. *Pharmacology, Biochemistry & Behavior* 1980; 13: 9–16.

Schuckit, M. A., and Gold, E. O.: A simultaneous evaluation of multiple markers of ethanol/placebo challenges in sons of alcoholics and controls. *Archives of General Psychiatry* 1988; 45: 211–216.

Schuckit, M. A., Goodwin, D. W., et al.: A study of alcoholism in half-siblings. *American Journal of Psychiatry* 1972; 128: 122–126.

Schuckit, M. A., and Rayses, V.: Ethanol ingestion: Differences in blood acetaldehyde concentrations in relatives of alcoholics and controls. *Science* 1979; 203: 54–55.

Shive, W.: Development of lymphocyte culture methods for assessment of the nutritional and metabolic status of individuals. *Journal of the International Academy of Preventive Medicine* 1984; 8 (4): 5–16.

Steggerda, F. R., and Mitchell, H. H.: Variability in the calcium metabolism and calcium requirements of adult human subjects. *Journal of Nutrition* 1946; 31: 407–422.

Thacker, S. B., Veech, R. L., et al.: Genetic and biochemical factors relevant to alcoholism. *Alcoholism: Clinical and Experimental Research* 1984; 8 (4): 375–383.

Williams, R. J.: *Biochemical Individuality.* New York: John Wiley & Sons, 1956.

Williams, R. J.: Biochemical individuality and its implications. *Chemical Engineering News* 1947; 25: 112–113.

Williams, R. J.: Clinical implications of biochemical differences between individuals. *Modern Medicine* 1958; 26: 134–159.

Williams, R. J., and Deason, G.: Individuality in vitamin C needs. *Proceedings of the National Academy of Science* 1967; 57: 1,638–1,641.

Williams, R. J., et al.: *Individual Metabolic Patterns and Human Disease.* University of Texas Publication #5109; Austin, TX, 1951.

Williams, R. J., et al.: Metabolic peculiarities in normal young men as revealed by repeated blood analysis. *Proceedings of the National Academy of Science* 1955; 41: 615–620.

Willoughby, J.: Primal prescription. *Eating Well* 1991; May/June: 52–59.

Chapter 10: Putting It Together

Goldbeck, N., and Goldbeck, D.: *The Supermarket Handbook: Access to Whole Foods.* New York: Signet Books, 1976.

Julien, R. M.: *A Primer of Drug Action* (5th ed). New York: W. H. Freeman, 1988.

Ketcham, K., and Mueller, A.: *Eating Right to Live Sober.* Seattle, WA: Madrona Publishers, 1983.

Lefferts, L.: Water, treat it right. *Nutrition Action Health Letter* 1990; 17 (9): 5–7.

Liska, K.: *The Pharmacist's Guide to the Most Misused and Abused Drugs in America.* New York: Collier Books, 1988.

Reuben, C., and Priestley, J.: *Essential Supplements for Women.* New York: Perigee Books, 1988.

Weil, A., and Rosen, W.: *From Chocolate to Morphine: Understanding Mind-Active Drugs.* New York: Houghton Mifflin Co., 1993.

Williams, R.: *The Prevention of Alcoholism Through Nutrition.* New York: Bantam Books, 1981.

Winter, R.: *A Consumer's Dictionary of Food Additives.* New York: Crown Publishers, Inc., 1989.

Chapter 11: Whole Foods and Their Importance

Buist, R.: *Food Chemical Sensitivity.* Garden City Park, NY: Avery Publishing Group, 1988.

Center for Science in the Public Interest (eds.): Is it safe? *Nutrition Action Health Letter* 1990; 17 (8): 1, 4–9.

Claypool, J., and Nelson, C. D.: *Food Trips & Traps.* Minneapolis: Compcare Publishers, 1983.

Colbin, A.: *Food and Healing.* New York: Ballantine Books, 1986.

Coon, C. S.: *The Hunting Peoples.* Boston: Little, Brown & Co., 1971.

Erasmus, U.: *Fats and Oils.* Vancouver: Alive Books, 1986.

Griggs, B.: *The Food Factor.* London: Penguin Books, 1988.

Liebman, B.: Lessons from China. *Nutrition Action Health Letter* 1990; 17 (10): 3–5.

Loveglo, A. W.: *Why Panic? Eat Organic.* Tempe, AZ: Loveglo & Comfort, 1989.

Mann, J. D., et al.: Seed of hope. *Solstice* 1989; 38: 10–23.

Perlmutter, C., and Gardey, T.: Diet and immunity. *Prevention* 1989; October: 46–52, 124–128.

Price, W.: *Nutrition and Physical Degeneration.* New Canaan, CT: Keats Publishing, 1989.

Rodale Press (eds.): *The Good Fats.* Emmaus, PA: Rodale Press, 1988.

Schmid, R. F.: *Traditional Foods Are Your Best Medicine.* New York: Ballantine Books, 1987.

Wood, C. T.: *Organically Grown Food: A Consumer's Guide.* Los Angeles: Wood Publishing, 1990.

World Resources Institute: *The 1992 Information Please Environmental Almanac.* Boston: Houghton Mifflin Co., 1992.

Chapter 12: Nutrient-Dense Foods

Arasaki, S., and Arasaki, T.: *Vegetables from the Sea.* Tokyo: Japan Publications, 1983.

Balch, P. A., and Balch, J. F.: *Prescription for Cooking.* Greenfield, IN: PAB Books, 1993.

Ballantine, R.: *Diet & Nutrition.* Honesdale, PA: Himalayan International Institute, 1978.

Bellem, J.: Natural soy sauce. *Solstice* 1989; Sept./Oct.: 25–30.

Bradford, P., and Bradford, M.: *Cooking with Sea Vegetables.* Rochester, VT: Healing Arts Press, 1988.

Center for Science in the Public Interest (eds.): Cereals: Playing the grain game. *Nutrition Action Health Letter* 1992; 19 (2): 10–11.

East West Journal (eds.): *Shopper's Guide to Natural Foods.* Garden City Park, NY: Avery Publishing Group, 1987.

Fox, A., and Fox, B.: Keeping your immune system strong. *Let's Live* 1989; August: 26–33.

Jensen, B.: *Foods That Heal.* Garden City Park, NY: Avery, 1988.

McGee, H.: *On Food and Cooking: The Science and Lore of the Kitchen.* New York: Collier Books, 1984.

Micozzi, M. S.: Does your diet prevent or promote cancer? *Executive Health Report* 1991; 27 (4): 1, 4–5.

Rinzler, C. A.: *The Complete Food Book.* NY: World Almanac, 1987.

Robertson, L., Flindus, C., and Godfrey, B.: *Laurel's Kitchen.* Petaluma, CA: Nilgiri Press, 1981.

Shurtleff, W., and Aoyagui, A.: *The Book of Miso.* New York: Ballantine Books, 1979.

Shurtleff, W., and Aoyagui, A.: *The Book of Tempeh.* New York: Harper & Row, 1977.

Shurtleff, W., and Aoyagui, A.: *The Book of Tofu.* New York: Ballantine Books, 1979.

Williams, X.: *What's in My Food?* London: Nature & Health Books/ Prism Press, 1988.

Wood, R.: *The Whole Foods Encyclopedia.* NY: Prentice Hall, 1988.

Chapter 13: Going Shopping: Fruits and Vegetables

Brody, J.: *The Good Food Book.* New York: Bantam Books, 1985.

Carper, J.: *The Food Pharmacy.* New York: Bantam Books, 1988.

Council on Economic Priorities: *Shopping for a Better World.* New York: Ballantine Books, 1989.

East West Journal (eds.): *Shopper's Guide to Natural Foods.* Garden City Park, NY: Avery Publishing Group, 1987.

Garland, A. W.: *For Our Kids' Sake.* New York: Mothers and Others for Pesticide Limits/National Resources Defense Council, 1989.

Goldbeck, N., and Goldbeck, D.: *The Goldbecks' Guide to Good Food.* New York: New American Library, 1987.

Liebman, B.: Fresh fruit. *Nutrition Action Health Letter* 1992; 19 (4): 10–11.

Makower, J.: *The Green Consumer Supermarket Guide.* New York: Penguin Books, 1991.

Marquardt, S.: *Exporting Banned Pesticides: Fueling the Circle of Poison.* Washington, DC: Greenpeace, 1989.

Mott, L., and Snyder, K.: *Pesticide Alert: A Guide to Pesticides in Fruits and Vegetables.* San Francisco: Sierra Club Books/National Resources Defense Council, 1987.

Powledge, F.: Toxic shame. *The Amicus Journal* 1991; 13 (1): 38–44.

Root, W.: *Food: An Authoritative Visual History and Dictionary of the Foods of the World.* New York: Fireside Books, 1980.

Wittenberg, M. M.: *Experiencing Quality: A Shopper's Guide to Wholefoods.* Austin, TX: Wholefoods Market, Inc., 1987.

Wood, R.: *The Whole Foods Encyclopedia.* NY: Prentice Hall, 1988.

Chapter 14: Fish, Poultry, Eggs, Meats, and Dairy

Center for Science in the Public Interest (eds.): *Chemical Cuisine.* Washington, DC: CSPI, 1989.

Center for Science in the Public Interest (eds.): Eating green. *Nutrition Action Health Letter* 1992; 19 (1): 5–7.

Gilbert, S.: America tackles the pesticide crisis. *The New York Times Magazine* 1989; October 8: 22–25, 51–57.

Hall, R. H.: *Food for Naught*. New York: Vintage Books, 1976.

Jacobson, M. F., Lefferts, L. Y., and Garland, A. W.: *Safe Food*. Washington, DC: Center for Science in the Public Interest, 1991.

Loomis, S. H.: *The Great American Seafood Cookbook*. New York: Workman Publishing Co., 1988.

Nettleton, J. A.: *Seafood and Health*. New York: Osprey Books, 1987.

Robbins, J.: *Diet for a New America*. Walpole, NH: Stillpoint, 1987.

Smith, R.: Eating fish extends life. *Natural Healing Newsletter* 1990; 2 (2): 1, 3–4.

Steinman, D.: *Diet for a Poisoned Planet*. New York: Harmony, 1987.

Sunset Magazine (eds.): *Seafood Cook Book*. Menlo Park, CA: Lane Publishing, 1987.

Time Life Books (eds.): *The Good Cook Poultry*. Alexandria, VA: Time Life Books, 1979.

Chapter 15: Healthy Prepared Foods

Goldbeck, N., and Goldbeck, D.: *The Goldbecks' Guide to Good Food*. New York: New American Library, 1987.

Jacobson, M. F., and Fritschner, S.: *Fast Food Guide*. Washington, DC: Center for Science in the Public Interest, 1991.

Kilholm, C. S.: *The Bread & Circus Whole Food Bible*. Reading, MA: Addison-Wesley Publishing Co., Inc., 1991.

Malstrom, S.: *Own Your Own Body*. New Canaan, CT: Keats, 1977.

Marlin, J. T.: *The Catalogue of Healthy Foods*. NY: Bantam, 1990.

Restaurant Hospitality (eds.): *Make It Healthy: Restaurants and Healthy Menus in the 90s*. Cleveland: Penton Publishing, 1989.

Rodale Press (eds.): Eighteen emergency snacks. *Rodale's Food & Nutrition Letter* 1991; 5 (10): 11.

Rodale Press (eds.): Nine essential rules for healthy fast food dining. *Rodale's Food & Nutrition Letter* 1991; 5 (9): 6.

Winter, R.: *A Consumer's Dictionary of Food Additives*. New York: Crown Publishers, Inc., 1989.

World Resources Institute: *The 1992 Information Please Environmental Almanac*. Boston: Houghton Mifflin Co., 1992.

Chapter 16: Recovery Cooking: Getting Started

Beard, J.: *James Beard's Theory and Practice of Good Cooking*. New York: Knopf, 1984.

Blackman, J. F.: *The Working Chef's Cookbook for Natural Wholefoods*. Morrisville, VT: Central Vermont Publishers, 1989.

Brody, J.: *Jane Brody's Good Food Book*. NY: Bantam Books, 1985.

Herbst, S. T.: *The Food Lover's Companion*. Hauppauge, NY: Barron's Educational Series, Inc., 1990.

Hill, B.: *The Cook's Book of Essential Information*. NY: Dell, 1987.

Hullah, E.: *Cardinal's Handbook of Recipe Development*. Ontario: Cardinal Kitchens, 1984.

Lang, J. H.: *Larousse Gastronomique*. NY: Crown Publishers, 1988.

Leith, P.: *The Cook's Handbook*. Toronto: Stewart House, 1981.

McGee, H.: *On Food and Cooking: The Science and Lore of the Kitchen*. New York: Collier Books, 1984.

Riley, E.: *The Chef's Companion*. NY: Van Nostrand Reinhold, 1986.

Chapter 17: The Recipes

Crouch, D.: *Entertaining Without Alcohol*. Washington, DC: Acropolis Books, Ltd., 1985.

Hullah, E.: *Cardinal's Handbook of Recipe Development*. Ontario: Cardinal Kitchens, 1984.

King, P.: *Taste and See Allergy Relief Cooking*. Keene, NH: NMI Press, 1988.

Liebman, B.: From sweets to beets. *Nutrition Action Health Letter* 1991; 18 (10): 10–11.

Rodale Press (eds.): Garlic + selenium = super cancer fighter. *Rodale's Food & Nutrition Letter* 1992; 6 (1): 2.

Chapter 18: People and Food: Finding the Spiritual Connection

Baker, S., and Henry, R. R.: *Parent's Guide to Nutrition*. Reading, MA: Addison-Wesley Publishing Co., Inc., 1987.

Benson, H.: *Minding the Body, Mending the Mind*. Reading, MA: Addison-Wesley Publishing Co., Inc., 1987.

Bricklin, M.: How to buy a few extra years. *Prevention* 1990; April: 143.

David, M.: *Nourishing Wisdom*. New York: Bell Tower Books, 1990.

Douglas, M. (ed.): *Food in the Social Order*. New York: The Russell Sage Foundation, 1984.

Farb, P., and Armelagos, G.: *Consuming Passions: The Anthropology of Eating*. New York: Washington Square Press, 1983.

Hazelden Foundation: *Food for Thought*. San Francisco: Harper/ Hazelden, 1980.

Kanzaki, N.: *Understanding Japan*. Tokyo: The International Society for Educational Information, 1989.

Levi-Strauss, C.: *The Origin of Table Manners*. New York: Harper & Row, 1978.

Logue, A. W.: *The Psychology of Eating and Drinking*. New York: W. H. Freeman & Co., 1991.

Lorenz, K. J.: *The Foundation of Ethology*. New York: Simon & Schuster, 1981.

Mach, V. H., and Mach, J. P.: *Brain Power*. Boston: Houghton Mifflin Co., 1989.

Perera, P.: Ceremonies and sustenance. *Parabola* 1984; November.

Siegal, R., et al.: *The First Jewish Catalogue*. Philadelphia: The Jewish Publication Society of America, 1973.

Tannahill, R.: *Food in History*. New York: Crown Publishers, 1989.

Visser, M.: *Much Depends on Dinner*. New York: Grove Press, 1986.

INDEX

AA. *See* Alcoholics Anonymous
Absorption, of nutrients, 37–38
Abstinence, 9, 87, 88
Acetaldehyde, 45, 69
Acidosis, 30, 39
Acid rain, 80
Addiction
  behavior patterns/symptoms of, 324–27
  biological/psychological factors contributing to,
    6–7
  cross-addiction, 7, 78, 87, 168
  eating patterns correlated to, 95
  food allergies and food addiction, 56–63
  genetic factors, 6, 64–76
  impact on brain functioning, 51–52
  impact on nutrition, 41–47
  physical damage caused by, 4, 5–7, 32, 38, 39,
    62
  see also Alcohol and alcoholism; Drugs and
    drug abuse; Eating disorders; Recovery;
    Smoking; Treatment programs
Additives
  artificial/chemical, 6, 17, 77, 78, 80, 102–3,
    148
  in fast foods, 43
  list of most dangerous, 158–59, 355–56
  in prepared/processed foods, 78, 80, 109
  side effects caused by, 355–56
  sulfites, 143
Adrenaline, 21
Adverse food reactions. *See* Allergies/sensitivities,
  food
Aerobic exercise, 83–84
Agriculture Department. *See* Department of
  Agriculture
AIDS, 58
Air quality, 77, 82
  see also Oasis, establishing an
Alcohol and alcoholism
  allergies/immune system impairment, 60–
    62
  brain function impairment, 51–52
  cancer risks, 58
  cellular function and mineral loss, 30
  consumption amounts and diet, 8
  in ethnic groups, 64, 71–72
  genetic factors, 3, 68–72
  impact on glucose levels, 4
  medications, alcohol content of, 89, 319–21
  medications, alcohol free, 322–23
  metabolic effects, 70–72
  negative impact on nutrition, 44–46
  prostaglandins link, 71–72

  research on, 7–10, 61, 68–69, 70–72, 86
  sobriety/relapse factors, 3, 55
  in women, 64
  see also Addiction; Treatment programs
Alcoholic hypoglycemia, 4, 50, 53, 325
Alcoholics Anonymous (AA), 11, 61, 89, 332
Alkalosis, 30
Allergies/sensitivities
  and addictive/compulsive behavior, 6, 7
  and alcoholism, 60–62
  allergy/addiction cycle, 59–62
  allergy-free products, 81
  delayed reactions, 59
  and eating disorders, 62–63
  establishing an oasis, 81, 82, 344–46
  food, 4, 6, 56–63, 74–76, 109, 151, 338–40
  food families/related foods, 75–76, 341–44
  immediate reactions, 59
American Society of Addiction Medicine (ASAM),
  89, 332
Amino acids, 15, 19–20, 39, 54, 114
Amphetamines, 42
Anaerobic exercise, 83–84
Anaphylaxsis, 56
Anorexia
  behavior patterns/symptoms of, 328–29
  brain function impairment, 52
  cellular function and mineral loss, 30
  death rates from, 8
  genetic factors, 72–73
  negative impact on nutrition, 41–43
  physical damage caused by, 46–47
Anson, Barry, 67
Antibiotics, 62–63, 99, 148, 150, 151
Antibodies, 57–58, 61, 75
Antigens, 57
Antioxidant enzymes, 25
Anxiety, 4, 41, 53, 55
Appetite loss, 41
Arsenic, 19
Arterial plaque, 24, 25
Arthritis, 100
ASAM. *See* American Society of Addiction
  Medicine
Asia/Asians, 14, 151
Asthma, 82, 100
Atherosclerosis, 82, 95, 100, 151
Autoimmune disorders, 60

Bacteria, 145, 146, 148–49; *see also* Salmonella
Baked goods, 159–60
  recipes, 193–95
Beans. *See* Legumes

367